HEALTHCARE TECHNOLOGIES SERIES 33

Electromagnetic Waves and Antennas for Biomedical Applications

Other volumes in this series:

Volume 1	**Nanobiosensors for Personalized and Onsite Biomedical Diagnosis** P. Chandra (Editor)
Volume 2	**Machine Learning for Healthcare Technologies** D.A. Clifton (Editor)
Volume 3	**Portable Biosensors and Point-of-Care Systems** S.E. Kintzios (Editor)
Volume 4	**Biomedical Nanomaterials: From design to implementation** T.J Webster and H. Yazici (Editors)
Volume 6	**Active and Assisted Living: Technologies and Applications** F. Florez-Revuelta and A.A. Chaaraoui (Editors)
Volume 7	**Semiconductor Lasers and Diode-Based Light Sources for Biophotonics** P.E. Andersen and P.M. Petersen (Editors)
Volume 9	**Human Monitoring, Smart Health and Assisted Living: Techniques and technologies** S. Longhi, A. Monteriù and A. Freddi (Editors)
Volume 13	**Handbook of Speckle Filtering and Tracking in Cardiovascular Ultrasound Imaging and Video** C.P. Loizou, C.S. Pattichis and J. D'hooge (Editors)
Volume 14	**Soft Robots for Healthcare Applications: Design, modelling, and control** S. Xie, M. Zhang and W. Meng
Volume 16	**EEG Signal Processing: Feature extraction, selection and classification methods** W. Leong
Volume 17	**Patient-Centered Digital Healthcare Technology: Novel applications for next generation healthcare systems** L. Goldschmidt and R.M. Relova (Editors)
Volume 19	**Neurotechnology: Methods, advances and applications** V. de Albuquerque, A. Athanasiou and S. Ribeiro (Editors)
Volume 20	**Security and Privacy of Electronic Healthcare Records: Concepts, paradigms and solutions** S. Tanwar, S. Tyagi and N. Kumar (Editors)
Volume 23	**Advances in Telemedicine for Health Monitoring: Technologies, design and applications** Tarik A. Rashid, Chinmay Chakraborty and Kym Fraser
Volume 24	**Mobile Technologies for Delivering Healthcare in Remote, Rural or Developing Regions** P. Ray, N. Nakashima, A. Ahmed, S. Ro and Y. Soshino (Editors)
Volume 26	**Wireless Medical Sensor Networks for IoT-Based eHealth** Fadi Al-Turjman (Editor)
Volume 29	**Blockchain and Machine Learning for e-Healthcare Systems** Balamurugan Balusamy, Naveen Chilamkurti, Lucia Agnes Beena and Poongodi T (Editors)
Volume 39	**Digital Tools and Methods to Support Healthy Ageing** Pradeep Kumar Ray, Siaw-Teng Liaw and J Artur Serano (Editors)

Electromagnetic Waves and Antennas for Biomedical Applications

Edited by
Lulu Wang

The Institution of Engineering and Technology

Published by The Institution of Engineering and Technology, London, United Kingdom

The Institution of Engineering and Technology is registered as a Charity in England & Wales (no. 211014) and Scotland (no. SC038698).

First published 2021

The Institution of Engineering and Technology
Michael Faraday House
Six Hills Way, Stevenage
Herts, SG1 2AY, United Kingdom

www.theiet.org

British Library Cataloguing in Publication Data
A catalogue record for this product is available from the British Library

ISBN 978-1-83953-167-5 (hardback)
ISBN 978-1-83953-168-2 (PDF)

Typeset in India by MPS Limited
Printed in the UK by CPI Group (UK) Ltd, Croydon

Contents

About the editor

Lulu Wang is currently a Distinguished Professor of Biomedical Engineering at Shenzhen Technology University in China. She received the M.E. (First class Hons.) and Ph.D. degrees from the Auckland University of Technology, New Zealand, in 2009 and 2013, respectively. From 2013 to 2015, she was a Research Fellow with the Institute of Biomedical Technologies, Auckland University of Technology, New Zealand. In June 2015, Dr Wang became an Associate Professor of biomedical engineering with the Hefei University of Technology. In June 2019, she became a Distinguished Professor of Biomedical Engineering at Shenzhen Technology University. In 2020 May, she became the director of the Biomedical Device Innovation Center at Shenzhen Technology University. Her research interests include medical devices, electromagnetic sensing and imaging, and computational mechanics. Over the past five years, Dr Wang has authored more than 70 peer-reviewed publications, 2 ASME books, 6 book chapters, and 4 issued patents. Dr Wang is a member of ASME, IEEE, MRSNZ, AAAS, PSNZ, and IPENZ. She is an active reviewer of numerous journals, books, and conferences. She has edited three books and two special issues of international journals. She has received multiple National and International Awards from various professional societies and organizations. She is an active topic/track organizer of several international conferences include ASME IMECE, ICCES.

Chapter 1

Point-spread functions in inverse scattering and image reconstruction with microwaves and millimeter waves

Daniel Tajik[1], Romina Kazemivala[1] and Natalia K. Nikolova[1]

1.1 Introduction

Real-time microwave and millimeter-wave (MMW) imaging is the workhorse in applications ranging from a synthetic aperture radar (SAR), which operates with far-field data, to nondestructive testing and medical imaging, which employ near-field measurements. Research in this field is intensifying with expansion into numerous applications enabled by the advances in high-frequency electronics (from microwaves through millimeter waves to THz). Advances in the flexible programmable platforms, also known as field-programmable gate arrays, provide the critical capability to control and reconfigure very complex high-frequency sensor networks and arrays. This chapter is an attempt to explain, categorize, compare, and contrast real-time MMW reconstruction methods within a common mathematical framework, thus making this interdisciplinary subject more comprehensible and accessible to the wider research community. The discussion is supported by many examples aiding, understanding, and highlighting important performance metrics such as spatial resolution and computational efficiency. The examples are based on two distinctly different real-time quantitative reconstruction methods: quantitative microwave holography (QMH) [1–3] and scattered-power mapping (SPM) [1,4,5]. The impact of approximations that stem from the assumed models of scattering and the practical limitations of the MMW imaging systems are also discussed.

There are two particulars to the discussion here. First, the focus is on real-time imaging methods. These are methods that reconstruct an image quickly, practically without any delay after the measurements are taken. Such short reconstruction times are achieved with mathematical techniques and scattering models, which differ substantially from those in nonlinear reconstructions methods. Nonlinear iterative reconstruction is common in biomedical imaging with microwaves, but it

[1]Department of Electrical and Computer Engineering, McMaster University, Hamilton, Canada

will not be discussed here except where a comparison with real-time reconstruction is made.

Second, the central theme of this chapter is the system (or data) point-spread function (PSF) and how it is used in real-time reconstruction. The use of measured PSFs is critical to the success of image reconstruction with data from near-field measurements. The biomedical applications of MMW imaging necessarily employ near-field data since the sensing antennas are placed in close proximity (sometimes in almost direct contact) with the imaged tissue in order to maximize signal strength.

1.2 System point-spread function (PSF)

In the context of inverse scattering, the PSF describes the system's response to a point scatterer. The concept comes from optical (e.g., photographic) imaging systems where it describes the image obtained with a point source. Depending on how well the lens is focused, the image does not show a perfect point at the location of the source but rather a smeared spot, hence the term "point-spread."

There are two types of PSFs used in MMW imaging: system (or data) and image. The data PSF is the set of responses acquired when measuring a point scatterer, also referred to as the scattering probe (SP), embedded in the background medium. The overall object consisting of the background and the SP is referred to as the *calibration object* (CO) [1] since it is used to calibrate the system for optimal image reconstruction. The PSF data in MMW imaging come in the form of scattering (S) parameters (in the case of frequency-sweep or stepped-frequency measurements) or various types of voltage waveforms such as pulses or frequency-modulated signals. These responses are functions of the position on the acquisition (or observation) aperture. For example, in planar scanning with step-frequency measurements, the PSF data sets are functions of the frequency ω and position (x, y) on the acquisition plane. Figure 1.1 shows an illustration of a CO measurement setup in a planar imaging system where two antennas (oriented for orthogonal polarization) scan each plane (on opposing sides of the imaged volume). If each antenna is capable of operating in both transmitting (Tx) and receiving (Rx) modes, then a total of 16 types of PSF responses can be acquired (4 reflections and 12 transmission responses) at each scan position (x, y) and at each frequency ω or time instance t. The SP is usually positioned at the center of the imaged volume where the origin of the coordinate system resides. As the antennas scan the acquisition apertures, their respective position vectors ($\mathbf{r}_{Tx}$, $\mathbf{r}_{Rx}$) change relative to the SP.

On the other hand, the image PSF is the image produced by a reconstruction algorithm operating on the data PSF. Note that the data PSF has nothing to do with the reconstruction algorithm but rather describes the hardware performance. It is typically used to estimate the data signal-to-noise ratio (SNR) [6] and the system sensitivity to the presence of weak scatterers, i.e., scatterers that are electrically very small and/or have very low contrast to the background. In contrast, the image PSF is typically used to evaluate the performance of a reconstruction algorithm in

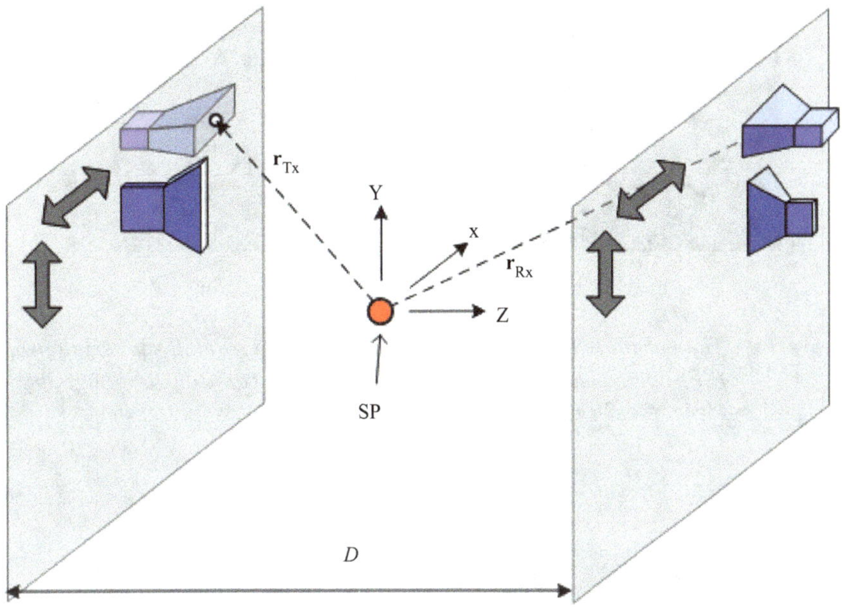

Figure 1.1 *Illustration of a measurement setup to acquire the PSFs in a planar imaging system where two antennas (oriented for mutually orthogonal polarization) scan each plane (on opposing sides of the imaged volume)*

terms of (i) the spatial resolution limit, which is represented by the width of the main lobe in the image PSF [1], and (ii) the PSF side-lobe level, which represents the ability of the algorithm to produce artifact-free images and to clearly separate targets in close proximity to each other. Ideally, the image PSF should be obtained from noise-free PSF data such as those obtained from simulations, so that hardware errors and noise are excluded from the performance analysis of a reconstruction algorithm. In the absence of measurement noise, the image PSF side-lobe level sets the fundamental "noise floor" in the image, which is expected to only worsen when imaging with measured data.

To depict the difference between data and image PSF, consider the following example of a simulated CO; see Figure 1.2, which shows the true distribution of the complex relative permittivity of the CO in a $z =$ const. plane. A small cubical SP, 1 cm on a side, with relative permittivity $\tilde{\varepsilon}_{r,SP} = 1.2 - i0.0$, is placed in a background of air $\left(\tilde{\varepsilon}_{r,b} = 1.0 - i0.0\right)$. This CO is then measured using reflection *S*-parameters and reconstructed using QMH to generate the data PSF and the image PSF. Figure 1.3 shows a typical data PSF acquired on a planar aperture at one frequency (8 GHz). The PSF magnitude is shown in Figure 1.3(a) whereas its phase is shown in Figure 1.3(b). This is a simulated PSF, which is practically noise-free except for the negligible numerical errors. The distribution of the PSF depicts well the scattering from a very small (point-like) scatterer, the field of which features

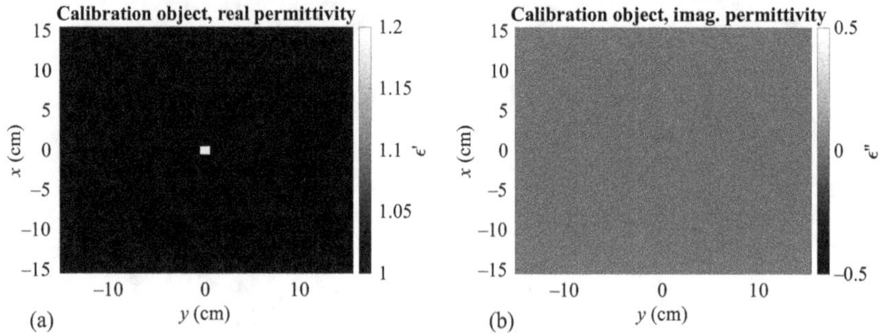

Figure 1.2 The permittivity of the CO, which consists of a small scattering probe (SP) embedded in the background medium: (a) real, (b) imaginary. Here, the SP is a cube of size 1 cm^3 and relative permittivity $\widetilde{\varepsilon}_{r,SP} = 1.2 - i0.0$. *It is immersed in air*

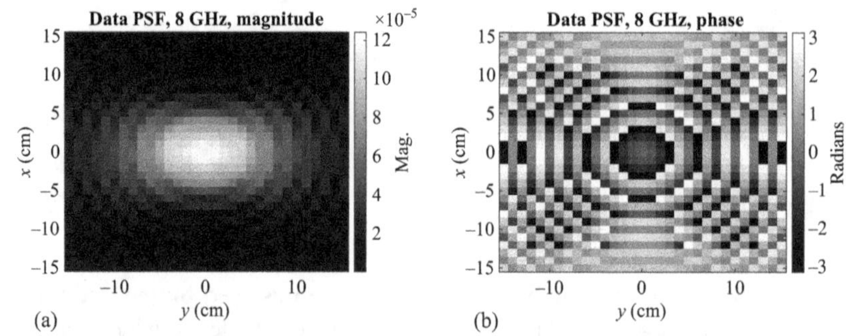

Figure 1.3 The data PSF for the reflection S-parameter at 8 GHz in the measurement of the CO shown in Figure 1.2: (a) magnitude, (b) phase

near-spherical symmetry. The scattered-field symmetry, however, is usually affected by the directional and polarization properties of the Rx antenna and the PSF itself often departs from a perfect spherical symmetry.

The image PSF obtained using QMH with several added filters (see discussion in Section 1.8) is shown in Figure 1.4. Here, the filters are added intentionally to reduce the amount of spatial and frequency information provided by the simulation, mimicking a realistic scenario. Note that without filtering, QMH reconstructs the object shown in Figure 1.2 perfectly due to the highly accurate noise-free data and the fact that the PSF is *not* an analytical approximation—it is obtained by simulating the measurement of the CO that is also the reconstructed object. The real part of the reconstructed complex relative permittivity (with the filters applied) is plotted in Figure 1.4(a) whereas its imaginary part is shown in Figure 1.4(b). We see that the reconstruction is not perfect. Side lobes and ripples limit the image spatial resolution that exceeds the selected voxel size.

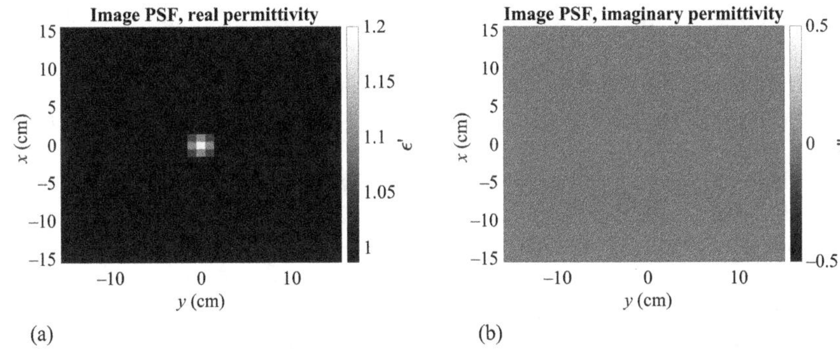

Figure 1.4 The image PSF of the CO shown in Figure 1.2 generated with quantitative microwave holography (QMH): (a) real part of the relative permittivity, (b) imaginary part of the relative permittivity. Several filters are enabled to demonstrate the impact on the spatial resolution

It is worth elaborating on the CO, the measurements of which provide the data PSF. The CO requires a physical embodiment of a point scatterer (i.e., SP) and a choice of background medium (usually homogeneous within the imaged volume). The SP is embedded in the background medium, the electromagnetic (EM) properties of which are assumed known. It is this background in which the object under test (OUT) is also embedded during measurements. For example, in imaging for security screening (whole-body scanners), the background is assumed to be open air. In medical imaging, the background is typically a specially designed coupling medium, the EM properties of which usually mimic the averaged properties of the tissues or organs to be imaged.

The SP has a small but finite volume Ω_{SP}. Ideally, the size of the SP must be much smaller than the shortest wavelength of the radiation, i.e., $\lambda_{min}/8$ or smaller, because an assumption is made that within Ω_{SP} the EM field is constant. In [7,8], metallic SPs are used to reconstruct the qualitative images of both metallic and dielectric targets in very close-range measurements. Also there, it is demonstrated that high-contrast dielectric SPs made of microwave ceramics are suitable as well. In biomedical imaging, the interest is on the scattering from (lossy) dielectric bodies. Often the goal is to detect regions of pathological changes or malignancies. These are characterized by their complex permittivity $\widetilde{\varepsilon}$, or, equivalently, the relative permittivity ε_r and the effective conductivity σ_e. In these cases, it is preferable to use a dielectric SP of known permittivity that is made of microwave ceramics [2,5,6] or a small fruit such as a blueberry [3,9]. In the former case, the manufacturers provide accurate permittivity values (and the loss is usually negligible), whereas in the latter case, the complex permittivity of the fruit must be measured. The reason why a dielectric SP is preferable to a metallic one is that modern real-time imaging can produce quantitative images (images of the real and imaginary parts of the permittivity of the object) but the best quantitative estimates are achieved at locations where the permittivity in the lossy dielectric object is similar to that of the SP [4]. For instance, if breast malignancy is to be detected, it is desirable to have an SP, which has permittivity and conductivity close to those of cancerous breast tissue. In the frequency range from 1 to 8 GHz, where most breast imaging prototypes work [10,11], the averaged (over frequency) relative permittivity values of breast-cancer samples range approximately from 40 to 60 whereas the conductivity is in the range of 1–5 S/m [12]. In comparison, the averaged measured relative permittivity of a blueberry is about 55 whereas its conductivity is about 4 [3,9]. The alternative presented by a probe made of microwave ceramics [2,5,6] features a relative complex permittivity $\tilde{\varepsilon}_r = 50.00 + i0.05$, which is practically constant in the previous frequency range. The respective effective conductivity averaged over all frequencies is about 12.5 mS/m.

1.3 Models of scattering in terms of point-spread functions

In the following discussion, we focus on the use of the data PSF in real-time MMW imaging and, for brevity, we refer to it simply as “PSF.” The PSF is the impulse response of a linear system. It therefore provides a valuable system-level description and allows for the prediction of a response due to any complex input through convolution.

1.3.1 Scattering models using convolution

PSFs have been used widely in optical, acoustic, and microwave imaging to de-blur images and to take advantage of near-field information when measurements are taken at a very close range [13–18]. The underlying model is inherently linear in the unknown imaged quantity, typically the target reflectivity $\rho(\mathbf{r}')$. Here, $\mathbf{r}'$ is the position in the imaged volume. It assumes that the acquired data with the OUT are a convolution of the reflectivity with the PSF. In the language of scattering, this means that the OUT is viewed as a collection of independent point scatterers. As a consequence, the OUT response is viewed as the superposition (a convolution integral) of the scattering from each point scatterer.

For example, if the responses are collected on a planar acquisition aperture (similar to what is shown in Figure 1.1) at $z = z_{\text{Rx}}$, they are expressed as [18]

$$s(x, y, z_{\text{Rx}}; \mathbf{r}_{\text{Tx}}; t) = \rho(x, y, t) * h(x, y, z_{\text{Rx}}; \mathbf{r}_{\text{Tx}}; t), \tag{1.1}$$

where $s(x, y, z_{\text{Rx}}; \mathbf{r}_{\text{Tx}}; t)$ is the response at the receiver (Rx) position $\mathbf{r}_{\text{Rx}} \equiv (x, y, z_{\text{Rx}})$, $\mathbf{r}_{\text{Tx}}$ is the position of the transmitter (Tx), t is time, $h(x, y, z_{\text{Rx}}; \mathbf{r}_{\text{Tx}})$ is the PSF for a point scatterer, and $*$ denotes convolution over x, y, and t. Note that (1.1) assumes that $\mathbf{r}_{\text{Tx}}$ is fixed while the Rx position sweeps along x and y at the acquisition aperture. However, it also can easily accommodate measurement setups where the Rx and Tx antennas are in a fixed configuration while scanning together over x and y. Mathematically, this means that $\mathbf{r}_{\text{Tx}}$ is defined through $\mathbf{r}_{\text{Rx}}$ and it is not an independent variable. In this case, $\mathbf{r}_{\text{Rx}} \equiv (x, y, z_{\text{Rx}})$ describes both the Rx and the Tx positions and $\mathbf{r}_{\text{Tx}}$ can simply be omitted from the expression in (1.1).

We notice three important features of the model in (1.1). First, it is *linear* in the unknown target reflectivity ρ. Second, it is only qualitative in the sense that the reflectivity has, in general, unknown (and, in fact, nonunique) relation to the target's permittivity, conductivity, and permeability. Third, reflectivity is a function of time t whereas the image reconstruction algorithms usually assume that the target EM properties are time-invariant, i.e.,

$$\rho(\mathbf{r}',t) = \rho(\mathbf{r}') \cdot \delta(t), \tag{1.2}$$

where δ denotes Dirac's δ-function and $\mathbf{r}' \equiv (x',y',z')$ is the position in the imaged volume. Note that here we have used primed coordinates for the position inside the imaged volume V' (these are the integration variables in the convolution integral) in order to distinguish those from the observation position, which is expressed with non-primed coordinates in the same coordinate system. The time dependence of $\rho(x,y,t)$ in (1.1) stems from the time being an implicit function of position $\mathbf{r}'$ through the speed of light v_b in the background—the distance from the Tx antenna to the point scatterer and back to the Rx antenna determines the time of arrival of the signal $s(x,y,z_{Rx};t)$, i.e.,

$$t(\mathbf{r}') = \frac{|\mathbf{r}' - \mathbf{r}_{Tx}| + |\mathbf{r}' - \mathbf{r}_{Rx}|}{v_b}. \tag{1.3}$$

In the frequency domain, the model in (1.1) can be expressed as a two-dimensional (2-D) convolution in (x,y) space:

$$S(x,y,z_{Rx};\mathbf{r}_{Tx};\omega) = \iint_{x'y'} \rho(x',y',\omega) \cdot H(x-x',y-y',z_{Rx};\mathbf{r}_{Tx};\omega)dx'dy', \tag{1.4}$$

where the frequency ω is now an implicit function of $\mathbf{r}'$. We discuss this implicit dependence later in the chapter.

1.3.2 Field-based electromagnetic scattering models

In contrast to the convolution models of scattering in (1.1) and (1.4), the rigorous formulation of EM scattering in terms of a PSF has not been available until recently. The field-based mathematical model of EM scattering is vectorial in nature since it is derived from Maxwell's equations and is cast in terms of the EM field vectors $\mathbf{E}$ and $\mathbf{H}$ [1,19]. It is also nonlinear with respect to the unknown properties (permittivity and/or permeability) of the OUT. For example, in the case of the scattering from a dielectric body in an unbounded background, the frequency-domain equation for the scattered electric field vector $\mathbf{E}^{sc}$ at the Rx position $\mathbf{r}_{Rx}$ is

$$\mathbf{E}^{sc}(\mathbf{r}_{Rx},\mathbf{r}_{Tx};\omega) = k_0^2 \iiint_{V'} \Delta\tilde{\varepsilon}_r(\mathbf{r}') \cdot \bar{\mathbf{G}}_b(\mathbf{r}_{Rx},\mathbf{r}';\omega) \cdot \mathbf{E}^{tot}(\mathbf{r}',\mathbf{r}_{Tx};\omega;\Delta\tilde{\varepsilon}_r)d\mathbf{r}', \tag{1.5}$$

where $\mathbf{r}_{Tx}$ is the Tx position, $\mathbf{r}' \in V'$ is the position inside the OUT, V' is the volume of the OUT, ω is the frequency in radians, k_0 is the free-space wavenumber, and $\Delta\tilde{\varepsilon}_{\mathrm{r}}$ is the relative permittivity contrast of the OUT,

$$\Delta\tilde{\varepsilon}_{\mathrm{r}} = \tilde{\varepsilon}_{\mathrm{r}} - \tilde{\varepsilon}_{\mathrm{r,b}}, \tag{1.6}$$

with $\tilde{\varepsilon}_{\mathrm{r}}$ and $\tilde{\varepsilon}_{\mathrm{r,b}}$ being the relative permittivities of the OUT and the background, respectively. Green's dyadic function $\bar{\mathbf{G}}_{\mathrm{b}}(\mathbf{r}_{\mathrm{Rx}}, \mathbf{r}'; \omega)$ is that of the background. The field $\mathbf{E}^{\mathrm{tot}}$ is the *total* field at $\mathbf{r}'$ due to the Tx antenna at $\mathbf{r}_{\mathrm{Tx}}$. The term *total* indicates that the field is taken in the presence of the OUT; therefore, it depends implicitly on the permittivity contrast $\Delta\tilde{\varepsilon}_{\mathrm{r}}$. It is now clear that (1.5) is *nonlinear* in the unknown contrast unlike (1.4). We should also mention that the term *scattered* in $\mathbf{E}^{\mathrm{sc}}$ indicates that this response is due entirely and only to the scattering from the OUT. This scattering response is part of the total field $\mathbf{E}^{\mathrm{tot}}(\mathbf{r}_{\mathrm{Rx}}, \mathbf{r}_{\mathrm{Tx}}; \omega)$, which also contains the *incident* field $\mathbf{E}^{\mathrm{inc}}(\mathbf{r}_{\mathrm{Rx}}, \mathbf{r}_{\mathrm{Tx}}; \omega)$, i.e., the contribution that would exist in the absence of the OUT. We discuss strategies of extracting $\mathbf{E}^{\mathrm{sc}}$ from $\mathbf{E}^{\mathrm{tot}}$ later in the chapter.

From a practical standpoint, there are several drawbacks in the model presented by (1.5). First, the measurement of vector fields such as $\mathbf{E}^{\mathrm{sc}}(\mathbf{r}_{\mathrm{Rx}}, \mathbf{r}_{\mathrm{Tx}}; \omega)$ is difficult and impractical. It requires calibrated field probes, which are expensive as well as relatively large and narrowband. The actual data format is either *S*-parameters (in step-frequency measurements) or voltage waveforms (in time-domain measurements). Furthermore, as previously mentioned, what we measure is the *total* response, not the *scattering* one. Second, Green's dyadic function $\bar{\mathbf{G}}_{\mathrm{b}}(\mathbf{r}_{\mathrm{Rx}}, \mathbf{r}'; \omega)$ is analytically available only for a homogeneous unbounded (isotropic) background [1,19]. Such analytical approximations cannot capture the complexities of a measurement system (especially in near-field measurements) where reflections from system components and uncertainties in the background constitutive parameters may be significant. Third, the total field $\mathbf{E}^{\mathrm{tot}}(\mathbf{r}', \mathbf{r}_{\mathrm{Tx}}; \omega; \Delta\tilde{\varepsilon}_r)$ inside the OUT is not known since it depends on the unknown contrast $\Delta\tilde{\varepsilon}_{\mathrm{r}}$, leading to the nonlinear nature of the EM inverse-scattering problem. This nonlinearity can be avoided with Born's approximation [1,19],

$$\mathbf{E}^{\mathrm{tot}}(\mathbf{r}', \mathbf{r}_{\mathrm{Tx}}; \omega; \Delta\tilde{\varepsilon}_{\mathrm{r}}) \approx \mathbf{E}^{\mathrm{inc}}(\mathbf{r}', \mathbf{r}_{\mathrm{Tx}}; \omega), \tag{1.7}$$

but this approximation is subject to limitations in the size and contrast of the scatterer. Even still, $\mathbf{E}^{\mathrm{inc}}(\mathbf{r}', \mathbf{r}_{\mathrm{Tx}}; \omega)$ is unknown and in many conventional imaging algorithms must be approximated analytically. In near-field measurements, such analytical approximations are inadequate.

On the other hand, in the iterative methods of (nonlinear) inverse scattering, simulations are often used to obtain $\mathbf{E}^{\mathrm{tot}}(\mathbf{r}', \mathbf{r}_{\mathrm{Tx}}; \omega; \Delta\tilde{\varepsilon}_r)$ inside the OUT since, at each iteration, an estimate of the OUT is available. Unfortunately, simulations, too, suffer from large *modeling errors* [7,20], which are much more difficult to reduce compared to numerical errors. The modeling errors are rooted in the inability to predict all influencing factors arising in the measurement setup: fabrication tolerances of the antennas and the positioning components, uncertainties in the constitutive parameters of the materials (especially the absorbers), aging of the materials and the connectors, deformations due to temperature or humidity, etc. In addition, the simulation models often ignore complexities in the cables, the connectors, and the fine structural components such as screws, brackets, and thin supporting plates.

1.3.3 Electromagnetic scattering in terms of S-parameters

We turn next to the more recent mathematically rigorous models of EM scattering exploiting the system PSF [1,7,8,21]. These models not only have established the mathematical link between convolution and EM-field models—see (1.4) and (1.5)—but also have paved the way to real-time quantitative imaging [2–5]. The latter capability arises from the quantitatively accurate equations relating the measured scattered response to the electrical properties of the OUT through the PSF.

Starting from Maxwell's equations in the frequency domain, the EM scattering model in terms of S-parameters is derived as [1,8]

$$S_{jk}^{\mathrm{sc}}(\mathbf{r}_{\mathrm{Rx}}, \mathbf{r}_{\mathrm{Tx}}; \omega) = \frac{-i\omega\varepsilon_0}{2a_j a_k} \iiint\limits_{V'} \Delta\widetilde{\varepsilon}_{\mathrm{r}}(\mathbf{r}') \cdot \mathbf{E}_j^{\mathrm{inc}}(\mathbf{r}_{\mathrm{Rx}}, \mathbf{r}'; \omega) \cdot \mathbf{E}_k^{\mathrm{tot}}(\mathbf{r}', \mathbf{r}_{\mathrm{Tx}}; \omega; \Delta\widetilde{\varepsilon}_{\mathrm{r}}) d\mathbf{r}', \tag{1.8}$$

where j and k ($j, k = 1, \ldots, N_{\mathrm{p}}$) are the Rx and Tx port indices, respectively, N_{p} is the number of ports in the microwave network formed by the OUT and the antennas, a_ξ ($\xi \equiv j, k$) is the incoming root-power wave at the ξ th port, $\mathbf{E}_j^{\mathrm{inc}}(\mathbf{r}_{\mathrm{Rx}}, \mathbf{r}'; \omega)$ is the incident field due to the Rx antenna at the jth port if this antenna were to operate in a Tx mode excited by a_j, and $\mathbf{E}_k^{\mathrm{tot}}(\mathbf{r}', \mathbf{r}_{\mathrm{Tx}}; \omega; \Delta\widetilde{\varepsilon}_r)$ is the total field at $\mathbf{r}'$ due to the Tx antenna (at $\mathbf{r}_{\mathrm{Tx}} \notin V'$) excited by a_k. The root-power waves a_ξ ($\xi \equiv j, k$) are determined from the power of the incident wave at the respective excitation port, i.e., $a_\xi = (P_\xi^{\mathrm{inc}})^{1/2}$ W$^{1/2}$, provided $\mathbf{E}_j^{\mathrm{inc}}$ and $\mathbf{E}_k^{\mathrm{tot}}$ are root-mean-square phasors [22]. If they are magnitude phasors, $a_\xi = (2P_\xi^{\mathrm{inc}})^{1/2}$ W$^{1/2}$. Figure 1.5 illustrates an imaging experiment where the antenna at the kth port is excited with the incoming wave a_k and the outgoing waves b_k and b_j are measured at their respective ports, which allows for the calculation of the respective S-parameters, e.g., $S_{jk} = b_j/a_k$.

In comparison with (1.5), (1.8) offers two critical advantages. First, the response is now an S-parameter, which is exactly what is being measured in step-frequency experiments. Note that the relation between $\mathbf{E}^{\mathrm{sc}}(\mathbf{r}_{\mathrm{Rx}}, \mathbf{r}_{\mathrm{Tx}}; \omega)$ and the respective S-parameter is neither straightforward nor analytically available even if the Rx antenna design is known. This is because $\mathbf{E}^{\mathrm{sc}}$ is a point-like response whereas the antenna "collects" the entire E-field distribution in its vicinity (the antenna aperture). Second, Green's dyadic function $\bar{\mathbf{G}}_{\mathrm{b}}$ is now replaced by $\mathbf{E}_j^{\mathrm{inc}}$, which is in essence Green's vector function that allows the expression of the complex-scalar response S_{jk}^{sc} as a function of the vector-field excitation $\mathbf{E}_k^{\mathrm{tot}}$. $\mathbf{E}_j^{\mathrm{inc}}$ is sometimes replaced by analytical approximations. With far-zone measurements, this approximation can take the form

$$\mathbf{E}_j^{\mathrm{inc}}(\mathbf{r}_{\mathrm{Rx}}, \mathbf{r}'; \omega); \widehat{\mathbf{p}}_j(\mathbf{r}_{\mathrm{Rx}}, \mathbf{r}'; \omega) \cdot G_j(\mathbf{r}_{\mathrm{Rx}}, \mathbf{r}'; \omega) \cdot \frac{e^{-ik_{\mathrm{b}}|\mathbf{r}'-\mathbf{r}_{\mathrm{Rx}}|}}{|\mathbf{r}' - \mathbf{r}_{\mathrm{Rx}}|}, \tag{1.9}$$

where $\widehat{\mathbf{p}}_j$ and G_j are the polarization vector and the gain pattern of the antenna attached to the jth port. Both of these antenna parameters are functions of the position $\mathbf{r}'$ of the scattering center relative to the antenna as well as the frequency. Alternatively, when the far-zone approximations do not hold, $\mathbf{E}_j^{\mathrm{inc}}$ can be found

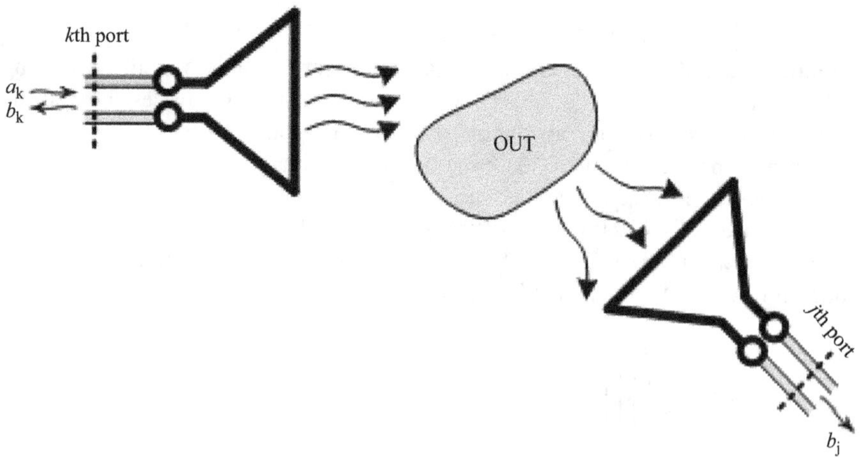

Figure 1.5 Illustration of a measurement setup showing a pair of antennas attached to the jth and kth ports along with the imaged object. The kth port is excited by the incident root-power wave a_k and the outgoing waves b_k and b_j are measured at their respective ports. These measurements are performed with a vector network analyzer [23,24]

through a simulation where the *j*th antenna transmits in the absence of an OUT. Finally, it can also be measured if the background medium allows for the placement of an SP in the form of a short wire [8].

Furthermore, using the approaches in [8,25], (1.8) can be generalized to include the scattering from magnetic bodies as

$$S_{jk}^{\text{sc}}(\mathbf{r}_{\text{Rx}},\mathbf{r}_{\text{Tx}};\omega) = \frac{i\omega}{2a_j a_k}\iiint_{V'}\Big[\Delta\tilde{\mu}(\mathbf{r}')\cdot\mathbf{H}_j^{\text{inc}}(\mathbf{r}_{\text{Rx}},\mathbf{r}';\omega)\cdot\mathbf{H}_k^{\text{tot}}(\mathbf{r}',\mathbf{r}_{\text{Tx}};\omega;\Delta\tilde{\mu}) - \Delta\tilde{\varepsilon}(\mathbf{r}')\cdot\mathbf{E}_j^{\text{inc}}(\mathbf{r}_{\text{Rx}},\mathbf{r}';\omega)\cdot\mathbf{E}_k^{\text{tot}}(\mathbf{r}',\mathbf{r}_{\text{Tx}};\omega;\Delta\tilde{\varepsilon})\Big]\,d\mathbf{r}', \quad (1.10)$$

where $\Delta\tilde{\mu} = \tilde{\mu} - \tilde{\mu}_b$ and $\Delta\tilde{\varepsilon} = \tilde{\varepsilon} - \tilde{\varepsilon}_b$ are the absolute permeability and permittivity contrasts, respectively. The background permeability and permittivity are denoted as $\tilde{\mu}_b$ and $\tilde{\varepsilon}_b$, respectively, whereas those of the OUT are $\tilde{\mu}$ and $\tilde{\varepsilon}$. The case of magnetic scattering is of interest in medical imaging with microwaves because significant research effort is currently dedicated to the possibility of using magnetic nanoparticles as contrast agents [26–28].

The *S*-parameter scattering model (1.10) is quite general in the sense that it is valid even in the case of an inhomogeneous background. It is quantitatively accurate and is strictly based on Maxwell's equations in isotropic media. In fact, the contrasts $\Delta\tilde{\varepsilon}$ and $\Delta\tilde{\mu}$ can also depend on frequency. While this frequency dependence is often ignored in real-time imaging, this is only because it simplifies the inversion algorithms, i.e., this is not a limitation of the scattering model.

1.3.4 Electromagnetic scattering models for real-time inversion

The scattering models used in real-time imaging are a compromise between two opposing requirements: speed and accuracy. To gain speed, approximations are made. One such approximation is Born's approximation of the total internal field (1.7), which can be applied to $\mathbf{E}_k^{\text{tot}}(\mathbf{r}', \mathbf{r}_{\text{Tx}}; \omega; \Delta\tilde{\varepsilon}_r)$ in (1.8). It linearizes the scattering equation thus eliminating the need for (i) an iterative solution of the inherently nonlinear inverse problem and (ii) solving Maxwell's equations for the total internal field. The price to pay is accuracy, which quickly deteriorates if the OUT contrast $\Delta\tilde{\varepsilon}_r(\mathbf{r}')$ and size violate the limitations of Born's approximation [1,19].

1.3.4.1 Frequency-domain scattering models in terms of PSF

With Born's approximation (1.7), the linearized form of the frequency-domain scattering model in (1.8) is

$$S_{jk}^{\text{sc}}(\mathbf{r}_{\text{Rx}}, \mathbf{r}_{\text{Tx}}; \omega) \approx a \iiint_{V'} \Delta\tilde{\varepsilon}_r(\mathbf{r}') \cdot \mathbf{E}_j^{\text{inc}}(\mathbf{r}_{\text{Rx}}, \mathbf{r}'; \omega) \cdot \mathbf{E}_k^{\text{inc}}(\mathbf{r}', \mathbf{r}_{\text{Tx}}; \omega) d\mathbf{r}', \tag{1.11}$$

where $a = (-i\omega\varepsilon_0)/(2a_j a_k)$ is a known constant. The linearized inverse problem in (1.11) can now be solved directly (i.e., without iterations). These inversion methods, referred to as *linear* or *direct*, are very fast and capable of real-time reconstruction of three-dimensional (3-D) images containing hundreds of millions of voxels.

To establish the link between the linearized scattering model in (1.11) and the convolution model in (1.4), let us first express (1.11) in terms of Cartesian coordinates to accommodate a planar scan along x and y while z_{Rx} is fixed. To simplify the notations, we introduce a single subscript ξ ($\xi = 1, \ldots, N_{\text{T}}$), which indicates the *response type* and which combines all system parameters that determine how a response is acquired, namely, the port indices j and k ($j, k = 1, \ldots, N_{\text{p}}$), and the position of the observation plane z_{Rx} (which may change from one experiment to another). Equation (1.11) is now written as

$$S_\xi^{\text{sc}}(x, y; \omega) \approx a \iiint_{x'y'z'} \Delta\tilde{\varepsilon}_r(x', y', z') \cdot \mathbf{E}_{\xi\text{Rx}}^{\text{inc}}(x, y; x', y', z'; \omega) \cdot \mathbf{E}_{\xi\text{Tx}}^{\text{inc}}(x', y', z'; x, y; \omega) dx'dy'dz', \quad \xi = 1, \ldots, N_{\text{T}}. \tag{1.12}$$

The subscripts in $\mathbf{E}_{\xi\text{Rx}}^{\text{inc}}$ and $\mathbf{E}_{\xi\text{Tx}}^{\text{inc}}$ indicate by which antenna the respective incident field is generated. The reader is reminded that the incident field $\mathbf{E}_{\xi\text{Rx}}^{\text{inc}}$ is generated by the Rx antenna if this antenna were to operate in a transmitting mode in the absence of an OUT.

Note that we have allowed the incident field of the Tx antenna $\mathbf{E}_{\xi\mathrm{Tx}}^{\mathrm{inc}}$ to depend on the observation position (x, y). This is necessary for scenarios where the Tx and Rx antennas are in a fixed configuration, moving together relative to the OUT. In this case, $\mathbf{r}_{\mathrm{Tx}}$ depends on $\mathbf{r}_{\mathrm{Rx}} \equiv (x, y, z_{\mathrm{Rx}})$. One typical example is a monostatic radar where $\mathbf{r}_{\mathrm{Tx}} \equiv \mathbf{r}_{\mathrm{Rx}}$. If $\mathbf{r}_{\mathrm{Tx}}$ is independent of $\mathbf{r}_{\mathrm{Rx}}$, $\mathbf{E}_{\xi\mathrm{Tx}}^{\mathrm{inc}}$ is constant with respect to (x, y), which does not affect the analysis that follows.

Next, we find the PSF predicted by (1.12) for an SP at (x', y', z') :

$$H_{\xi}^{\mathrm{sc}}(x, y; x', y', z'; \omega) \approx a\Delta\tilde{\varepsilon}_{\mathrm{r,SP}}\,\Omega_{\mathrm{SP}} \cdot$$
$$\mathbf{E}_{\xi\mathrm{Rx}}^{\mathrm{inc}}(x, y; x', y', z'; \omega) \cdot \mathbf{E}_{\xi\mathrm{Tx}}^{\mathrm{inc}}(x', y', z'; x, y; \omega), \tag{1.13}$$

where Ω_{SP} is the volume of the SP and $\Delta\tilde{\varepsilon}_{\mathrm{r,SP}}$ is its relative-permittivity contrast. We can now express the kernel of (1.12) through the PSF as

$$\xi(x, y; x', y', z'; \omega) = \mathbf{E}_{\xi\mathrm{Rx}}^{\mathrm{inc}}(x, y; x', y', z'; \omega) \cdot \mathbf{E}_{\xi\mathrm{Tx}}^{\mathrm{inc}}(x', y', z'; x, y; \omega)$$
$$\approx \frac{H_{\xi}^{\mathrm{sc}}(x, y; x', y', z'; \omega)}{a\Delta\tilde{\varepsilon}_{\mathrm{r,SP}}\Omega_{\mathrm{SP}}}. \tag{1.14}$$

Let us assume that the background medium is homogeneous or layered in x and y. In this case, the PSF is translationally invariant with respect to x and y, i.e., a shift of the SP from $(0, 0, z')$ to (x', y', z') simply causes the respective coordinate shift of the PSF (see Figure 1.6). Assume that we have the PSF for an SP at $x' = 0$, $y' = 0$ in the plane $z' =$ const.:

$$H_{\xi 0}^{\mathrm{sc}}(x, y; z'; \omega) \equiv H_{\xi}^{\mathrm{sc}}(x, y; 0, 0, z'; \omega). \tag{1.15}$$

Then, the PSF for a probe at any other position (x', y') in the plane $z' =$ const. can be written as

$$H_{\xi}^{\mathrm{sc}}(x, y; x', y', z'; \omega) = H_{\xi 0}^{\mathrm{sc}}(x - x', y - y', z'; \omega). \tag{1.16}$$

With (1.14) and (1.16) in mind, the scattering model in (1.12) can be expressed in terms of the PSF as

$$S_{\xi}^{\mathrm{sc}}(x, y; \omega) \approx \frac{1}{\Delta\tilde{\varepsilon}_{\mathrm{r,SP}}\Omega_{\mathrm{SP}}} \iiint\limits_{x'y'z'} \Delta\tilde{\varepsilon}_{r}(x', y', z') \cdot H_{\xi 0}^{\mathrm{sc}(x - x', y - y', z'; \omega) dx' dy' dz'}$$
$$\xi = 1, \ldots, N_{\mathrm{T}}. \tag{1.17}$$

It is now clear that the S-parameter response $S_{\xi}^{\mathrm{sc}}(x, y; \omega)$ is a 2-D convolution (in x and y) of the unknown contrast $\Delta\tilde{\varepsilon}_{\mathrm{r}}(x', y', z')$ and the PSF $H_{\xi 0}^{\mathrm{sc}}(x, y; z'; \omega)$ corresponding to an SP in the center of the plane $z' =$ const.. This establishes the link between the convolution models of scattering, such as (1.4), and EM-based quantitatively accurate models such as (1.17). It is clear that the convolution models are

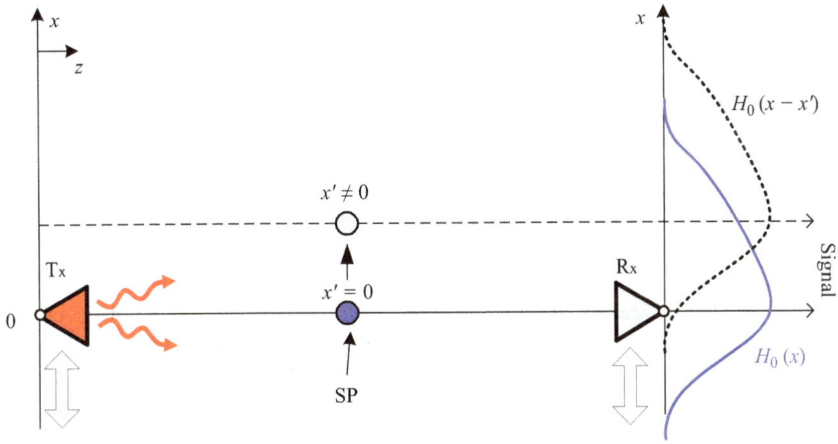

Figure 1.6 Illustration of the translational invariance of a data PSF along x. A Tx antenna on the left illuminates the scattering probe (SP) and the signal scattered by the SP is recorded by the Rx antenna on the right. The Tx and Rx antennas scan together (in a fixed mutual configuration) along the x-axis. With the probe at $x' = 0$, the centered PSF $H_0(x)$ is obtained (solid blue line). Since the medium is uniform, if the probe is at $x' \neq 0$, the PSF is a shifted (along x) version of the centered PSF, i.e., $H(x; x') = H_0(x - x')$ (dash black line)

rooted in Born's linearizing approximation for the total internal field. Until now, they have been capable only of qualitative imaging due to the lack of quantitative means to account for system specifics such as excitation power, antenna, and gain. In contrast, quantitatively accurate linearized models such as (1.17) allow for extracting the complex permittivity distribution of the OUT (quantitative imaging) while taking an advantage of the remarkable speed of the convolution-based real-time imaging.

Quantitative real-time imaging depends critically on a quantitatively accurate PSF $H^{sc}_{\xi 0}(x, y; z'; \omega)$ in (1.17), which can account for (i) the specifics of the measurement setup, including the antennas and (ii) the impact of the scatterer's electrical properties on the magnitude and phase of the received scattered signal. Such PSFs are provided by measurements only that are performed on the CO; see Figure 1.1. A measured PSF is particularly important in biomedical imaging, where the antennas are placed very close to the tissue or organ, often in practically direct contact with the skin surface; see, e.g., [10,29–31]. Such placement optimizes the energy coupling into the tissue and the scattered signal strength. When the imaged object is that close to the antenna, only a measured PSF can capture well the near-field effects specific to the antenna. In [7], a near-field nondestructive testing experiment demonstrates that even PSFs computed from simulated near-field distributions using (1.13) fail to capture the complexities of the overall measurement setup. Yet, the image reconstruction is successful with a measured PSF.

Analytical approximations of the PSF are common with far-zone measurements, e.g., in a SAR for remote sensing or in millimeter-wave whole-body scanners for concealed weapon detection. However, the resulting images are only qualitative. For example, the qualitative analytical PSF used in monostatic radar is [32,33]

$$\begin{aligned} &H(x, y, z_{\mathrm{Rx}}; x', y', z'; \omega) \\ &= exp\left(-2ik_0\sqrt{(x'-x)^2 + (y'-y)^2 + (z'-z_{\mathrm{Rx}})^2}\right), \end{aligned} \tag{1.18}$$

where k_0 is the wavenumber in vacuum. It is clear that this PSF takes into account only the round-trip phase delay of the signal. In another example, the PSF of a multi-static radar takes into account not only the phase delay but also the free-space amplitude decay as [34]

$$H(\mathbf{r}_{\mathrm{Rx}}; \mathbf{r}_{\mathrm{Tx}}; \mathbf{r}'; \omega) = \frac{e^{-ik_0 R_{\mathrm{Tx}}} \cdot e^{-ik_0 R_{\mathrm{Rx}}}}{R_{\mathrm{Tx}} R_{\mathrm{Rx}}}, \tag{1.19}$$

where $R_{\cdot\mathrm{x}} = \sqrt{(x'-x_{\cdot\mathrm{x}})^2 + (y'-y_{\cdot\mathrm{x}})^2 + (z'-z_{\cdot\mathrm{x}})^2}$ with the subscript $_{\cdot\mathrm{x}}$ indicating both Tx and Rx.

1.3.4.2 Time-domain scattering models in terms of PSF

In the following discussion, we focus on methods for real-time reconstruction based on the frequency-domain model in (1.17). Nonetheless, it is worth delineating briefly the analogous PSF-based models for time-dependent scattering signals. In the time domain, the assumption of frequency-independent contrast is essential in simplifying the scattering model. A further assumption is made that the **E**-field and, therefore, the scattered signals are governed by the scalar wave equation, which is true only if the background medium is homogeneous. With these assumptions, the received scattered signal (e.g., voltage) is expressed as [1]

$$\begin{aligned} s^{\mathrm{sc}}(\mathbf{r}_{\mathrm{Rx}}, \mathbf{r}_{\mathrm{Tx}}, t) = &\iiint_{V'} \kappa(\mathbf{r}') \cdot \\ &\left[h_{\mathrm{Rx}}^{\mathrm{inc}}(\mathbf{r}'; \mathbf{r}_{\mathrm{Rx}}, t) * h_{\mathrm{Tx}}^{\mathrm{tot}}(\mathbf{r}'; \mathbf{r}_{\mathrm{Tx}}, t; \kappa) * w''(t)\right] d\mathbf{r}', \end{aligned} \tag{1.20}$$

where $*$ denotes convolution in time, v_b is the speed of light in the background medium, $h_{\mathrm{Rx}}^{\mathrm{inc}}(\mathbf{r}'; \mathbf{r}_{\mathrm{Rx}}, t)$ is the incident-field impulse response to excitation at the Rx antenna, $h_{\mathrm{Tx}}^{\mathrm{tot}}(\mathbf{r}'; \mathbf{r}_{\mathrm{Rx}}, t)$ is the total-field impulse response to excitation at the Tx antenna, $w(t)$ is the excitation waveform submitted to the Tx antenna, $w''(t)$ is its second derivative in time, and $\kappa(\mathbf{r}')$ is the *contrast function* defined as

$$\kappa(\mathbf{r}') = \mu(\mathbf{r}')\varepsilon(\mathbf{r}') - \mu_b \varepsilon_b, \tag{1.21}$$

where $\mu(\mathbf{r}')$ and $\varepsilon(\mathbf{r}')$ are the (real-valued) permeability and permittivity, respectively, in the OUT whereas μ_b and ε_b are those of the background. Note that the last convolution term in (1.20) relates to the total field $u_{\mathrm{Tx}}^{\mathrm{tot}}$ due to the Tx antenna when excited with $w(t)$:

$$h_{\mathrm{Tx}}^{\mathrm{tot}}(\mathbf{r}', t, \mathbf{r}_{\mathrm{Tx}}; \kappa) * w''(t) = \frac{\partial^2}{\partial t^2} u_{\mathrm{Tx}}^{\mathrm{tot}}(\mathbf{r}', t, \mathbf{r}_{\mathrm{Tx}}; \kappa). \tag{1.22}$$

Using the same approach as in the case of the S-parameter scattering model, a PSF-based linearized time-domain model of scattering can be obtained as

$$s(\mathbf{r}_{\mathrm{Rx}}, \mathbf{r}_{\mathrm{Tx}}, t) = \frac{1}{\kappa_{\mathrm{SP}} \Omega_{\mathrm{SP}}} \iiint_{V'} \kappa(\mathbf{r}') h^{\mathrm{sc}}(\mathbf{r}_{\mathrm{Rx}}, \mathbf{r}_{\mathrm{Tx}}, \mathbf{r}', t) d\mathbf{r}', \tag{1.23}$$

where $h^{\mathrm{sc}}(\mathbf{r}_{\mathrm{Rx}}, \mathbf{r}_{\mathrm{Tx}}, \mathbf{r}', t)$ is the system PSF obtained with the SP being at $\mathbf{r}'$. Similarly to (1.16), this PSF is obtained from a "central" or reference PSF, $h_0^{\mathrm{sc}}(\mathbf{r}_{\mathrm{Rx}}, \mathbf{r}_{\mathrm{Tx}}, t)$, which is obtained with the SP being at $\mathbf{r}' = 0$. With the assumption of a homogeneous loss-free unbounded medium and neglecting the signal's amplitude decay with distance, adjusting the PSF $h_0^{\mathrm{sc}}(\mathbf{r}_{\mathrm{Rx}}, \mathbf{r}_{\mathrm{Tx}}, t)$ to represent scattering from any other SP position ($\mathbf{r}' \neq 0$) amounts to a time shift that reflects the changing distances from the Tx antenna to the SP and from the SP to the Rx antenna:

$$h^{\mathrm{sc}}(\mathbf{r}_{\mathrm{Rx}}, \mathbf{r}_{\mathrm{Tx}}, \mathbf{r}', t) \approx h_0^{\mathrm{sc}}(\mathbf{r}_{\mathrm{Rx}}, \mathbf{r}_{\mathrm{Tx}}, t - \Delta t(\mathbf{r}')), \Delta t = \frac{\Delta r_{\mathrm{Tx}}(\mathbf{r}') + \Delta r_{\mathrm{Rx}}(\mathbf{r}')}{v_{\mathrm{b}}}, \tag{1.24}$$

where

$$\begin{aligned} \Delta r_{\mathrm{Tx}} &= |\mathbf{r}' - \mathbf{r}_{\mathrm{Tx}}| - |\mathbf{r}_{\mathrm{Tx}}|, \\ \Delta r_{\mathrm{Rx}} &= |\mathbf{r}' - \mathbf{r}_{\mathrm{Rx}}| - |\mathbf{r}_{\mathrm{Rx}}|. \end{aligned} \tag{1.25}$$

Figure 1.7 illustrates the shift in the SP position that leads to the time shift $\Delta t(r')$ in (1.24). It shows two antennas (Tx and Rx) measuring the PSF in two scenarios: when the SP is at the origin ($\mathbf{r}' = 0$) and the SP is shifted to $\mathbf{r}' \neq 0$.

Equation (1.24) can easily be modified to account for an amplitude free-space decay with distance ($\sim 1/r_{\mathrm{Rx}}$) in the wave scattered by the SP. Bearing in mind that the PSF $h_0^{\mathrm{sc}}(\mathbf{r}_{\mathrm{Rx}}, \mathbf{r}_{\mathrm{Tx}}, t)$ is a signal due to a point scatterer, such decay exists and its impact may be significant depending on the shape and size of the acquisition aperture. We must also keep in mind that the PSF's strength is proportional to the product of the strengths of the incident-field impulse response of the Rx antenna $h_{\mathrm{Rx}}^{\mathrm{inc}}$ (which by reciprocity represents the wave scattered by the SP) and the field $u_{\mathrm{Tx}}^{\mathrm{tot}}$ due to the Tx antenna as per (1.20) and (1.22). In the linearized equation (Equation (1.23)), Born's approximation implies that $u_{\mathrm{Tx}}^{\mathrm{tot}} \approx u_{\mathrm{Tx}}^{\mathrm{inc}}$. The amplitude free-space decay in $u_{\mathrm{Tx}}^{\mathrm{inc}}$ may or may not be significant depending on the Tx antenna and its position relative to the SP. If the losses in the background medium are not negligible, they, too, can be accounted for by including the respective exponential decay over the total distance travelled by the signal from the Tx antenna to the SP and on to the Rx antenna.

1.4 Extracting the scattering signals from measured data

As mentioned before, it is rarely possible to measure the scattered-field portion of a signal (e.g., S_{jk}^{sc}) directly because there is a significant incident-field contribution

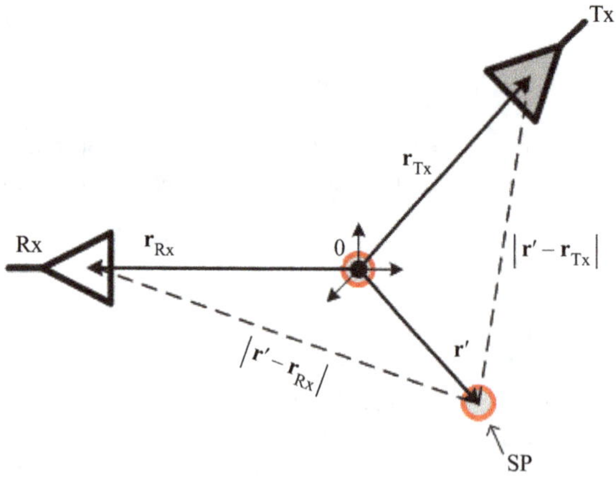

Figure 1.7 Illustration of a measurement setup showing a pair of antennas measuring the PSF when the scattering probe (SP) is at the origin ($\mathbf{r}' = 0$) *and when it is shifted to* $\mathbf{r}' \neq 0$

(e.g., S_{jk}^{inc}) to the total measured response (e.g., S_{jk}^{tot}). Hereafter, we omit details regarding the type of response (e.g., frequency- or time-domain and reflection or transmission coefficient) and we refer to it simply as the *signal* S. We are concerned only whether the signal is *total*, *incident*, or *scattered*, which is reflected by the superscript.

By definition, the incident signal S^{inc} is the one measured in the absence of an OUT; see Figure 1.8(a). The measurement setup (antennas, positioning mechanism, etc.) together with the respective background medium forms the *reference object* (RO). The RO measurement is also referred to as the background or baseline measurement. It is part of the system calibration, i.e., it has nothing to do with the subsequently imaged objects. It is often performed immediately before the measurement of the CO (see Figure 1.8(b)) or that of the OUT (see Figure 1.8(c)) to make sure that possible hardware changes in the system are accounted for. The CO measurement provides the total-field response H_0^{tot} to an SP embedded in the background medium, usually at the center of the imaged volume. The CO is identical to the RO except for the embedded SP. The OUT measurement provides the total-field OUT signal S^{tot}.

The scattered-field response S^{sc} is extracted from S^{tot} and S^{inc}. The collection of all OUT scattered-field responses forms the *data* submitted to the reconstruction algorithm. Similarly, the system PSF H_0^{sc} is extracted from H_0^{tot} and S^{inc}. The PSF data are independent from the OUT but they are critical for the reconstruction algorithm because they describe the system-specific response to point scatterers. In fact, the PSF is not always measured; it is often approximated analytically, especially in far-zone qualitative imaging. In such cases, the calibration measurement of the CO depicted in Figure 1.8(b) is omitted.

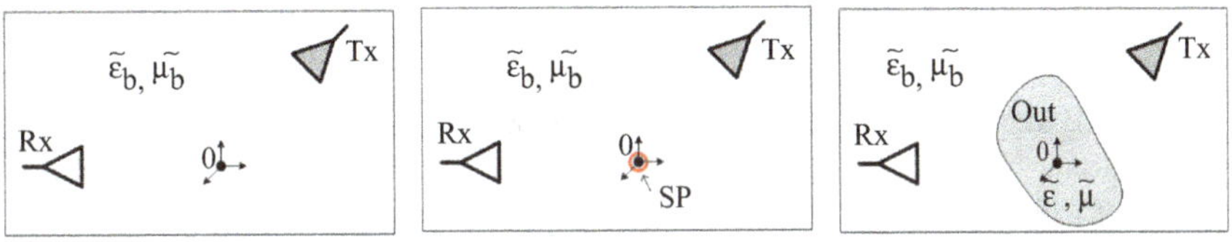

(a) (b) (c)

Figure 1.8 Illustration of the three measurements involved in an imaging procedure. (a) Measurement of the reference object (RO), which provides the incident-field response S^{inc}. The background medium is void of any scattering objects. Its constitutive parameters are $\tilde{\varepsilon}_b$ and $\tilde{\mu}_b$. (b) Measurement of the calibration object (CO), which provides the total-field PSF response H_0^{tot}. The CO consists of the scattering probe (SP) at the origin of the coordinate system, which is typically at the center of the imaged volume. The SP is embedded in the same background medium as that of the RO. (c) Measurement of the object under test (OUT), which provides total-field OUT response S^{tot}. The OUT is placed in the same background medium as that of the RO. The constitutive parameters of the OUT, $\tilde{\varepsilon}$, and $\tilde{\mu}$, are functions of position in general. The measurements in (a) and (b) are part of the system calibration

There are two approaches to accomplish the extraction. The most common approach is based on Born's first-order approximation of the total response, which is viewed as a superposition of the incident and scattered signal components. It then follows that S^{sc} can be obtained as

$$S_{\text{B}}^{\text{sc}} \approx S^{\text{tot}} - S^{\text{inc}}. \tag{1.26}$$

In view of the limitations of Born's approximation as applied to the data [1], the errors arising in (1.26) are associated with (i) large permittivity/permeability contrast and size of scattering regions inside the OUT, and (ii) significant coupling between the antennas and the OUT, including multiple scattering between the antennas and the OUT. These errors are usually negligible when H_0^{sc} is extracted using

$$H_{0\text{B}}^{\text{sc}} \approx H_0^{\text{tot}} - S^{\text{inc}}, \tag{1.27}$$

because the SP is electrically very small.

The less common approach is based on Rytov's approximation [1,19]. It can be shown that the extraction formula based on Rytov's approximation is [2,5]

$$S_{\text{R}}^{\text{sc}} \approx S^{\text{inc}} \cdot \ln\left(\frac{S^{\text{tot}}}{S^{\text{inc}}}\right). \tag{1.28}$$

The extraction of $H_{0\text{R}}^{\text{sc}}$ is analogous, with S^{tot} being replaced by H_0^{tot}. Unlike Born's approximation, Rytov's approximation is limited only by the permittivity contrast (in dielectric objects) and it is not sensitive to the size of the scattering object [1,19]. This is an important advantage in certain cases, e.g., in breast imaging, where the electrical size of the OUT is large but the contrast between malignant and healthy tissues is low. On the other hand, Rytov's approximation is sensitive to phase wrapping [3], which is not a factor in Born's approximation. Consider (1.28) written in terms of magnitude and phase:

$$S_{\mathrm{R}}^{\mathrm{sc}} \approx S^{\mathrm{inc}} \cdot \left\{ \ln \frac{|S^{\mathrm{tot}}|}{|S^{\mathrm{inc}}|} + \mathrm{i}\left[\angle S^{\mathrm{tot}} - \angle S^{\mathrm{inc}}\right] \right\}. \tag{1.29}$$

The imaginary part of (1.29) is different depending on whether the signal is phase wrapped or unwrapped. Thus, in order to generate a valid reconstruction, it is recommended that all responses are phase unwrapped (along the spatial coordinates of the acquisition surface) before applying Rytov's approximation.

1.5 Reconstruction with quantitative microwave holography

1.5.1 Microwave holography with analytical PSFs

Modern MMW holographic image reconstruction was introduced at the end of the last century by Sheen *et al.* [32,35,36] who describe it as "a combination of the holographic (backward-wave) image reconstruction with an SAR image-reconstruction algorithm developed by Soumekh" [37–39]. Holography needs magnitude and phase information in the scattered data. Another hallmark of MMW holography is that the inversion is done in k-space, i.e., the spatial Fourier space.

The scattering model used in the original work of Sheen *et al.* [32,33] is a qualitative monostatic-radar version of (1.17) with the PSF in (1.18). The reconstruction is 3-D and highly efficient numerically as it employs only 2-D and 3-D fast Fourier transforms (FTs). It is worth summarizing the reconstruction process in order to appreciate the differences with QMH in the near-field scenario of medical imaging. In the case of planar acquisition (along x and y), the reconstruction formula is [32]

$$\rho(x', y', z') = \mathrm{FT}_{3\mathrm{D}}^{-1}\{\mathrm{SM}\{\mathrm{FT}_{2\mathrm{D}}[S^{\mathrm{sc}}(x, y, \omega)]\} \cdot e^{-\mathrm{i}k_z \bar{z}}\}, \tag{1.30}$$

where $\rho(x', y', z')$ is the reconstructed reflectivity of the OUT, $S^{\mathrm{sc}}(x, y, \omega)$ are the monostatic data acquired at the plane $z_{\mathrm{R}x} = z_{\mathrm{T}x} = \bar{z}$, and the wavenumber k_z is given by

$$k_z = \sqrt{4k_{\mathrm{b}}^2 - k_x^2 - k_y^2} = \sqrt{4\omega^2/c^2 - k_x^2 - k_y^2}, \tag{1.31}$$

where (k_x, k_y) are the Fourier variables corresponding to (x, y) and c is the speed of light in vacuum. Note that only propagating modes in a loss-free background are assumed so that $k_x^2 + k_y^2 \leq 4k_{\mathrm{b}}^2$. The imaged position (x', y', z') and the observation one $(x, y, \bar{z})$ are defined in a common coordinate system. Further, notice that the 2-D FT

(FT_{2D}) casts the data $S^{sc}(x,y,\omega)$ into the space (k_x,k_y,ω). Meanwhile, the 3-D inverse FT (IFT) (FT_{3D}^{-1}) operates in the space (k_x,k_y,k_z) where k_z relates to ω through the nonlinear dispersion relation in (1.31). To facilitate the use of the fast Fourier transform (FFT) on a uniform grid in (k_x,k_y,k_z) space, resampling is needed on the data in the (k_x,k_y,ω) space, known as Stolt's mapping (or Stolt's interpolation) [40]. This is indicated in (1.30) as SM. The reconstruction with (1.30) produces 3-D images of domains containing millions of voxels within seconds.

A Fourier reconstruction formula has been developed for the PSF in (1.19), too [34]. Moreover, its application extends to include multiple receivers and transmitters (multi-static radars). For a planar aperture, it is stated as [34]

$$\rho(x',y',z') = FT_{3D}^{-1}\{SM\{k_{zTx}k_{zRx}\cdot FT_{4D}[S^{sc}(x_{Rx},y_{Rx},\bar{z}_{Rx};x_{Tx},y_{Tx},\bar{z}_{Tx};\omega)]\}\}, \tag{1.32}$$

where FT_{3D}^{-1} operates on (k_x,k_y,k_z). On the other hand, the 4-D Fourier transform FT_{4D} casts the data from the space defined by $(x_{Rx},y_{Rx},x_{Tx},y_{Tx},\omega)$ into the space $(k_{xRx},k_{yRx},k_{xTx},k_{yTx},\omega)$. Here, the subscripts Rx and Tx indicate the positions of the Rx and Tx antennas, respectively, which scan their respective apertures located at z_{Rx} and z_{Tx}. Stolt's mapping is used to interpolate the data from the uniform grid in $(k_{xRx},k_{yRx},k_{xTx},k_{yTx},\omega)$ to that in (k_x,k_y,k_z) using

$$k_x = k_{xTx} + k_{xRx} \tag{1.33}$$

$$k_y = k_{yTx} + k_{yRx} \tag{1.34}$$

$$k_z = \sqrt{k_b^2 - k_{xTx}^2 - k_{yTx}^2} + \sqrt{k_b^2 - k_{xRx}^2 - k_{yRx}^2},\ k_b = \omega/c. \tag{1.35}$$

1.5.2 Basics of quantitative microwave holography (QMH)

The Fourier inversion of the more general PSF-based scattering model in (1.17) has been first proposed in [2,7] and has since been developed into a real-time quantitative imaging method [1,3,9,41] suitable for the near-field scenario of biomedical imaging.

Applying FT to $S_\xi^{sc}(x,y;\omega)$ in (1.17) with respect to x and y leads to

$$\tilde{S}_\xi^{sc}(k_x,k_y,\omega) \approx b\int_{z'} \tilde{F}(k_x,k_y;z')\cdot \tilde{H}_{\xi 0}^{sc}(k_x,k_y;z';\omega)\,dz', \tag{1.36}$$

where $\tilde{F}(k_x,k_y,z')$ is the 2-D FT of the unknown $\Delta\tilde{\varepsilon}_r(x',y',z')$, $\tilde{H}_{\xi 0}^{sc}$ is the 2-D FT of the PSF, and

$$b = \frac{\Delta x'\Delta y'}{(\Delta\tilde{\varepsilon}_{r,SP}\Omega_{SP})} \tag{1.37}$$

is a known constant with $\Delta x'$ and $\Delta y'$ being the voxel extents along x and y.

The algorithm proceeds to discretize the integral along z' into a sum, leading to a linear equation in the unknown $\tilde{F}$ values along z' at each point $\boldsymbol{\kappa} = (k_x,k_y)$ in

k-space. Such equation is available for each frequency sample ω_m ($m = 1, \ldots, N_\omega$) and each response type $\xi = 1, \ldots, N_\mathrm{T}$:

$$\widetilde{S}^{\,\mathrm{sc}}_{\xi}(\boldsymbol{\kappa}, \omega_m) \approx \sum_{n=1}^{N_z} \widetilde{f}(\boldsymbol{\kappa}; z'_n)\left[\widetilde{H}^{\,\mathrm{sc}}_{\xi 0}(\boldsymbol{\kappa}; z'_n; \omega_m)\right], m = 1, \ldots, N_\omega$$

$$\xi = 1, \ldots, N_\mathrm{T}, \tag{1.38}$$

where $\widetilde{f}(\boldsymbol{\kappa}; z'_n) = b\Delta z'_n \cdot \widetilde{F}(\boldsymbol{\kappa}; z'_n)$ is a scaled form of $\widetilde{F}$, $n = 1, \ldots, N_z$ is the index of an image slice along range at z'_n, and $\Delta z'_n$ is the discretization step along z centered on the nth image slice. The availability of multiple data points along frequency ω and data type ξ allows for "stacking" all these equations into a relatively small linear system of equations at each grid-point in Fourier space $\boldsymbol{\kappa}_{ij} = (i\Delta k_x, j\Delta k_y)$:

$$A(\boldsymbol{\kappa}_{ij}) \cdot f(\boldsymbol{\kappa}_{ij}) = d(\boldsymbol{\kappa}_{ij}). \tag{1.39}$$

With 2-D FFT, the number of grid point in Fourier space is the same as that in real space; therefore, $i = 1, \ldots, N_x$ and $j = 1, \ldots, N_y$, where N_x and N_y are the number of samples along x and y, respectively, on the acquisition aperture. The data vector $d(\boldsymbol{\kappa}_{ij})$ in (1.39) is the vectorized arrangement of all N_T responses at all N_ω frequencies, i.e.,

$$d(\boldsymbol{\kappa}_{ij}) = [d_1^T(\boldsymbol{\kappa}_{ij}) \cdots d_{N_\mathrm{T}}^T(\boldsymbol{\kappa}_{ij})]^T_{N_\mathrm{T}N_\omega \times 1}, i = 1, \ldots, N_x, j = 1, \ldots, N_y, \tag{1.40}$$

where the superscript T denotes a transposed vector and

$$d_\xi(\boldsymbol{\kappa}_{ij}) = \left[\widetilde{S}^{\,\mathrm{sc}}_{\xi}(\boldsymbol{\kappa}_{ij}, \omega_1) \cdots \widetilde{S}^{\,\mathrm{sc}}_{\xi}(\boldsymbol{\kappa}_{ij}, \omega_{N_\omega})\right]^T, \xi = 1, \ldots, N_\mathrm{T}. \tag{1.41}$$

The vectors,

$$f(\boldsymbol{\kappa}_{ij}) = [\widetilde{f}(\boldsymbol{\kappa}_{ij}; z'_1) \cdots \widetilde{f}(\boldsymbol{\kappa}_{ij}, z'_{N_z})]^T, i = 1, \ldots, N_x, j = 1, \ldots, N_y, \tag{1.42}$$

contain the values of the FT of the unknown contrast at all N_z range positions. Finally, the system matrix $A(\boldsymbol{\kappa}_{ij})$ is constructed from the PSFs as

$$A(\boldsymbol{\kappa}_{ij}) = \begin{bmatrix} A_1(\boldsymbol{\kappa}_{ij}) \\ \vdots \\ A_{N_\mathrm{T}}(\boldsymbol{\kappa}_{ij}) \end{bmatrix}_{N_\mathrm{T}N_\omega \times N_z}, i = 1, \ldots, N_x, j = 1, \ldots, N_y, \tag{1.43}$$

where

$$A_\xi(\boldsymbol{\kappa}_{ij}) = \begin{bmatrix} \widetilde{H}^{\,\mathrm{sc}}_{\xi 0}(\boldsymbol{\kappa}_{ij}; \omega_1; z'_1) & \cdots & \widetilde{H}^{\,\mathrm{sc}}_{\xi 0}(\boldsymbol{\kappa}_{ij}; \omega_1; z'_{N_z}) \\ \vdots & \ddots & \vdots \\ \widetilde{H}^{\,\mathrm{sc}}_{\xi 0}(\boldsymbol{\kappa}_{ij}; \omega_{N_\omega}; z'_1) & \cdots & \widetilde{H}^{\,\mathrm{sc}}_{\xi 0}(\boldsymbol{\kappa}_{ij}; \omega_{N_\omega}; z'_{N_z}) \end{bmatrix}_{N_\omega \times N_z}, \tag{1.44}$$

for each $\xi = 1, \ldots, N_\mathrm{T}$.

From (1.44) it is clear that the size of each system solved at a point in k-space is $N_T N_\omega \times N_z$. Typical values for N_T are from 1 to 5, for N_ω from 10 to 100, and for N_z from 3 to 10. Thus, the systems are small and the system matrix is "tall." All $N_x N_y$ such systems are solved very fast, typically using pseudoinverse solvers.

Once $f(k_x, k_y; z'_n)$ at each $n = 1, \ldots, N_z$ is found, the FT of the object's contrast $\widetilde{F}(k_x, k_y, z'_n)$ is recovered using the proper scaling factor:

$$\widetilde{F}(k_x, k_y, z'_n) = \frac{\Delta\widetilde{\varepsilon}_{r,SP}\Omega_{SP}}{\Delta x' \Delta y' \Delta z'_n} \widetilde{f}(k_x, k_y; z'_n), \quad n = 1, \ldots, N_z. \tag{1.45}$$

Finally, the inverse 2-D FT is applied to $\widetilde{F}(k_x, k_y, z'_n)$ to reconstruct a 2-D slice of the contrast $\Delta\widetilde{\varepsilon}_r(x', y', z')$ at each z'_n plane:

$$\Delta\widetilde{\varepsilon}_r(x', y', z'_n) = \mathrm{FT}_{2D}^{-1}\left\{\widetilde{F}(k_x, k_y, z'_n)\right\}, n = 1, \ldots, N_z. \tag{1.46}$$

The result for $\Delta\widetilde{\varepsilon}_r(x', y', z'_n)$ can be displayed in separate images for its real and imaginary parts. Instead of the OUT contrast, the images can display the real and imaginary parts of the OUT complex permittivity:

$$\widetilde{\varepsilon}_r(x', y', z'_n) = \widetilde{\varepsilon}_{r,b} + \Delta\widetilde{\varepsilon}_r(x', y', z'_n), n = 1, \ldots, N_z. \tag{1.47}$$

Finally, a qualitative contrast image can also be displayed by plotting the normalized contrast function:

$$I(x', y', z'_n) = \frac{|\Delta\widetilde{\varepsilon}_r(x', y', z'_n)|}{|\Delta\widetilde{\varepsilon}_r|_{\max}}, n = 1, \ldots, N_z. \tag{1.48}$$

Below is the summary of the basic steps of the reconstruction algorithm of QMH.

Quantitative microwave holography: summary

Calibration

1. Measure incident-field responses $S^{\mathrm{inc}}(x, y, z_{\mathrm{Rx}})$ with the RO (see Figure 1.8(a)).
2. Measure total-field PSF responses $H_0^{\mathrm{tot}}(x, y, z_{\mathrm{Rx}})$ with the CO (see Figure 1.8(b)) where the SP is positioned at the center of each desired range location z'_n, $n = 1, \ldots, N_z$. As a minimum, $H_0^{\mathrm{tot}}(x, y, z_{\mathrm{Rx}})$ is measured with an SP at the $z' = 0$ plane. At all other desired range locations ($z' = 0$), the PSF can be derived from H_0^{tot} at $z' = 0$ through an analytical transformation (range translation).
3. Extract scattered-field PSF $H_0^{\mathrm{tot}}(x, y, z_{\mathrm{Rx}})$ using either Born's approximation (1.27) or Rytov's approximation (1.28).
4. Perform 2-D FT to find $\widetilde{H}_0^{\mathrm{sc}}(k_x, k_y, z_{\mathrm{Rx}})$.

Object under test

1. Measure total-field responses $S^{\text{tot}}(x, y, z_{\text{RX}})$ with the OUT (see Figure 1.8(c)).
2. Extract scattered-field data $S^{\text{sc}}(x, y, z_{\text{Rx}})$ using either Born's approximation (1.26) or Rytov's approximation (1.28).
3. Perform 2-D FT to find $\tilde{S}^{\text{sc}}(k_x, k_y, z_{\text{Rx}})$.
4. Construct the system of equations (Equation (1.39)) at each point in k-space $\boldsymbol{\kappa}_{ij}$ $(i = 1, \ldots, N_x, j = 1, \ldots, N_y)$ and solve for the contrast vectors $f(\boldsymbol{\kappa}_{ij})$ (1.42).
5. Construct k-space contrast function $\tilde{f}(k_x, k_y; z'_n)$ at each range slice z'_n, $n = 1, \ldots, N_z$ and apply proper scaling fact to obtain $\tilde{F}(k_x, k_y, z'_n)$ using (1.45).
6. At each slice z'_n, $n = 1, \ldots, N_z$, apply 2-D IFT to $\tilde{F}(k_x, k_y, z'_n)$ to recover the contrast $\Delta\tilde{\varepsilon}_{\text{r}}(x', y', z'_n)$ in real space; see (1.46).
7. Compute the complex relative permittivity of the OUT $\tilde{\varepsilon}_{\text{r}}(x', y', z'_n)$ using (1.47).
8. Generate images for the real and imaginary parts of $\tilde{\varepsilon}_{\text{r}}(x', y', z'_n)$. If desired, the imaginary-part plot can be converted to that of the effective conductivity using $\sigma_{\text{e}} = \omega\varepsilon_0 \text{Im}\tilde{\varepsilon}_{\text{r}}$.

1.6 Basics of scattered power mapping (SPM)

SPM is rooted in early work on image reconstruction with response sensitivities [42,43]. Unlike holography, it can perform reconstruction with data acquired at any configuration of observation points [4], i.e., it does not require apertures of canonical shapes (plane, cylinder, sphere), which holography needs in order to apply FFTs. However, it does benefit if the data are measured on such apertures because then it can employ fast deconvolution in k-space [1,5]. It is the k-space implementation of SPM that is described later. This implementation offers the best computational efficiency of the SPM image reconstruction.

The SPM is a two-stage image-reconstruction algorithm. The first stage is the generation of the scattered-power map $M(\mathbf{r}')$. It is a (complex-valued) qualitative estimate of the OUT. For a set of observation (Rx) points $\mathbf{r}_p$, $p = 1, \ldots, N_{\text{Rx}}$, source (Tx) points $\mathbf{r}_q$, $q = 1, \ldots, N_{\text{Tx}}$, frequency samples ω_m, $m = 1, \ldots, N_\omega$, and types of responses $\xi = 1, \ldots, N_{\text{T}}$, it is expressed as [1,4]

$$M(\mathbf{r}') = \sum_{\xi=1}^{N_{\text{T}}} \sum_{p=1}^{N_{\text{Rx}}} \sum_{q=1}^{N_{\text{Tx}}} \sum_{m=1}^{N_\omega} S_\xi^{\text{sc}}(\mathbf{r}_p, \mathbf{r}_q; \omega_m) \cdot \left[H_\xi^{\text{sc}}(\mathbf{r}_p, \mathbf{r}_q; \omega_m; \mathbf{r}')\right]^*, \tag{1.49}$$

where $S_\xi^{\text{sc}}(\mathbf{r}_p, \mathbf{r}_q, \omega_m)$ is the ξth scattered signal whereas $H_\xi^{\text{sc}}(\mathbf{r}_p, \mathbf{r}_q; \omega_m; \mathbf{r}')$ is the respective PSF for a point scatterer at $\mathbf{r}'$. At this stage, a qualitative OUT image can be obtained by plotting $|M(\mathbf{r}')|$ or its normalized version,

$$I(\mathbf{r}') = \frac{|M(\mathbf{r}')|}{|M(\mathbf{r}')|_{\max}}. \tag{1.50}$$

In [1], it is shown that, under conditions of weak scattering, the contrast solution provided by (1.49) minimizes the squared ℓ_2 norm of the data error function,

$$e(p) = 0.5|R(p) - R|_2^2, \tag{1.51}$$

where p is the vector of the contrast values across the imaged domain V', $R(p)$ is the vector of responses for a given estimate of p, and R is the vector of measured responses.

Note that each term in (1.49) can be weighted to control its impact on the image. For example, normalization across a data set at each frequency may be beneficial [4,5] if the signal strengths are strongly frequency dependent. The frequency normalization procedure is described in Section 1.8. Further, just like holography, (1.49) admits the use of analytical PSFs in the form of (1.18) or (1.19), if the measurements are taken in the antenna's far zone.

The reconstruction with (1.49) is fast since it uses only multiplications and summations. It is also very fast if processing in Fourier space is possible, e.g., with data acquired on a planar surface (along x and y) with uniform sampling. In this case, we take the advantage of the translational invariance of the PSFs along and to compute the scattered-power map as [1,5]

$$M(x', y', z') = \mathrm{FT}_{2\mathrm{D}}^{-1}\left\{\sum_{\xi=1}^{N_\mathrm{T}}\sum_{m=1}^{N_\omega} \widetilde{S}_\xi^{\mathrm{sc}}(k_x, k_y, \omega_m) \cdot \left[\widetilde{H}_{\xi 0}^{\mathrm{sc}}(k_x, k_y; \omega_m; z')\right]^*\right\}, \tag{1.52}$$

where $\widetilde{S}_\xi^{\mathrm{sc}}(k_x, k_y, \omega_m)$ is the 2-D FT of the data $S_\xi^{\mathrm{sc}}(x, y, \omega_m)$ with respect to x and y, and $\widetilde{H}_{\xi 0}^{\mathrm{sc}}(k_x, k_y; \omega_m; z')$ is the 2-D FT of the respective PSF response $H_{\xi 0}^{\mathrm{sc}}(x, y; \omega_m; z')$ for an SP located at $x' = 0, y' = 0$, in the plane $z' = \mathrm{const}$. Similarly to holography, the PSF $H_{\xi 0}^{\mathrm{sc}}(x, y; \omega_m; z')$ can be measured or analytically approximated. However, for SPM to produce a quantitative result in its second stage, it is best if the PSF is measured. Further, the PSFs at the various range locations $\widetilde{H}_{\xi 0}(k_x, k_y; \omega_m; z')$ can be obtained from that at $z' = 0$ through an analytical transformation (range translation).

With quantitatively accurate measured PSFs, SPM can proceed with a second stage of reconstruction, which provides a quantitative image. In [4] (see also [1]), it is shown that the scattered-power map of the OUT $M(\mathbf{r}')$ relates to the scattered-power map of an SP at $\mathbf{r}''$, $M_H(\mathbf{r}', \mathbf{r}'')$, as

$$M(\mathbf{r}') = \frac{1}{\Delta\widetilde{\varepsilon}_{\mathrm{r,SP}}\Omega_{\mathrm{SP}}} \iiint_{V'} \Delta\widetilde{\varepsilon}_\mathrm{r}(\mathbf{r}'') \cdot M_H(\mathbf{r}', \mathbf{r}'') dv''. \tag{1.53}$$

The SP maps $M_H(\mathbf{r}', \mathbf{r}'')$ are nothing but the qualitative image PSFs when the imaged object is the SP located at $\mathbf{r}''$. Explicitly, they are calculated using (49) as

$$M_H(\mathbf{r}', \mathbf{r}'') = \sum_{\xi=1}^{N_\mathrm{T}}\sum_{p=1}^{N_\mathrm{Rx}}\sum_{q=1}^{N_\mathrm{Tx}}\sum_{m=1}^{N_\omega} H_\xi^{\mathrm{sc}}(\mathbf{r}_p, \mathbf{r}_q; \omega_m; \mathbf{r}'') \cdot \left[H_\xi^{\mathrm{sc}}(\mathbf{r}_p, \mathbf{r}_q; \omega_m; \mathbf{r}')\right]^*. \tag{1.54}$$

In the case of planar acquisition in x and y, (1.52) is used for both the OUT and the SP scattered-power maps. The quantitative reconstruction in k-space works directly with the 2-D FTs of the OUT map, $\widetilde{M}(k_x, k_y, z')$, and the PSF map (for an SP in the center of the range slice $z'' = \text{const.}$), $\widetilde{M}_{H0}(k_x, k_y, z'; z'')$. Their respective expressions follow from (1.52) and are explicitly written as

$$\widetilde{M}(k_x, k_y, z') = \sum_{\xi=1}^{N_\mathrm{T}} \sum_{m=1}^{N_\omega} \widetilde{S}_\xi^{\mathrm{sc}}(k_x, k_y, \omega_m) \cdot \left[\widetilde{H}_{\xi 0}(k_x, k_y; \omega_m; z')\right]^*, \tag{1.55}$$

and

$$\widetilde{M}_{H0}(k_x, k_y, z'; z'') = \sum_{\xi=1}^{N_\mathrm{T}} \sum_{m=1}^{N_\omega} \widetilde{H}_{\xi 0}^{\mathrm{sc}}(k_x, k_y, \omega_m; z'') \cdot \left[\widetilde{H}_{\xi 0}(k_x, k_y; \omega_m; z')\right]^*. \tag{1.56}$$

To solve (1.53) for the unknown contrast $\Delta\widetilde{\varepsilon}_\mathrm{r}(\mathbf{r}'')$ efficiently in k-space, we cast it in the form of a convolution. To achieve that, we exploit the assumption that the background medium is either homogeneous or layered in x and y. In this case, the image PSFs $M_H(\mathbf{r}', \mathbf{r}'')$ are translationally invariant in x and y, i.e.,

$$M_H(x', y', z'; x'', y'', z'') = M_{H0}(x' - x'', y' - y'', z'; z''), \tag{1.57}$$

where

$$M_{H0}(x', y', z'; z'') \equiv M_H(x', y', z'; 0, 0, z'') \tag{1.58}$$

is the scattered-power map of an SP located at $(0, 0, z'')$. Equation (1.57) is simply a statement that the image of the SP at (x'', y'', z'') is a shifted (along x and y) version of the image of the SP at $(0, 0, z'')$. This allows for writing (1.53) as

$$M(x', y', z') = \frac{1}{\Delta\widetilde{\varepsilon}_{\mathrm{r,SP}}\Omega_{\mathrm{SP}}} \cdot \iiint_{x''y''z''} \Delta\widetilde{\varepsilon}_\mathrm{r}(x'', y'', z'') \cdot M_{\mathrm{H0}}(x' - x'', y' - y'', z'; z'') dx'' dy'' dz''. \tag{1.59}$$

This is a 2-D convolution in (x', y') and it can be written in Fourier space as

$$\widetilde{M}(k_x, k_y, z') = \frac{\Delta x' \Delta y'}{\Delta\widetilde{\varepsilon}_{\mathrm{r,SP}}\Omega_{\mathrm{SP}}} \int_{z''} \Delta\widetilde{\varepsilon}(k_x, k_y, z'') \cdot \widetilde{M}_{H0}(k_x, k_y, z'; z'') dz'', \tag{1.60}$$

where $\Delta x'$ and $\Delta y'$ are the lateral dimensions of the voxel size. Representing the integral along z'' as a sum leads to

$$\widetilde{M}(k_x, k_y, z_p) = \frac{\Delta\Omega}{\Delta\widetilde{\varepsilon}_{\mathrm{r,SP}}\Omega_{\mathrm{SP}}} \cdot \sum_{q=1}^{N_z} \Delta\widetilde{\varepsilon}_\mathrm{r}(k_x, k_y, z_q) \cdot \widetilde{M}_{H0}(k_x, k_y, z_p; z_q), \quad p = 1, \ldots, N_z, \tag{1.61}$$

where $\Delta\Omega = \Delta x'\Delta y'\Delta z'$ is the voxel's volume, $\Delta z'$ is the voxel size along z, and N_z is the number of image slices along z. We can now solve a small square ($N_z \times N_z$) linear system of equations at each point in Fourier space $\boldsymbol{\kappa}_{ij} = (i\Delta k_x, j\Delta k_y)$:

$$M(\boldsymbol{\kappa}_{ij}) \cdot x(\boldsymbol{\kappa}_{ij}) = m(\boldsymbol{\kappa}_{ij}),\, i = 1,\ldots,N_x, j = 1,\ldots,N_y, \tag{1.62}$$

where

$$x(\boldsymbol{\kappa}_{ij}) = \frac{\Delta\Omega}{\Delta\tilde{\varepsilon}_{\mathrm{r,SP}}\Omega_{\mathrm{SP}}}\left[\Delta\tilde{\varepsilon}_{\mathrm{r}}(\boldsymbol{\kappa}_{ij}, z_1) \quad \cdots \quad \Delta\tilde{\varepsilon}_{\mathrm{r}}(\boldsymbol{\kappa}_{ij}, z_{N_z})\right]^T, \tag{1.63}$$

$$m(\boldsymbol{\kappa}_{ij}) = \left[\widetilde{M}(\boldsymbol{\kappa}_{ij}, z_1) \quad \cdots \quad \widetilde{M}(\boldsymbol{\kappa}_{ij}, z_{N_z})\right]^T, \tag{1.64}$$

$$M(\boldsymbol{\kappa}_{ij}) = \begin{bmatrix} \widetilde{M}_{H0}(\boldsymbol{\kappa}_{ij}, z_1; z_1) & \cdots & \widetilde{M}_{H0}(\boldsymbol{\kappa}_{ij}, z_1; z_{N_z}) \\ \widetilde{M}_{H0}(\boldsymbol{\kappa}_{ij}, z_2; z_1) & \cdots & \widetilde{M}_{H0}(\boldsymbol{\kappa}_{ij}, z_2; z_{N_z}) \\ \vdots & \ddots & \vdots \\ \widetilde{M}_{H0}(\boldsymbol{\kappa}_{ij}, z_{N_z}; z_1) & \cdots & \widetilde{M}_{H0}(\boldsymbol{\kappa}_{ij}, z_{N_z}; z_{N_z}) \end{bmatrix}. \tag{1.65}$$

Once we have $\Delta\tilde{\varepsilon}_{\mathrm{r}}(\boldsymbol{\kappa}_{ij}, z_p)$ for $\forall\boldsymbol{\kappa}_{ij}$ and for all $p = 1,\ldots,N_z$, the 3-D contrast is recovered through 2-D IFT slice by slice:

$$\Delta\tilde{\varepsilon}_{\mathrm{r}}(x', y', z'_p) = \mathrm{F}T_{2D}^{-1}\left\{\Delta\tilde{\varepsilon}_{\mathrm{r}}(k_x, k_y, z'_p)\right\}, \quad p = 1,\ldots,N_z. \tag{1.66}$$

Finally, the relative complex permittivity of the OUT is calculated as

$$\tilde{\varepsilon}_{\mathrm{r}}(x', y', z'_p) = \tilde{\varepsilon}_{\mathrm{b,r}} + \Delta\tilde{\varepsilon}_{\mathrm{r}}(x', y', z'_p). \tag{1.67}$$

The summary of the basic steps of the reconstruction algorithm of quantitative SPM is given in the following.

Scattered-power mapping: summary
Calibration

1. Measure incident-field responses $S^{\mathrm{inc}}(x, y, z_{\mathrm{Rx}})$ with the RO (see Figure 1.8(a)).
2. Measure total-field PSF responses $H_0^{\mathrm{tot}}(x, y, z_{\mathrm{Rx}})$ with the CO (see Figure 1.8(b)) where the SP is positioned at the center of each desired range location z'_p, $p = 1,\ldots,N_z$. As a minimum, $H_0^{\mathrm{tot}}(x, y, z_{\mathrm{Rx}})$ is measured with an SP at the $z' = 0$ plane. At all other desired range locations ($z' \neq 0$), the PSF can be derived from H_0^{tot} at $z' = 0$ through range translation.
3. Extract scattered-field PSF $H_0^{\mathrm{tot}}(x, y, z_{\mathrm{Rx}})$ using either Born's approximation (1.27) or Rytov's approximation (1.28).
4. Perform 2-D FT to find $\widetilde{H}_0^{\mathrm{sc}}(k_x, k_y, z_{\mathrm{Rx}})$.

5. Compute the 3-D scattered-power maps $\widetilde{M}_H(k_x, k_y, z'; z_p)$ for each range position of the SP z_p, $p = 1, \ldots, N_z$; see (1.56).

Object under test

1. Measure total-field responses $S^{\text{tot}}(x, y, z_{\text{RX}})$ with the OUT (see Figure 1.8(c)).
2. Extract scattered-field data $S^{\text{sc}}(x, y, z_{\text{Rx}})$ using either Born's approximation (1.26) or Rytov's approximation (1.28).
3. Perform 2-D FT to find $\widetilde{S}^{\text{sc}}(k_x, k_y, z_{\text{Rx}})$.
4. Compute the 3-D scattered-power map $\widetilde{M}(k_x, k_y, z')$; see (1.55).
5. If desired, plot the OUT qualitative image $|M(x', y', z')|$ where $M(x', y', z') = FT_{2D}^{-1}\left\{\widetilde{M}(k_x, k_y, z')\right\}$.
6. Construct the system of equations (Equation (1.62)) at each point in k-space $\boldsymbol{\kappa}_{ij}$ $(i = 1, \ldots, N_x,\ j = 1, \ldots, N_y)$ and solve for the contrast vectors $x(\boldsymbol{\kappa}_{ij})$; see (1.63).
7. Construct k-space contrast function $\Delta\widetilde{\varepsilon}_{\text{r}}(k_x, k_y; z'_p)$ at each range slice z'_p, $p = 1, \ldots, N_z$.
8. At each slice z'_p, $p = 1, \ldots, N_z$, apply 2-D IFT to $\Delta\widetilde{\varepsilon}_{\text{r}}(k_x, k_y; z'_p)$ in order to recover the contrast $\Delta\widetilde{\varepsilon}_{\text{r}}(x', y', z'_p)$ in real space.
9. Compute the complex relative permittivity of the OUT $\widetilde{\varepsilon}_{\text{r}}(x', y', z'_p)$ using (1.67).
10. Generate images for the real and imaginary parts of $\widetilde{\varepsilon}_{\text{r}}(x', y', z'_p)$. If desired, the imaginary-part plot can be converted to that of effective conductivity using $\sigma_{\text{e}} = \omega\varepsilon_0 \text{Im}\widetilde{\varepsilon}_{\text{r}}$.

1.7 Examples of QMH and SPM

To demonstrate the ability of QMH and SPM to reconstruct the permittivity of imaged objects, a simulation example similar to the one shown in [2] is performed. The data acquisition is performed on an RO, three COs, (with an SP at three desired range locations) and an OUT. The OUT is constructed of several dielectric objects. The largest object of relative permittivity $\widetilde{\varepsilon}_{\text{r}} = 1.5 - \text{i}0.0$ is shaped to form the letter “C.” Three smaller cube-shaped objects are placed nearby the C-shaped object. Their relative permittivity is $\widetilde{\varepsilon}_{\text{r}} = 1.1 - \text{i}0.0$. These three cubes are offset along z to provide benchmark targets in 3-D imaging. The background medium is vacuum (relative permittivity $\widetilde{\varepsilon}_{\text{r,b}} = 1.0 - \text{i}0.0$). The completed structure is shown in Figure 1.9.

The three COs have the same background (vacuum) with a small SP placed at the center $(x' = 0, y' = 0)$ of three different range (z') planes. The three range locations ($z' = 30$, $z' = 40$, $z' = 50$ mm) enable QMH and SPM to reconstruct a respective 2-D image slice, thereby providing a 3-D image. The SP is a cube

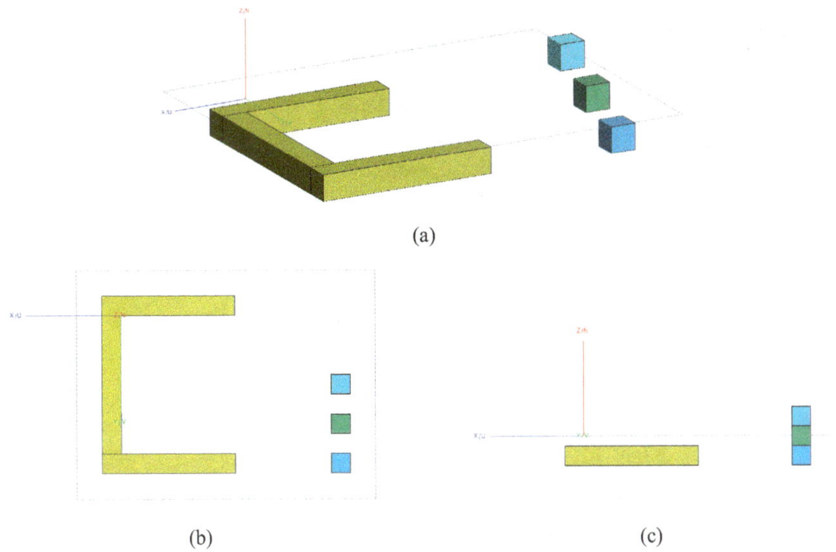

Figure 1.9 *The OUT in the simulation example used to demonstrate the ability of QMH and SPM to generate 3-D images: (a) isometric view, (b) top view, (c) side view. The C-shape and the three cuboid objects reside in three range "slices," where the PSFs are available. The C-shape is 7 cm by 9 cm by 1 cm, and the cubes are all 1 cm^3*

(1 cm^3) of relative permittivity $\tilde{\varepsilon}_{r,SP} = 1.1 - i0.0$. Finally, the RO involves a background of vacuum with no embedded objects.

To measure these structures, two half-wavelength (at the center frequency of 5 GHz) dipole antennas are positioned 80 mm apart. The dipoles are positioned so that the OUT is centered between them, forming a 2-port network. Each dipole performs a reflection measurement to acquire S_{11} and S_{22} data. They sweep a frequency range of 3–8 GHz in 1-GHz increments, and across a 300 mm by 300 mm acquisition plane in 10-mm increments.

The quantitative images reconstructed utilizing QMH and SPM are shown in Figures 1.10 and 1.11, respectively. The results are similar to one another. The C-shape is clearly visible and detected in the $z = 30$ mm slice, with its permittivity well estimated. However, the three small cubes are somewhat masked by ringing artifacts, which appear in each layer. In tissue measurements, these artifacts can become so pronounced that the entire image is obscured (see Section 1.9) [3,6,9].

The astute reader will also notice that nonphysical permittivity values ($\varepsilon'_r < 1$ and $\varepsilon''_r > 0$) are generated. There are two major reasons leading to such nonphysical values. The first is due to the fact that the inversion takes place in Fourier space with numerical artifacts arising from the direct and IFTs. The resolution of these issues is discussed in Section 1.8. The second reason is the violation of the limitations imposed by the linear approximation of scattering [1]. This problem can strictly be resolved only if nonlinear

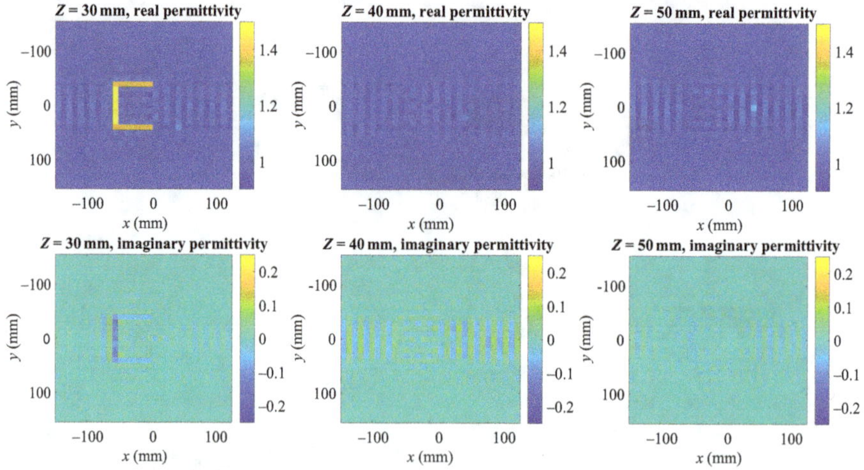

*Figure 1.10 Quantitative reconstruction of the OUT shown in Figure 1.9 utilizing **QMH**. The top row of images shows the real part of the relative permittivity whereas the bottom row shows its imaginary part. The images in each column correspond to a given slice along range*

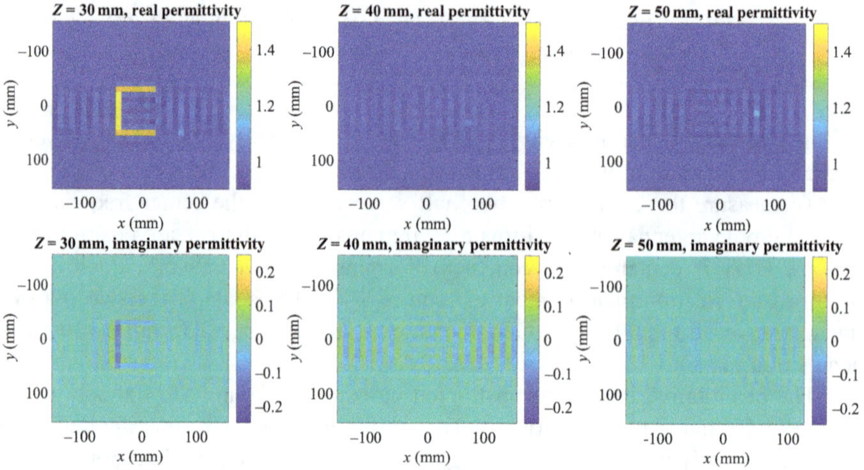

*Figure 1.11 Quantitative reconstruction of the OUT shown in Figure 1.9 utilizing **SPM**. The top row of images shows the real part of the relative permittivity whereas the bottom row shows its imaginary part. The images in each column correspond to a given slice along range*

iterative methods for enhancing the quantitative images are used. These optimization-based methods are not discussed here. We only mention that such methods are inherently suited for imposing constraints on the physical range of permittivity values.

1.8 Advanced signal processing for improved image reconstruction

A number of filtering and normalization techniques are available to attempt to reduce the impact of the artifacts that appear in Figures 1.10 and 1.11. The usefulness of these techniques depends on (a) the physics of the EM scattering and (b) the specifics of the experimental setup and procedure.

1.8.1 Apodization filtering

One issue that arises in Fourier-based image reconstruction is the generation of artifacts that are caused by the signals at the edge of the acquisition aperture. When applying the discrete FT, an assumption is made that the signal is periodic. In imaging, this assumption is valid when the edges of the measured space align well with one another in terms of signal values.

Consider a sample *S*-parameter measurement of the OUT used in Section 1.7, taken at 5 GHz and shown in Figure 1.12(a). Note that the signal scattered by the C-shaped object reaches the edge of the acquisition aperture. A small point-like artifact is also added artificially to the corner of the data set to emphasize the difference in the signal values at the aperture edges. Now, consider Figure 1.12(b), which shows the same data set as in Figure 1.12(a) but copied four times. We highlight the conspicuous boundaries indicating sharp changes in the signal magnitude. This boundary of signal discontinuity, when transformed into the 2-D Fourier domain, generates spurious high-frequency responses, which reduce the quality of the resultant reconstruction. Figure 1.14(a) shows the unsatisfactory result of the reconstructed image slice where

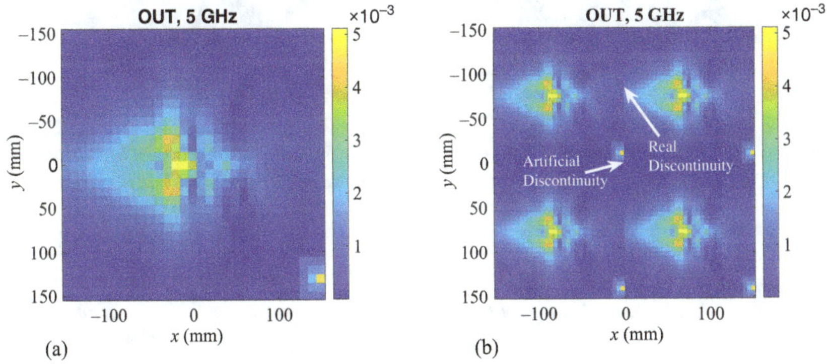

Figure 1.12 *S-parameter measurements of the OUT used in [2] at 5 GHz: (a) typical map of the* S*-parameter magnitude with the addition of a manually inserted artifact in the bottom right corner and (b) the map shown in (a) repeated four times. Note that two discontinuities appear here, one at the artifact location and the other along the center vertical boundary. These discontinuities lead to artifacts appearing in k-space after the 2-D Fourier transform is applied*

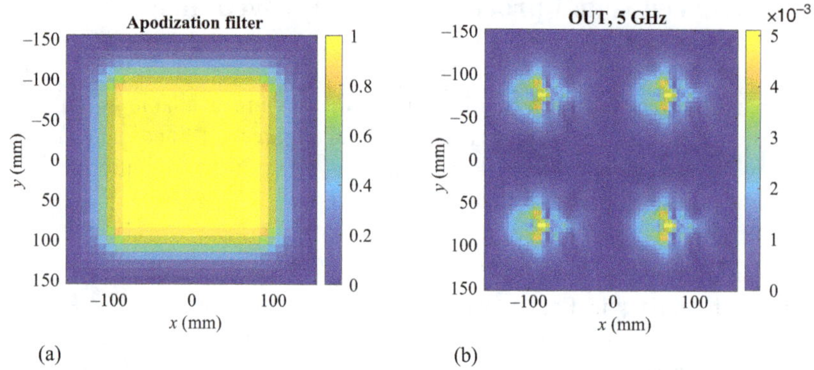

Figure 1.13 (a) The 2-D Tukey apodization filter applied to Figure 1.11 and (b) The resultant S*-parameter magnitude map is repeated four times. The apodization filter has effectively removed the data discontinuity at the borders between the four copies of the data set*

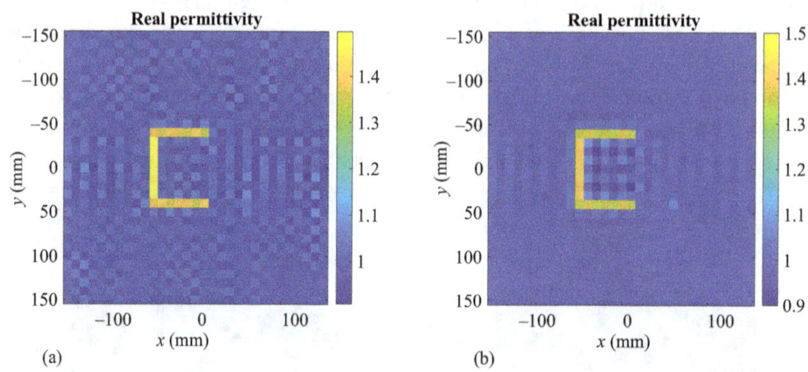

Figure 1.14 QMH reconstruction of the C-shape when (a) an edge artifact has been added to the 5-GHz OUT response and (b) an apodization filter has been applied to remove the impact of the edge discontinuities. Speckling artifacts cover the entire space of (a), but are substantially removed in (b). However, the overall permittivity estimate of the C-shape in (b) has decreased in accuracy due to the impact of the filter

the C-shape resides. The ringing artifacts are significantly stronger in comparison with the top-left image in Figures 1.10 and 1.11.

In order to suppress such artifacts, an apodization (or windowing) filter is applied. This filter reduces the edge values of the data sets to near zero, thereby ensuring that no high-frequency components in k-space are artificially generated by the FT. An example of such an apodization filter (a Tukey filter) is shown in Figure 1.13(a), which is applied to the data shown in Figure 1.12(a). Figure 1.13(b) shows the four copies (side by side) of the data set from Figure 1.12(a) with the apodization filter applied. Now, there are no discernible signal discontinuities. The reconstruction of the C-shape with the application of the apodization filter is shown in Figure 1.14(b). The ringing artifacts are suppressed significantly, allowing for the small and weak cubic scatterer to the right of the C-shape to become visible.

There is an important trade-off to consider when applying apodization filters. They effectively remove data at the edges of the acquisition aperture, thus reducing the aperture extent. The size of the aperture affects the image spatial resolution—the smaller the aperture, the poorer the lateral resolution [1]. In addition, the reduction of the overall signal power collected over the aperture leads to an observable decrease in the reconstructed permittivity distribution. Therefore, the apodization filter must be designed to reduce the signal at the boundary of the aperture while minimizing the effect on the image spatial resolution and its quantitative accuracy. Looking closely at Figure 1.14(b), the reader will notice that the estimate of the C-shape permittivity has somewhat decreased in value compared to Figure 1.14(a), particularly on the vertical bar of the C (from $\varepsilon_r = 1.5$ to $\varepsilon_r = 1.4$). This is an expected yet-undesirable consequence of the apodization data preprocessing.

The best approach to avoid over-filtering is to increase the size of the acquisition aperture. This reduces the signal strength at the edges naturally. In such cases, the image accuracy is less sensitive to the choice of the apodization filter and its parameters. In fact, with a sufficiently large aperture, apodization may not be necessary. However, hardware restrictions always put limits on the size of the aperture. Moreover, real-world experimental setups inevitably suffer from reflections and EM interactions with mechanical supports, enclosures, cabling, etc., leading to unwanted signals at the edges of the aperture.

1.8.2 Low-pass filtering in the Fourier domain

Fourier-based image reconstruction algorithms are known to suffer from spurious (spatial) high-frequency artifacts [2]. These artifacts are due to numerical errors generated during the inversion process in k-space. They can appear in the final reconstruction as speckling artifacts, such as those shown in Figure 1.15(b).

To understand how this noise is generated, first consider the maximum spatial frequency for which information can be collected at a given wavelength. As shown in [1], in the absence of evanescent field information, the maximum possible spatial frequency along the acquisition aperture arises in reflection (monostatic radar) measurements and it is given by

$$k_\xi^{\max} \approx \frac{4\pi}{\lambda_{\min}} \quad (\text{rad/m}), \qquad \xi = x, y, \tag{1.68}$$

where $\lambda_{\min}$ is the shortest wavelength of the radiation used to measure the OUT. The maximum spatial frequency of the data determines the *fundamental resolution limit* that an imaging algorithm can achieve. For example, (1.68) dictates a lateral spatial resolution limit of $\delta_\xi \approx \lambda_{\min}/4$, $\xi \equiv x, y$.

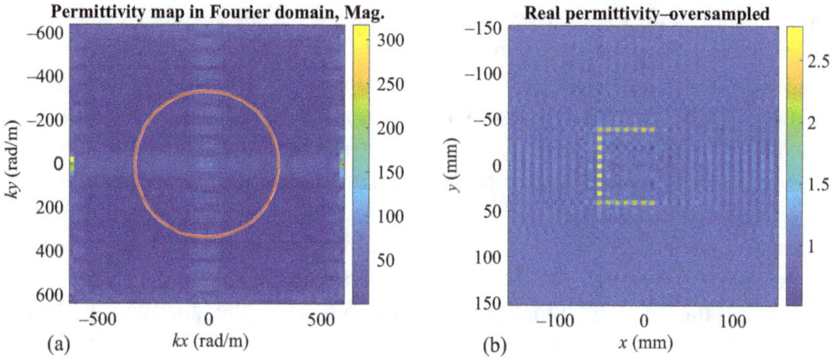

Figure 1.15 Reconstructions of the C-shaped object from [2]: (a) the Fourier domain permittivity of the C-shaped object (magnitude), with a red circle highlighting the $k_\xi^{\max}$ boundary and (b) the real domain permittivity of the C-shaped object, with a significant amount of rippling degrading the reconstruction. The signals shown in (a) beyond the red circle are not physical responses and can be filtered out

On the other hand, the minimum recommended sampling step is selected in accordance with the requirement that the phase shift from one sample to the next does not exceed π rad (Nyquist sampling criterion). The shortest recommended sampling step in far-field measurements Δ_ξ $(\xi \equiv x, y)$ arises in reflection measurements where the signal travels to/from the target at grazing angles [1]:

$$\Delta_\xi \approx \frac{\lambda_{\min}}{4}, \qquad \xi \equiv x, y. \tag{1.69}$$

Since practical apertures are finite, the angles of signal travel are rarely grazing. Thus, a sampling step on the order of $\lambda_{\min}/2$ is a common choice. Note that measurement time scales up with the number of samples. So, sampling is kept to the required minimum. With near-field measurements, however, the spatial signal behavior is *not* governed by the wavelength alone. Rapid changes occur due to evanescent and quasi-static modes, which lead to much higher spatial frequencies of the signal at the acquisition aperture. To capture such near-field behavior, the sampling rate must increase. Thus, the choice of sampling step is an interplay of two conflicting requirements: fewer samples for faster measurement and more samples for better utilization of high spatial frequency signal components at the aperture.

When the inversion process takes place in Fourier space, one has to consider the fact that the SNR of the data becomes poor as the spatial frequency increases. This is due to the fact that high spatial frequency components of the data are associated either with very weak evanescent-field signals or signals arriving at grazing angles. The latter are often associated with unwanted reflections from the environment, and even if they are due to the imaged object, the longer signal path leads to reduced signal strength, especially in the high-loss scenario of tissue imaging.

Biomedical imaging employs near-field measurements. Thus, dense sampling is beneficial in capturing evanescent field information. However, there must also be a strategy to deal with poor SNR at the high spatial frequencies. When a finer sampling step is used, the Fourier domain region extends beyond $k_\xi^{\max}$ in (1.68) (the limit dictated by propagation modes) where high levels of noise exist. To avoid the detrimental effect of these high frequencies on the reconstruction, a filter can be applied with a cutoff set to $k_\xi^{\max}$. As an example, Figure 1.15(a) shows the magnitude of the reconstructed C-shape permittivity in Fourier space whereas Figure 1.15(b) shows the real part of this permittivity in real (xy) space. Here, the reconstruction is carried out with QMH using intentionally oversampled data ($\Delta_\xi \approx \lambda_{min}/8$). A red circle in Figure 1.15(a) highlights the $k_\xi^{\max}$ boundary. Note that large spikes appear at the high-frequency values $k_x \approx \pm 628$ rad/m. These large spikes lead to speckling artifacts throughout the reconstructed image shown in Figure 1.15(b).

A fourth-order Butterworth low-pass filter with a 3-dB cutoff at $k_\xi^{\max}$ (see Figure 1.16(a)) is applied to the C-shape complex permittivity in Fourier domain (see Figure 1.15(a)) before performing the IFT. The resultant reconstruction after the IFT is shown in Figure 1.16(b). It has no speckling artifacts and is more quantitatively accurate compared to Figure 1.15(b). Nonetheless, the image is blurrier compared to the top left image in Figure 1.10. Similar to the apodization filters discussed in Section 1.8.1, a trade-off must be found between spatial resolution and noise suppression.

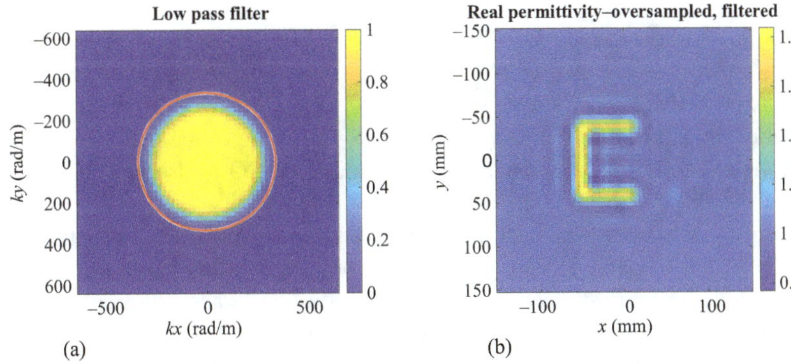

Figure 1.16 Images of (a) a low-pass filter in k-space with a cutoff frequency slightly below the $k_\xi^{\max}$ boundary and (b) the permittivity (real part) in real space of the C-shaped object after filtering has been applied in k-space. Now, the C-shape permittivity is estimated more accurately, and the small cube becomes visible. Note that the trade-off in using k-space filtering is the reduction of the high spatial-frequency information, leading to reduced image sharpness

1.8.3 PSF translation

Measured PSFs offer superior accuracy in comparison with analytical approximations or incident-field simulations. However, a critical challenge arises in 3-D imaging, where the PSF needs to be measured at each range (or depth) location where an image slice is desired. This may lead to a significant number of calibration (or CO) measurements. Note that the PSF $H^{sc}_{\xi 0}(x, y; z'; \omega)$ in (1.17) and (1.52) is acquired with a CO that contains an SP at the center of the z' range slice.

To reduce the calibration effort, one measurement of a CO is performed with the SP being at the range slice $z' = 0$, which is typically chosen in the middle of the imaged volume. With the PSF at $z' = 0$ known, the PSFs at all other range locations can be estimated accurately. This method for the PSF "range translation" employs the principles of the angular spectrum representation [13].

As an example, we consider the case of reflection measurements, where the Tx and Rx antennas coincide. It can be shown that the PSF translation can be efficiently done in k-space using

$$\widetilde{H}^{sc}_{\xi 0}(k_x, k_y; s; \omega) = \widetilde{H}^{sc}_{\xi 0}(k_x, k_y; z' = 0; \omega) \cdot e^{-ik_z s}, \tag{1.70}$$

where s is the shift in the z position of the SP from $z' = 0$ to $z' = s$, k_z is the spatial frequency along z, and $\widetilde{H}^{sc}_{\xi 0}(k_x, k_y; z' = 0; \omega)$ is the FT of the PSF measured with the SP at $z' = 0$. The expression in (1.70) assumes that positive s ($s > 0$) indicates that the SP position moves away from the Tx/Rx antenna pair whereas $s < 0$ indicates an SP shifted toward the Tx/Rx antenna pair. In the former case, the exponential factor results in a phase delay and (in a lossy medium) magnitude decay whereas with $s < 0$ it leads to a phase advance and a magnitude increase. In the case of reflection measurements, k_z is obtained as

$$k_z = \sqrt{(2k_b)^2 - k_x^2 - k_y^2}, \quad \Im\{k_z\} > 0, \tag{1.71}$$

where k_b is the background wavenumber.

An example of an analytically shifted PSF versus the exact PSF can be seen in Figure 1.17. These PSFs are obtained in simulations of CO measurements where the SP is a dielectric cube of volume 1 cm^3 and permittivity $\tilde{\varepsilon}_{r,b} = 1.1 + i0.0$ in a background of vacuum. The cube is aligned with the center of the acquisition plane $(x', y') = (0, 0)$. Two PSFs are acquired using Born's approximation (1.7). One PSF is acquired with the SP positioned 3 cm away from the Tx/Rx acquisition plane and the second one is obtained with the SP being at a distance of 4 cm. The PSF corresponding to a distance of 4 cm is then used as the baseline PSF and is analytically "shifted" by 1 cm, using (1.70), to obtain the estimate of the PSF for a probe at 3 cm.

The left column of Figure 1.17 depicts the exact (or "measured") PSF (top: real part, bottom: imaginary part) at 3 GHz. The center column of Figure 1.17 shows the respective estimated PSF. Finally, the right column shows the "measured" PSF (for a probe at 4 cm from the Tx/Rx antenna) used as a baseline for the analytical shift. We observe that the analytically shifted and the exact PSFs are in excellent agreement.

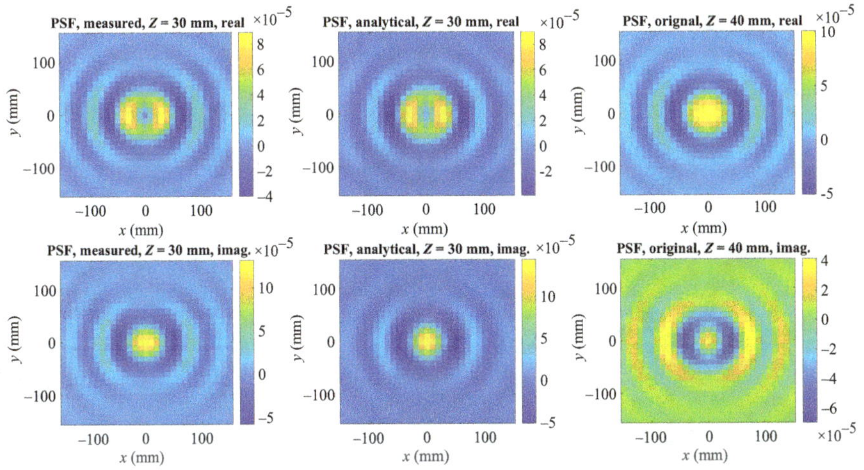

Figure 1.17 Plots of the real and imaginary parts of three PSFs based on reflection S*-parameter measurements with a scattering probe aligned with the center of the acquisition aperture,* $(x', y') = (0, 0)$*: real parts in the top row, imaginary parts in the bottom row. First column: PSF from a measurement where the probe is 30 mm away from the aperture. Second column: estimated PSF for a probe, which is 30 mm away from the aperture; the estimation uses a baseline PSF, which is measured with the probe being 40 mm away from the aperture. Third column: the baseline PSF measurement where the probe is 40 mm away from the aperture*

To evaluate the quality of the PSF translation in an imaging application, the example in Section 1.7 (an OUT including a C-shape with three small cubes) is repeated, but now only one measured PSF (for the central range slice) is assumed available whereas the PSFs at the other two range locations are analytically derived from the measured one. The resultant QMH and SPM reconstructions can be seen in Figures 1.18 and 1.19, respectively. The C-shape and the small cubes are reconstructed in the correct z-planes. In comparison with the reconstruction results based on exact PSFs (see Figures 1.10 and 1.11), a somewhat stronger artifact of the C-shape can be seen in the imaginary part of the middle layer ($z = 40$ mm) in both reconstructions. This is primarily due to the limitations associated with using the range-translation PSF approximation. The basic limitation stems from the fact that it is based on scalar wave theory where the scattered fields are governed by the Helmholtz equation. In reality, the EM field is governed by Maxwell's equations. Note that the simulations providing the data for this example employ a full 3-D EM simulator [44].

The scalar model of scattering cannot take into account the polarization properties of the employed dipole antennas and neither can they account for the polarization properties of the small dielectric cube used as an SP. Finally, the range

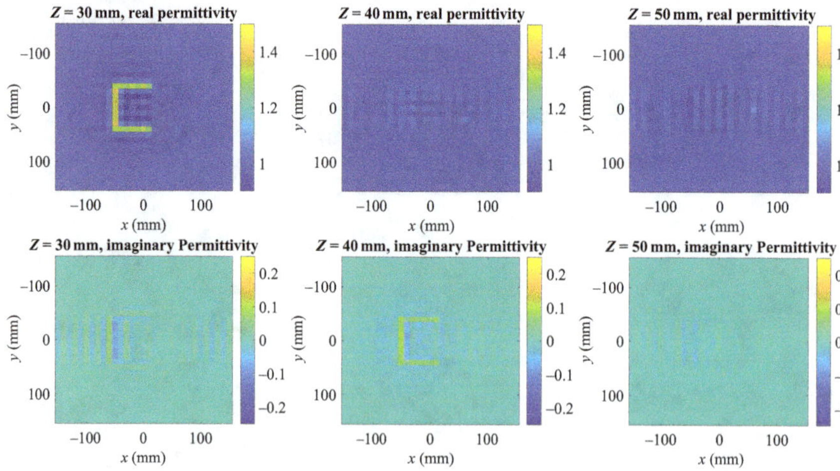

Figure 1.18 Reconstruction of the OUT shown in Figure 1.9 utilizing ***QMH*** *with* ***frequency normalization****, an* ***apodization filter****, and a* ***low-pass filter****. The top row shows the real part of the relative permittivity in three z slices, and the bottom row shows the respective imaginary parts. Each image column corresponds to a z-slice. The C-shape permittivity estimate is less accurate than previous, and some ghost images appear in the imaginary permittivity slice at* $z = 40 \ mm$

translation method of (1.70) cannot account for multiple reflections and mutual coupling between the antennas and the SP. Both limitations incur approximation errors that become increasingly prominent in near-field scenarios (probe being very close to the antennas), where multiple scattering and field polarization effects are not negligible.

While the analytical PSF range translation reduces the number of calibration measurements for 3-D imaging, its usefulness in medical imaging is limited. This is due to the high loss in tissue, which makes reflection measurements challenging. Transmission (or forward-scatter) measurements achieve a significantly higher SNR than the reflection (back-scatter) ones. On the other hand, the transmission measurements have poor range resolution [1], which in effect renders the modality 2-D. Accordingly, the forward-scatter PSFs are practically insensitive to the range position of the SP.

1.8.4 Frequency normalization

In order to reconstruct high-quality 2-D and 3-D images, broadband frequency measurements are required [5,7]. The selection of the frequency range depends on the application. As an example, breast cancer microwave imaging typically operates in the frequency range from about 1 to about 8 GHz [10]. Tissue loss depends strongly on the frequency. Lower frequency signals attenuate in tissue at a much

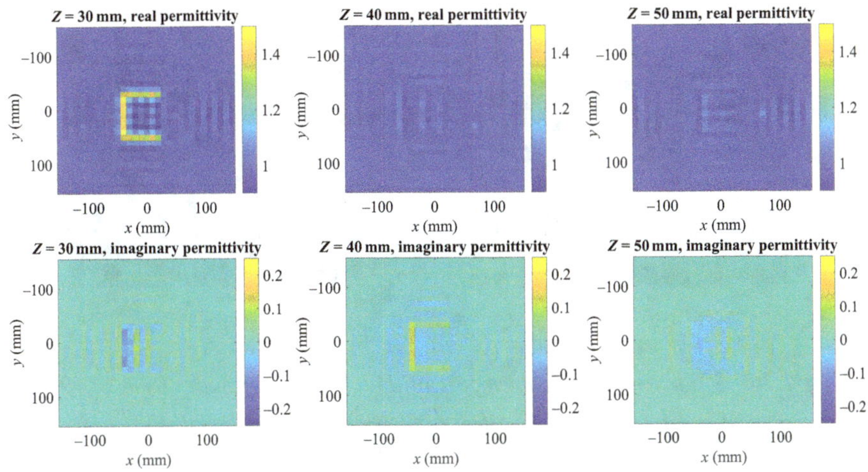

Figure 1.19 *Reconstruction of the OUT shown in Figure 1.9 utilizing* ***SPM*** *with* ***frequency normalization****, an* ***apodization filter****, and a* ***low-pass filter****. The top row of images shows the real part of the relative permittivity, and the bottom row shows the imaginary part of the relative permittivity. Each image column shows the range location (e.g., z-slice) being reconstructed. The C-shape permittivity estimate is somewhat less accurate than the results in Figures 1.10 and 1.11, which use exact PSFs. Some ghost image artifacts appear in the imaginary permittivity slice at* $z = 40\ \ mm$

slower rate than the high-frequency signals and thus they penetrate deeper. On the other hand, the high-frequency signals capture the most rapid spatial fluctuations in the propagation environment and thus provide the highest image resolution. Utilizing a wide frequency range provides a balance between penetration for a given SNR and image resolution [1].

When using such a wide bandwidth, it is important to consider the amount of attenuation that occurs at each measurement frequency. The dielectric attenuation constant (in dB/m) in a dielectric medium of significant loss can be estimated using

$$\alpha_{\rm d} \approx 8.686 \cdot \frac{1}{2} k_0 \sqrt{\mu_{\rm r}\varepsilon_{\rm r}} \cdot tan\delta_{\rm d} \quad ({\rm dB/m}), \tag{1.72}$$

where k_0 is the wavenumber in vacuum, $\mu_{\rm r}$ is the relative permeability (real part), $\varepsilon_{\rm r}$ is the relative permittivity (real part), and $tan\delta_{\rm d} = \varepsilon''/\varepsilon'$ is the dielectric loss tangent.

Utilizing a breast compression measurement as an example [9] ($\varepsilon'_{\rm r} \approx 10$, $\varepsilon''_{\rm r} \approx 5$, thickness $=$ 5 cm), we observe that at 3 GHz the signal on average attenuates by 23 dB, whereas at 8 GHz the signal on average attenuates by 61 dB. An example of this difference can be seen in Figure 1.20, which depicts *S*-parameter OUT measurements at 3 and 8 GHz from the breast phantom measurement

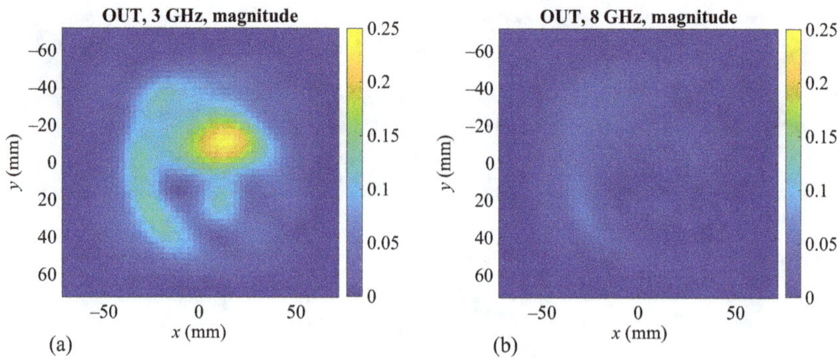

Figure 1.20 S-parameter measurements of the OUT (magnitude) used in [9] at (a) 3 GHz and (b) 8 GHz. The strength of the signal in (b) is substantially smaller than (a) due to the significant attenuation that occurs as the higher frequency signal travels through the tissue

used in [9]. This becomes an issue since the stronger responses dominate the image reconstruction, thus reducing the high spatial frequency information.

In order to ensure that the high-frequency data are adequately utilized, the signals are normalized with respect to the maximum signal in the PSF at each frequency:

$$\eta(\omega_m) = max\left(\left|H^{sc}_{\xi 0}(x, y; z'; \omega_m)\right|\right), \quad m = 1, \ldots, N_\omega, \tag{1.73}$$

$$\bar{H}^{sc}_{\xi 0}(x, y; z'; \omega_m) = \frac{H^{sc}_{\xi 0}(x, y; z'; \omega_m)}{\eta(\omega_m)}, \tag{1.74}$$

$$\bar{S}^{sc}_{\xi}(x, y; \omega_m) = \frac{S^{sc}_{\xi}(x, y; \omega_m)}{\eta(\omega_m)}, \tag{1.75}$$

where $\eta(\omega_m)$ is the normalization factor calculated at every frequency. $\bar{H}^{sc}_{\xi 0}$ and $\bar{S}^{sc}_{\xi}$ are the normalized PSF and OUT data sets, respectively. It is these normalized data sets (in (1.74) and (1.75)), which are used in (1.17) and (1.52) for QMH and SPM, respectively.

The impact of frequency normalization cannot be seen in the simulation example shown in the previous sections due to the absence of lossy materials. However, an example of frequency normalization will be seen in the following section.

1.9 Image reconstruction of breast phantom

To demonstrate the ability of QMH and SPM, as well as the techniques shown in Section 1.8, the experimental example from [9,45] is reconstructed. A compressed

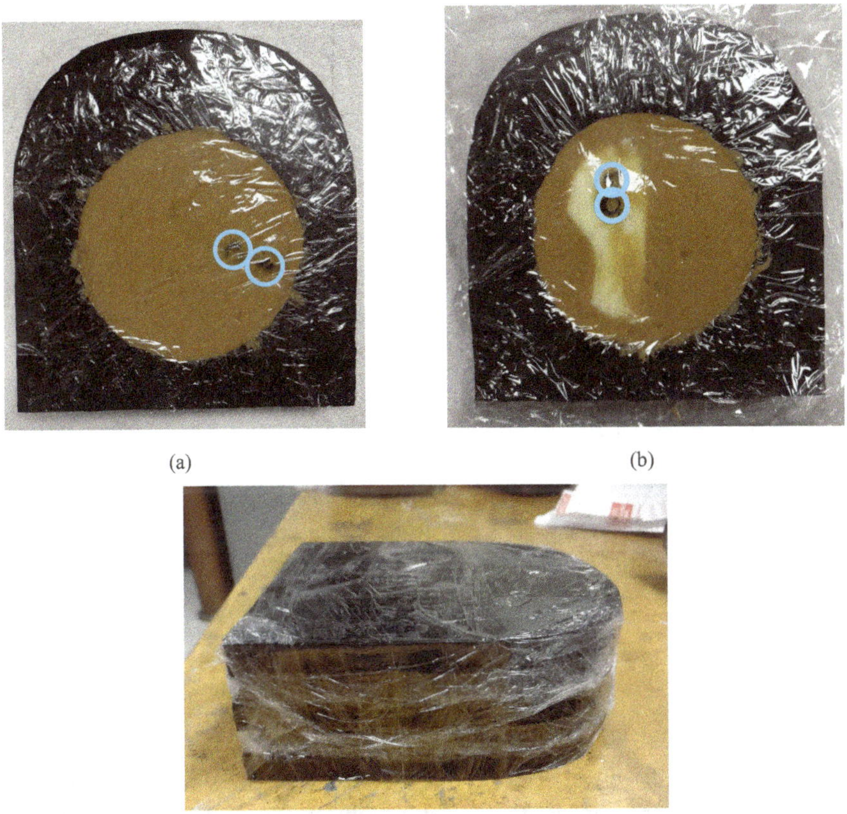

(a) (b) (c)

Figure 1.21 Photos of the breast phantom: (a) Layer 2 contains two tumor simulants (circled in photo) inside the embedding medium; (b) Layer 4 contains two tumor simulants (circled in photo) within the fibroglandular simulant surrounded by the embedding medium; and (c) the assembled phantom. Plastic wrap secures the phantom and protects it from the background medium. Photos taken from [45]

breast phantom is constructed utilizing five layers (1-cm thick) of carbon-rubber materials, which is designed to mimic averaged type-2 scattered fibroglandular breast tissue $\widetilde{\varepsilon}_{\mathrm{r}} \approx 11 - \mathrm{i}3$ [9] (see Figure 1.21). Inside the phantom, two separate layers (hereon labeled "Layer 2" and "Layer 4") have sections that are hollowed out. Several tumor simulants ($\widetilde{\varepsilon}_{\mathrm{r}} \approx 55 - \mathrm{i}17$) are inserted in both layers along with materials mimicking healthy breast tissues. More specifically, in Layer 4, two tumor simulants are embedded in a fibroglandular mimicking material ($\widetilde{\varepsilon}_{\mathrm{r}} \approx 24 - \mathrm{i}11$), which is in turn surrounded by an embedding medium representing averaged breast tissue of $\widetilde{\varepsilon}_{\mathrm{r}} \approx 10 - \mathrm{i}5$. The embedding medium is also used in

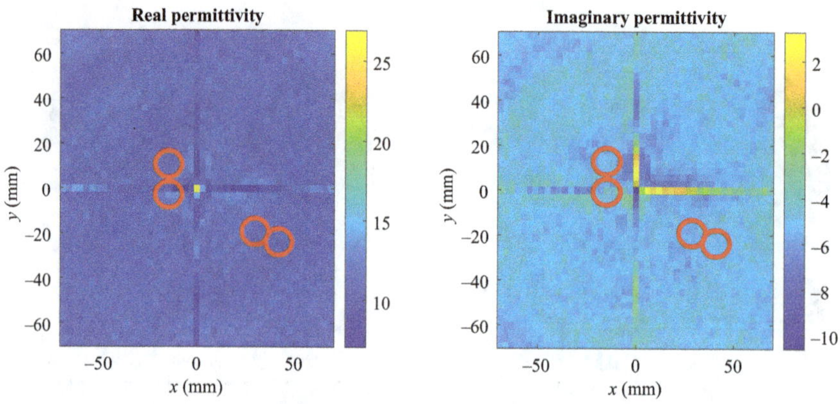

Figure 1.22 Reconstructions of the permittivity of the compressed breast phantom shown in [9,45] utilizing QMH with no filtering or image processing: real permittivity (left) and imaginary permittivity (right). The tumors and the phantom structure are not discernible due to the large cross-shaped artifacts as well as the speckling noise throughout the images

Layer 2 where two more tumor simulants are inserted. Once the two layers are fully assembled, they are stacked with other solid carbon-rubber layers to complete the phantom. Plastic wrap is used to ensure all embedded materials remain secured within the phantom.

This phantom is measured using the methods discussed in [45]. Only transmission measurements are used, which limits the reconstruction to 2-D images. Figure 1.22 shows the 2-D reconstruction of the breast phantom with QMH using Born's approximation without any additional filtering/processing techniques. These 2-D images are in essence projections of the phantom structure onto a plane, similar to mammography [46]. We observe that the reconstruction in Figure 1.22 lacks any diagnostic quality due to significant noise and artifacts. These are due to a number of factors, some of which can be handled utilizing the techniques described in Section 1.8.

To improve the image quality, an apodization filter, a low-pass filter, and frequency normalization are applied. The resultant images can be seen in Figure 1.23. In this reconstruction, the outline of the phantom can be discerned. The tumor locations, indicated by arrows, can be more easily identified, and they correspond to the true lateral position in the phantom. Note that the permittivity estimate should be viewed as an average of the permittivities across all the layers of the phantom.

Now consider the results shown in Figure 1.24. Here, the same filtering techniques are applied, but the frequency normalization is not performed. The resultant reconstructions have lost some of the high definition (or sharpness) that can be seen in Figure 1.23 where frequency normalization was used. However, the decrease in the resolution has led to an increase in the diagnostic quality, i.e., the tumor structures can

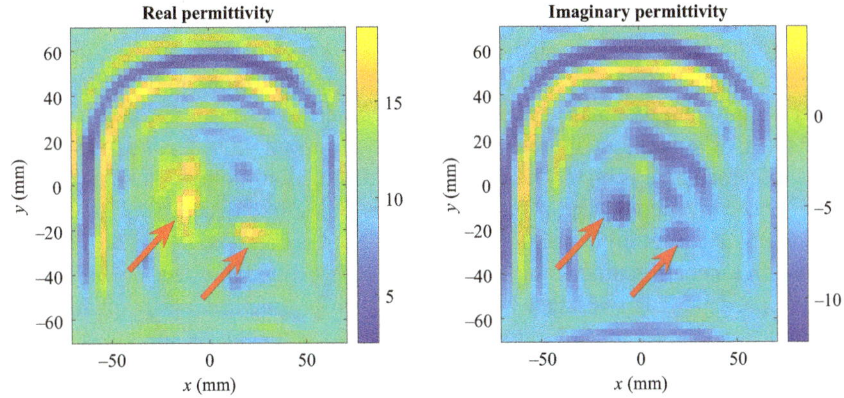

Figure 1.23 Reconstructions of the permittivity of the compressed breast phantom shown in [9,45] utilizing QMH with apodization filtering, low-pass filtering, and frequency normalization: real permittivity (left) and imaginary permittivity (right). The outline of the phantom can now be seen and the tumor structures are visible

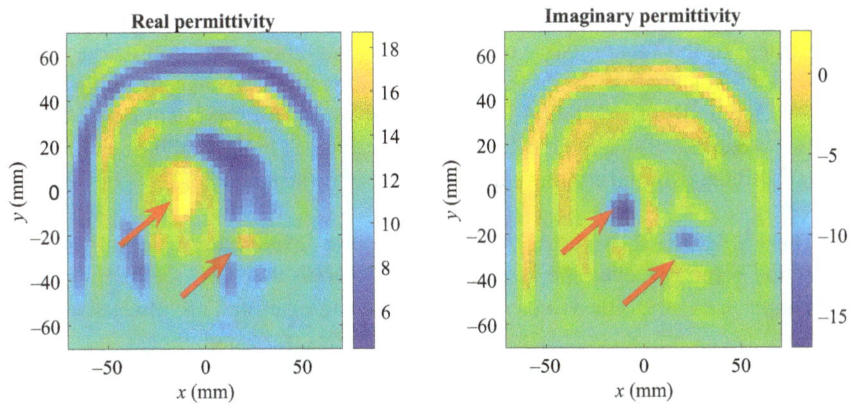

Figure 1.24 Reconstructions of the permittivity of the compressed breast phantom shown in [9,45] utilizing QMH with apodization filtering, low-pass filtering, but no frequency normalization: real permittivity (left) and imaginary permittivity (right). The sharpness of the image has decreased, but the outline of the phantom is still visible. The tumor locations appear more prominently, potentially indicating that the high-frequency data in this measurement is noisy

be more clearly identified, particularly in the imaginary part of the permittivity. The cause for the higher diagnostic quality when not applying frequency normalization is due to the lower SNR of the higher frequencies. Since the normalization increases the contribution of the high-frequency responses, more noise is added to the data processed by the reconstruction algorithm but, on the other hand, the image sharpness improves. Thus, the trade-off in utilizing frequency normalization in tissue imaging is between improving the image resolution and degrading the image SNR.

As a final remark, we must emphasize that the speed of all reconstruction algorithms discussed here is high. The presented reconstruction examples take a couple of seconds on conventional laptops with all codes being implemented in MATLAB® without any acceleration or parallel-computing approaches. The use of all discussed filtering and signal preprocessing approaches has a negligible effect on the computational speed. This is important because it allows for quick real-time tuning of the reconstruction process toward optimizing the diagnostic quality of the images.

1.10 Conclusions

QMH and scattered power mapping have both been demonstrated as options for performing real-time reconstructions for microwave and MMW biomedical imaging. These methods are able to generate quantitative estimates of the permittivity and conductivity in seconds [2,9]. With further optimization, and written with memory management in mind, these algorithms are expected to execute in milliseconds.

Critical to the functionality of these methods is the acquisition of the system PSF. The PSF captures the impulse response of the measurement setup to an SP, the dielectric properties of which are known. This allows for the quantitative estimation of the permittivity and the effective conductivity of biological tissues, which in turn carry diagnostic information about the type of the tissue and its pathology (if present).

The PSF can also be used as a quality control experiment to ensure that the acquisition setup achieves the desired SNR [6]. Note that PSF measurements are commonplace in most other medical imaging technologies and are also used to perform quality control and quality assurance evaluations of the equipment [47–49].

QMH and SPM also benefit from the application of several filtering and normalization techniques. These strategies are particularly important in biomedical imaging. Problems arising in the near-field imaging of the lossy tissue impact significantly the diagnostic quality of the reconstruction. It is important to understand that the techniques shown in this work are not perfect solutions; they have limitations, which require trade-offs and tuning. The most common trade-off is between the image resolution and its diagnostic quality (e.g., image SNR and image artifacts).

While QMH and SPM have been applied in several tissue phantom experiments [3,6,9], their implementation in real-life medical imaging remains to be evaluated. It is our experience that the main challenges of microwave biomedical imaging are not related to the reconstruction algorithms but rather the hardware. This hardware must be capable of sampling an acquisition space within milliseconds across a wide bandwidth of frequencies, while maintaining safe levels of microwave radiation dosage following the relevant regulations (e.g., Canada Safety Code 6 [50]). Though some developments regarding the design and testing of small antenna arrays has been performed [51], work still remains on the development of a fully functional microwave biomedical imaging system.

Acronyms

CO	calibration object
EM	electromagnetic
MMW	microwave and millimeter-wave
OUT	object under test
PSF	point-spread function
QMH	quantitative microwave holography
RO	reference object
Rx	receiver or receiving
SAR	synthetic aperture radar
SNR	signal-to-noise ratio
SP	scattering probe
SPM	scattered-power mapping
Tx	transmitter or transmitting

References

[1] Nikolova NK. *Introduction to Microwave Imaging*. Cambridge, United Kingdom: Cambridge University Press; 2017.

[2] Tajik D, Pitcher AD, and Nikolova NK. Comparative study of the Rytov and Born approximations in quantitative microwave holography. *Progress in Electromagnetic Research B*. 2017;79:1–19.

[3] Tajik D, Foroutan F, Shumakov DS, *et al.* Real-time microwave imaging of a compressed breast phantom with planar scanning. *IEEE Journal of Electromagnetics, RF, and Microwaves in Medicine and Biology*. 2018;2(3): 154–162.

[4] Tu S, McCombe JJ, Shumakov DS, *et al.* Fast quantitative microwave imaging with resolvent kernel extracted from measurements. *Inverse Problems*. 2015;31(4):045007.

[5] Shumakov DS and Nikolova NK. Fast quantitative microwave imaging with scattered-power maps. *IEEE Transactions on Microwave Theory and Techniques*. 2018;66(1):439–449.

[6] Tajik D, Trac J, and Nikolova NK. Quality control of microwave equipment for tissue imaging. *IEEE Journal of Electromagnetics, RF and Microwaves in Medicine and Biology*. 2019;4(1):52–60.

[7] Amineh RK, McCombe JJ, Khalatpour A, *et al.* Fast quantitative microwave imaging with resolvent kernel extracted from measurements. *IEEE Transactions on Instrumentation and Measurement*. 2015;64(2):403–417.

[8] Beaverstone AS, Shumakov DS, and Nikolova NK. Integral equations of scattering for scalar frequency-domain responses. *IEEE Transactions on Microwave Theory and Techniques*. 2015;64(4):1120–1132.

[9] Tajik D, Nikolova NK, and Noseworthy MD. Improving quantitative microwave holography through simultaneous use of the Born and Rytov approximations. In: 16th European Radar Conference (EuRAD); 2019 Oct; Paris, France; 2019.

[10] Nikolova NK. Microwave imaging for breast cancer. *IEEE Microwave Magazine*. 2011;12(7):78–94.

[11] O'Loughlin D, O'Halloran M, Moloney BM, *et al.* Microwave breast imaging: Clinical advances and remaining challenges. *IEEE Transactions on Biomedical Engineering*. 2018;65(11):2580–2590.

[12] Sugitani T, Kubota S-i, Kuroki S-i, *et al.* Complex permittivities of breast tumor tissues obtained from cancer surgeries. *Applied Physics Letters*. 2014;104(25):253702.

[13] Goodman JW. *Introduction to Fourier Optics*. New York, USA: McGraw-Hill; 1996.

[14] Schatzberg A and Devaney AJ. Super-resolution in diffraction tomography. *Inverse Problems*. 1992;8(1):149–164.

[15] Bertero M, Miyakawa M, Boccacci P, *et al.* Image restoration in chirp-pulse microwave CT (CP-MCT). *IEEE Transactions on Biomedical Engineering*. 2000;47(5):690–699.

[16] Diener L. Microwave near-field imaging with open-ended waveguide—Comparison with other techniques of nondestructive testing. *Research in Nondestructive Evaluation*. 1995;7(2–3):137–152.

[17] Zoughi R. *Microwave Nondestructive Testing and Evaluation*. Amsterdam, The Netherlands: Kluwer; 2000.

[18] Savelyev T and Yarovoy A. Fast imaging by 3-D deconvolution in short-range UWB radar for concealed weapon detection. In: 9th European Radar Conference (EuRAD 2012). IEEE; 2012. p. 26–29.

[19] Chew WC. *Waves and Fields in Inhomogeneous Media*. New York: IEEE Press; 1990.

[20] Ostadrahimi M, Mojabi P, Gilmore C, *et al.* Analysis of incident field modeling and incident/scattered field calibration techniques in microwave tomography. *IEEE Antennas and Wireless Propagation Letters*. 2011;10: 900–903.

[21] Nikolova NK, Shumakov DS, and Beaverstone AS. Obtaining system-specific Green's functions through measurements: theory and applications in microwave imaging. In: IEEE AP-S/URSI Int. Symp. on Antennas and Propagation; Fajardo, Puerto Rico; 2016.

[22] Pozar DM. *Microwave Engineering*. 4th ed. Hoboken, NJ: John Wiley & Sons; 2012.

[23] Hiebel M. *Fundamentals of Vector Network Analysis*. 5th ed. Columbia, MD: Rohde & Schwarz; 2011.
[24] Dunsmore JP. *Handbook of Microwave Component Measurements: with Advanced VNA Techniques*. New York: John Wiley & Sons; 2012.
[25] Dadash MS, Nikolova NK, and Bandler JW. Analytical adjoint sensitivity formula for the scattering parameters of metallic structures. *IEEE Transactions on Microwave Theory and Techniques*. 2012;60(9):2713–2722.
[26] Bellizzi G, Bellizzi GG, Bucci OM, *et al.* Optimization of the working conditions for magnetic nanoparticle-enhanced microwave diagnostics of breast cancer. *IEEE Transactions on Biomedical Engineering*. 2018;65(7):1607–1616.
[27] Sachs J, Ley S, Just T, *et al.* Differential ultra-wideband microwave imaging: Principle application challenges. *Sensors*. 2018;18(7):2136. Available from: http://dx.doi.org/10.3390/s18072136.
[28] Aknc MN, Çayören M, and Göse E. Qualitative microwave imaging of breast cancer with contrast agents. *Physics in Medicine & Biology*. 2019;64(11):115018.
[29] Amineh RK, Trehan A, and Nikolova NK. TEM horn antenna for ultra-wide band microwave breast imaging. *Progress in Electromagnetics Research B*. 2009;13:59–74.
[30] Klemm M, Gibbins D, Leendertz J, *et al.* Development and testing of a 60-element UWB conformal array for breast cancer imaging. In: Proc. 5th European Conf. Antennas & Propagation (EuCAP). IEEE; 2011. p. 3077–3079.
[31] Porter E, Bahrami H, Santorelli A, *et al.* A wearable microwave antenna array for time-domain breast tumor screening. *IEEE Transactions on Medical Imaging*. 2016;35(6):1501–1509.
[32] Sheen DM, McMakin DL, and Hall TE. Three-dimensional millimeter-wave imaging for concealed weapon detection. *IEEE Transactions on Microwave Theory and Techniques*. 2001;49(9):1581–1592.
[33] Sheen D, McMakin D, and Hall T. Near-field three-dimensional radar imaging techniques and applications. *Applied Optics*. 2010;49(19):E83–E93.
[34] Zhuge X and Yarovoy AG. Three-dimensional near-field MIMO array imaging using range migration techniques. *IEEE Transactions on Image Processing*. 2012;21(6):3026–3033.
[35] Collins HD, McMakin DL, Hall TE, *et al.*, *Real-Time Holographic Surveillance System*. Ancel Surgical R&D Inc.; 1995.
[36] Sheen DM, McMakin DL, Collins HD, *et al.* Concealed explosive detection on personnel using a wideband holographic millimeter-wave imaging system. In: Proc SPIE 2755, Signal Processing, Sensor Fusion, and Target Recognition V; 1996 Jun.
[37] Soumekh M. A system model and inversion for synthetic aperture radar imaging. *IEEE Transactions on Image Processing*. 1992;1(1):64–76.
[38] Soumekh M. *Fourier Array Imaging*. Englewood Cliffs, NJ, United States: Prentice-Hall; 1994.
[39] Soumekh M. *Synthetic Aperture Radar Signal Processing With MATLAB Algorithms*. Hoboken, NJ, United States: Wiley; 1994.

[40] Stolt RH. Migration by Fourier transform. *Geophysics.* 1978;1(63):23–48.

[41] Tajik D, Nikolova NK, and Noseworthy MD. Comparison between MR, CT, and quantitative microwave holography images of a compressed breast phantom. In: 14th European Conf. on Antennas & Propagation (EuCAP'2020); Copenhagen, Denmark; 2020.

[42] Song Y and Nikolova NK. Memory-efficient method for wideband self-adjoint sensitivity analysis. *IEEE Transactions on Microwave Theory and Techniques.* 2008;56(8):1917–1927.

[43] Liu L, Trehan A, and Nikolova N. Near-field detection at microwave frequencies based on self-adjoint response sensitivity analysis. *Inverse Problems.* 2010;26(10):105001.

[44] Altiar FEKO, Electromagnetic Simulation Software. Available from: https://altairhyperworks.com/product/FEKO. Accessed September 2021.

[45] Tajik D, Trac J, and Nikolova NK. Spatial resolution evaluation of a microwave system for breast cancer screening. In: 13th European Conference on Antennas and Propagation (EuCAP); 2019. p. 1–5.

[46] Helvie MA, Chan HP, Adler DD, *et al.* Breast thickness in routine mammograms: Effect on image quality and radiation dose. *American Journal of Roentgenology.* 1994;163(6):1371–1374.

[47] Firbank MJ, Harrison RM, Williams ED, *et al.* Quality assurance for MRI: Practical experience. *British Journal of Radiology.* 2000;73(868):376–383.

[48] Price RR, Axel L, Morgan T, *et al.* Quality assurance methods and phantoms for magnetic resonance imaging: Report of AAPM nuclear magnetic resonance Task Group No. 1. *Medical Physics.* 1990;17(2):287–295.

[49] Droege RT. A quality assurance protocol for CT scanners. *Radiology.* 1983;(146):244–246.

[50] Health Canada. Limits of human exposure to radiofrequency electromagnetic energy in the frequency range from 3 KHz to 300 GHz. Health Canada; 2015.

[51] Foroutan F and Nikolova NK. Dynamic range of an active radio sensor for bias-switched arrays for microwave tissue imaging. *IEEE International Symposium on Antennas and Propagation & USNC/URSI National Radio Science Meeting.* 2018;11–12. doi:10.1109/APUSNCURSINRSM.2018.8609147.

Chapter 2
Solving inverse scattering problems in biomedical imaging with contraction integral equation models

Kuiwen Xu[1], *Lu Zhang*[1] *and Yu Zhong*[2]

Microwave imaging methods can be generally classified into two categories: qualitative and quantitative. Qualitative imaging methods retrieve the shape and location of unknown scatterers within the domain of interest (DoI) and cannot carry out quantitative estimates of the material properties of unknown targets. In comparison, quantitative imaging methods reconstruct the values of electric and/or magnetic constitutive parameters of unknown scatterers. Although quantitative methods require more computational resources (CPU time, memory, etc.) to obtain the quantitative information than qualitative methods do, they are more robust compared with qualitative methods, as the latter usually need a much better quality of measured data (lower noise and wider measurement aperture). Both quantitative estimates and robustness are desired properties in many biomedical imaging problems. Thus, more and more attention has been paid onto solving biomedical imaging problems with quantitative approaches, especially with the availability of the ever-increasing computational power of modern computers. In biomedical imaging, the focus is to distinguish healthy tissues from abnormal tissues by virtue of the difference of the electromagnetic parameters, i.e., the permittivity, the electric conductivity, and magnetic permeability, the last of which might only be considered when there is such contrast between the normal and abnormal tissues. Here we only consider the first two physical constitutive parameters that are usually embedded within the complex permittivity in time-harmonic modeling.

The working principle of the microwave imaging is mainly based on the difference between the electrical properties (relative permittivity and conductivity) of different tissues. While an abnormal tissue has different electrical properties compared with the surrounding normal and healthy tissues, it can be reflected from the reconstructed permittivity distributions. As aforementioned, quantitative imaging methods are capable of finding these material differences within the concerned DoI

[1]Engineering Research Center of Smart Microsensors and Microsystems, Ministry of Education, Hangzhou Dianzi University, Hangzhou, China
[2]FINIAC Pte. Ltd., Singapore

and provide the quantitative estimates of permittivity as well. This provides valuable information to medical practices whether further actions are needed. Thus far, quantitatively microwave imaging based on inverse scattering problems (ISPs) techniques has been mainly investigated for breast cancer and brain stroke detections. To this concern, microwave imaging faces two main challenges: large contrast between different tissues and complex inhomogeneous background. Both are due to the large electrical permittivity of human tissues within the microwave frequency band, which is still a proper choice of frequency band considering the penetration depth and attenuations. Being able to detect the scattered fields, including the backscattered ones and transmitted ones, the burdens fall onto the inversion side, i.e., to retrieve the information about the unknown targets from the measured data. Nevertheless, having large contrasts between the unknown abnormal tissues and background tissues, significant nonlinearity could severely reduce the efficiency of solving the concerned ISPs, while, on the other hand, complex inhomogeneous background tissues could strongly interferer the inversions, making the problem more ill-posed and more nonlinear.

In this chapter, in order to tackle such inherited difficulties within the biomedical imaging with ISP techniques, we implement the recently proposed new integral equation (IE) inversion models, i.e., the contraction integral equation for inversion (CIE-I) and its difference version, the difference CIE-I (D-CIE-I). The CIE-I effectively reduces the multiple scattering effects within the inversions, which is the major reason of causing the nonlinearity of the ISPs. Based on the CIE-I, the D-CIE-I properly models the background media such that the inversions can majorly focus on the unknown tissues without compromising the computational efficiency and, most importantly, without bringing additional interferences from the background strong media.

In the following, we will first give a recap on the two new IE models and provide numerical tests to validate their properties. Given these, three examples for biomedical imaging with D-CIE-I models will be given and associated analyses as well.

2.1 Introduction to inverse scattering problems

When talking about the inverse problem, one has to mention its counterpart, the forward problem (or direct problem). Studies of electromagnetic ISPs need to include both forward problem modeling and inverse problem modeling. The electromagnetic forward scattering problem is to find out electromagnetic scattered fields generated by some obstacles or some inhomogeneous media. The inputs are the electromagnetic incident waves and the physical properties of scatterers, such as the geometric distribution, the permittivity, and permeability of every scatterer. If we reverse the solution and the conditions of the electromagnetic forward scattering problem, the electromagnetic ISP can be found, i.e., given the knowledge of scattered fields and the incidences, the electromagnetic ISPs need to find out the geometric supports, like the shapes and the locations, and physical constitutive parameters (permittivity, conductivity, and (or) permeability) of the unknown scatterers [1].

ISPs have been of interest for several decades, which have wide applications in the fields of geophysics, nondestructive evaluation, through-wall imaging, medical imaging, ground-penetrating radar, and so on [2–7]. Due to all these important applications, it is essential to develop precise and fast methods to solve various ISPs. However, because of the intrinsic nonlinearity and ill-posedness, the ISPs usually can only be solved within some precision and the computational cost is usually quite large [8–10].

Researchers in mathematical, physical, and engineering societies have dedicated great efforts in developing more stable and more efficient solvers for decades. This includes qualitative and quantitative methods, as mentioned at the beginning of the chapter. Quantitative methods that have been intensively discussed and used in practical scenarios could be cast into two large groups: methods based on the IE solver of Maxwell equations and methods based on the differential equation solver of Maxwell equations. These two kinds of methods have their own advantages and disadvantages due to the forward problem solver they adopt, e.g., the number of unknowns in methods based on differential equation solver is usually larger than the one in methods based on IE solver, but the former does not need the explicit knowledge of Green's function. In this chapter, the methods based on IEs solver are investigated.

The inversion is carried out based on scattering data measured outside DoI when the object is illuminated by a series of known incident waves. The ISPs are usually cast into optimization problems, which minimize the mismatches between the synthetic physical model and the measured data. It is well known that solving ISPs are challenging due to a large number of unknowns, ill-posedness, and nonlinearity. The nonlinearity physically comes from multiple scattering effects in the DoI and mathematically are due to the matrix inverse operator between the unknown constitutive parameters and the measured scattered fields [10]. When the physical dimensions of unknown scatterers are not small compared to the wavelength of the probing waves (for instance, larger than two wavelengths), and/or the contrasts of the unknown scatterers are no longer small (say, larger than one, as can be seen in the numerical tests), multiple scattering effects within the DoI become significant, and this results in highly nonlinear ISPs, and the associated ill-posedness is increased as well due to the compactness of the scattering operator from the DoI to the measurement domain. To alleviate the ill-posedness, different regularization techniques can be employed [1,9,11]. Nevertheless, the strong nonlinearity of the ISPs becomes a major bottleneck of efficiently solving the optimization type ISPs, which will be discussed in the following.

Until now, the ISPs with homogeneous background medium have been intensively studied in the literature [12–21], where a Green's function for the homogeneous medium is utilized in the inversion if the IE method is employed. To solve the ISPs, two types of optimization methods are usually employed, i.e., linear and nonlinear, corresponding to the weak scatterers and non-weak ones. For weak scatterers, in order to accelerate the convergence, save computation time and alleviate the nonlinearity of the model, some representative algorithms based on the Born or Rytov approximations allow an easy substitution for the (unknown) total field within the DoI [22,23], but they suffer from several limitations caused by the linear approximations [24]. For instance, the linear methods cannot handle problems with strong scatterers, e.g., those with high contrast and/or electrically large dimensions.

When dealing with strong scatterers, fully nonlinear optimization schemes counting in all multiple scattering effects are needed. Consequently, many nonlinear optimization methods have been developed, such as the distorted Born iterative method (DBIM) [21,22], the contrast source inversion (CSI) method [25,26], Newton-type inversion methods [27], and subspace-based optimization method (SOM) [28–30]. Adopting deterministic type of optimization schemes, these methods are efficient to find the local minimums of the ISPs, and, nevertheless, are very sensitive to initial guesses. Especially, when scatterers are with high contrasts and/or with electrically large dimensions, these methods usually fail to find the global solutions, meaning that the previous methods can only handle problems without strong nonlinearity (high contrast and/or electrically large dimensions). On the other hand, stochastic optimization methods have a better chance of finding the wanted global solutions [31,32]. However, when handling ISPs, which usually involves a large number of unknowns especially for the medium-type ISPs, using stochastic optimization schemes often consumes a very large amount of computational resources, including CPU/GPU time and memory. Most of these methods are based on IE-based modeling with traditional Lippmann–Schwinger IE (LSIE), in which the nonlinearity mainly comes from multiple scattering effects.

Recently, a family of new IEs, namely CIE-I, has been proposed to tackle the mentioned highly nonlinear ISP [33]. With such a new inversion model, the multiple scattering effects within inversion are effectively reduced. Doing so, the nonlinearity of the ISPs is therefore reduced compared with the case of using LSIE. Since the CIE-I is mathematically equivalent to the LSIE, there is no compromise in the accuracy of the physical model. On the other hand, to stabilize the inversions with the CIE-I, we need proper regularizations on the unknowns. The fast Fourier transform–twofold subspace-based optimization method (FFT-TSOM) and multiplicative total variation (TV) are used here. The regularization of FFT-TSOM introduces strong subspace constraints onto the induced secondary sources, which excludes those "high-frequency" components that could be vulnerable to noises. Otherwise, the multiplicative regularization (MR) is a TV-type technique on the contrast, and therefore, might release the subspace constraint from the TSOM.

2.2 Formulation of the forward problems

For the convenience of presentation, a two-dimensional (2-D) ISP with transverse magnetic polarization is considered for the forward model, and time-harmonic fields are assumed with $\exp(-i\omega t)$ (ω is the angular frequency) and suppressed as implicitly present, where scalar wave equations are involved. The model of 2-D problems consists of a bounded DoI D, which includes unknown scatterers of

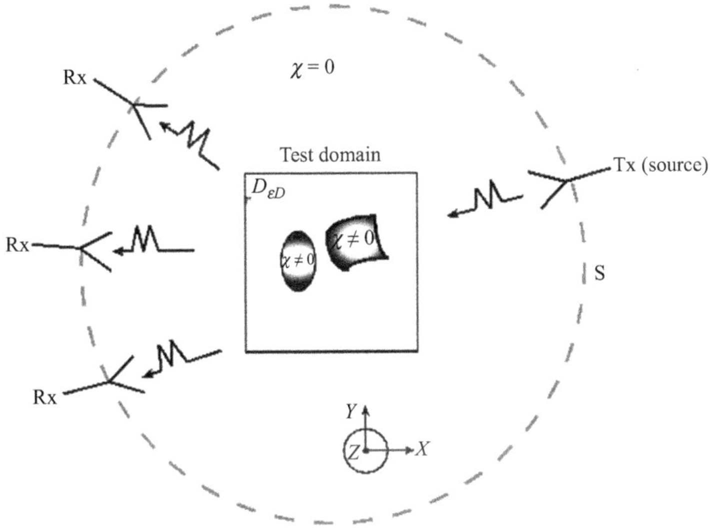

Figure 2.1 Geometrical model of the inverse scattering problems

interests. The background homogeneous medium is known with permittivity ε_b, permeability μ_b, and wavenumber $k_b=\omega(\varepsilon_b\mu_b)^{1/2}$. The unknown scatterers are assumed nonmagnetic with permittivity distribution $\varepsilon(r)$, $r\in D$. There are a total of N_i plane wave incidences at a single frequency located at r_l^i, $l=1, 2, \ldots, N_i$ in the domain (or on curve) S outside of D, and these incident fields are denoted as E_l^{inc}. For each incidence, the scattered electric fields are measured by N_r antennas located at r_q^s, $q=1, 2, \ldots, N_r$, as depicted in Figure 2.1.

The complex contrast in the DoI is defined as $\chi(r)=(\varepsilon(r)-\varepsilon_b)/\varepsilon_b$. In the inverse problem, we need to determine $\varepsilon(r)$, given a set of $N_i\times N_r$ scattering data, E_l^{sca}. The test domain D in the x–y plane is discretized into many small rectangular subdomains with one smaller than 1/10 wavelength dimension and centered at r_m. The total number of subdomains is M. The forward problem consists of the following two IEs. The governing equation inside the DoI is the LSIE [34]. The total electric fields $E_l^{tot}(r)$ in the DoI D for lth incidence can be expressed as

$$E_l^{tot}(r) = E_l^{inc}(r) + k_b^2\iint_D G(r,r')\chi(r')E_l^{tot}(r')\,dr', \tag{2.1}$$

which describes the wave-scattering and material interaction, and the second one describes the scattered fields $E_l^{sca}(r)$ on the measurement domain S as a reradiation of the induced contrast current,

$$E_l^{sca}(r) = k_b^2\iint_D G(r,r')\chi(r')E_l^{tot}(r')\,dr', \tag{2.2}$$

where G is the 2-D free-space Green's function $G(r,r') = (i/4)H_0^1(k_0|r-r'|)$, H_0^1 is zeroth-order Hankel function of the first kind, and the contrast function at r is defined as $\chi(r) = (\varepsilon(r) - \varepsilon_b)/\varepsilon_b$ with the relative permittivity $\varepsilon_r(r) = \varepsilon(r)/\varepsilon_b$. And the physical induced current $J(r)$ can be written as

$$J(r) = -i\omega\varepsilon_b(\varepsilon_r(r) - 1)E^{tot}(r). \tag{2.3}$$

However, in practice the contrast source that is a normalized induced current is usually used and can be formulated as $I(r) = (\varepsilon_r(r) - 1)E^{tot}(r) = \chi(r)E^{tot}(r)$. Then the previous electric IEs can be reformulated as

$$E_l^{tot}(r) = E_l^{inc}(r) + k_b^2 \iint_D G(r, r')I_l(r')\, dr'. \tag{2.4}$$

And

$$E_l^{sca}(r) = k_b^2 \iint_D G(r, r')I_l(r')\, dr'. \tag{2.5}$$

For convenience, two Green's functions are termed $G_S(J) = k_b^2 \iint_D G(r, r') I_l(r')dr', r \in S$ and $G_D(J) = k_b^2 \iint_D G(r, r')I_l(r')dr', r \in D$, G_S mapping the induced current to the scattered field in the measurement domain S and G_D mapping the induced current to the scattered field in the DoI D. Then the governing IEs can be written as this following compact form:

$$E^{tot}(r) = E^{inc}(r) + G_D(\chi(r)E^{tot}(r)), \tag{2.6}$$

$$E^{sca}(r) = G_S(\chi(r)E^{tot}(r)), \tag{2.7}$$

where only electric fields are involved in the two formulas. These two equations are denoted as a kind of field-type equations. And in virtue of the contrast source, the other type equations, termed source-type equations, are formulated as

$$I(r) = \chi(r)[E^{inc}(r) + G_D(I(r))], \tag{2.8}$$

$$E^{sca}(r) = G_S(I(r)), \tag{2.9}$$

where induced contrast source is involved in both equations. And (2.7) and (2.9) are referred to as the data equations, and (2.6) and (2.8) are referred to as object equations.

In the forward problem, the goal is to obtain the scattered field E^{sca} from the known scatterers distribution and the incident wave E^{inc}. In order to get the scattered field, the induced current or contrast source $I(r)$ should be obtained first, then the scattered field can be calculated by (2.9). By some mathematical manipulation of (2.8), the contrast source can be expressed as

$$I(r) = [\mathcal{I} - \chi(r)G_D]^{-1}(\chi(r)E^{inc}(r)), \tag{2.10}$$

where $\mathcal{I}$ is the identity operator. Consequently, we can get the induced contrast source $I_l(r)$ by the operation of the matrix inversion. The method of moments (MoM) is used to discretize the equations. The DoI is chosen to be rectangular to implement the conjugate gradient FFT (CG-FFT) scheme for the fast calculations of scattered fields within the domain.

The matrix inversion costs intensive computational burden especially when the DoI is electrically large. Herein, in order to implement the solution efficiently, the CG-FFT scheme is used to get the induced currents. After getting the induced currents, the scattered fields on the S can be calculated by formula (2.9) and can be expressed as by combining (2.9) and (2.10)

$$E_l^{sca} = G_S(I(r)) = G_S\left([\mathcal{I} - \chi(r)G_D]^{-1}\left(\chi(r)E_l^{inc}(r)\right)\right). \tag{2.11}$$

2.3 Formulation of the inverse problems

The DoI D is discretized into M small rectangular cells centered at $r_{m,n}$, with M_1 and M_2 being the number of cells along the x and y direction ($M = M_1 \times M_2$, $1 \leq m \leq M_1$, and $1 \leq n \leq M_2$). And within each subdomain, the induced current and the total electric field are assumed to be constants.

As stated in [9], casting the ISPs as optimization problems, the synthetic scattered electric fields on the measurement domain S can be denoted as the output of a nonlinear mapping,

$$E_l^{sca} = F\left(\chi, E_l^{inc}\right), \tag{2.12}$$

from the contrast χ and incidence field E_l^{inc}. Conventionally, we seek the solution of the optimization problem,

$$\text{Min}: f(\chi) = \sum_{l=1}^{N_i} \|E_l^{sca} - F\left(\chi, E_l^{inc}\right)\|_S^2, \tag{2.13}$$

where $\|\|_S$ denotes the Euclidian length of a function defined on measurement domain S. And to get a stable solution, a regularization technique is usually utilized so that the objective function can be formulated as

$$\text{Min}: f(\chi) = \sum_{l=1}^{N_i} \|E_l^{sca} - F\left(\chi, E_l^{inc}\right)\|_S^2 + \alpha R(\chi), \tag{2.14}$$

where $R(\chi)$ is a nonnegative penalty function. Such a regularized term is usually chosen on the basis of some a priori assumptions (or knowledge) on the unknown function.

After discretization, the unknown χ appears in the diagonal of a matrix, and the objective function involves the inversion of this matrix. Such an objective function is obviously nonlinear and nonconvex, which is well known to be difficult to solve, due to the presence of local minima. Roughly speaking, methods proposed for solving nonlinear optimization problems can be classified as deterministic algorithms and heuristic (or stochastic) ones [9]. In this chapter, we are instead using a different type of objective function than (2.14), considering both contrast and induced currents as unknowns. This will be discussed in detail later.

2.3.1 Inversions with LSIE and with CIE-I

Herein, in the inversion, the FFT-TSOM is used for reconstruction. As analyzed in [28–30], induced contrast sources in SOM methods can be decomposed into deterministic part of the induced current (DPIC) $\overline{\overline{I}}^d$ and ambiguous part of the induced current (APIC) $\overline{\overline{I}}^a$, where the double bar $=$ denotes a 2-D tensor and the double subscripts of such a 2-D tensor denote their corresponding element, such as $\overline{\overline{I}}^a_{m,n}$ for the (m,n)th element as for $r_{m,n}$. Therefore, the LSIE about the contrast sources, i.e., (2.8) can be discretized as

$$\overline{\overline{I}}^d_l + \overline{\overline{I}}^a_l = \overline{\overline{\chi}} \odot \left[\overline{\overline{E}}^{inc}_l + \overline{\overline{G}}_D\left(\overline{\overline{I}}^d_l\right) + \overline{\overline{G}}_D\left(\overline{\overline{I}}^a_l\right)\right], \tag{2.15}$$

where $\odot$ represents the element-wise multiplication of two tensors, while the scattered fields in the observation domain S can be written as matrix form,

$$\overline{E}^{sca}_l = \overline{\overline{G}}_S\left(\overline{I}^d_l + \overline{I}^a_l\right), \tag{2.16}$$

where $\overline{I}^d_l = \text{vec}\left\{\overline{\overline{I}}^d_l\right\}$ with $\text{vec}\{\cdot\}$ the vectorization manipulation. Also does the $\overline{I}^a_l$. And by the singular vector decomposition (SVD) of the compact operator $\overline{\overline{G}}_S$, i.e., $\overline{\overline{G}}_S \cdot \overline{v}^S_j = \sigma^S_j \overline{u}^S_j$, the induced contrast source is split into two parts, and the DPIC can be obtained as

$$\overline{I}^d_l = \sum_{j=1}^{L} \frac{\langle \overline{E}^{sca}_l, \overline{u}^S_j \rangle}{\sigma^S_j} \overline{v}^S_j, \tag{2.17}$$

where $\overline{u}^S_j$, $\overline{v}^S_j$, and σ^S_j are the left, right singular vectors, and singular values of the operator $\overline{\overline{G}}_S$ [28–30]. The value of L is chosen according to the singular values of $\overline{\overline{G}}_S$ and the level of noise [28]. And the APIC can be constructed as

$$\overline{I}^a_l = \overline{\overline{V}}^-_S \cdot \overline{\alpha}_1, \tag{2.18}$$

where $\overline{\overline{V}}^-_S = \left[\overline{v}^S_{L+1}, \ldots, \overline{v}^S_M\right]$, and $\overline{\alpha}_l$ as $(M-L) \times 1$ unknown vector that is determined by the optimization, as given in the SOM. On the other hand, as mentioned in the TSOM [29,30], we can express the APIC as

$$\overline{I}^a_l = \overline{\overline{V}}^{+'}_D \cdot \overline{\beta}_l, \tag{2.19}$$

where $\overline{\beta}_l$ is an M_0-dimensional vector ($M_0 \ll M$), and the corresponding current subspace $\overline{\overline{V}}^+_D$ can be expressed as

$$\overline{\overline{V}}^{+'}_D = \left(\overline{\overline{I}}_M - \overline{\overline{V}}^+_S \cdot \overline{\overline{V}}^{+*}_S\right) \cdot \overline{\overline{V}}^+_D, \tag{2.20}$$

where $\overline{\overline{I}}_M$ is the M-dimensional identity matrix, and $\overline{\overline{V}}^+_D = \left[\overline{v}^D_1, \overline{v}^D_2, \ldots, \overline{v}^D_{M_0}\right]$ is the current subspace spanned by the singular vectors to the largest M_0 singular values of the operator $\overline{\overline{G}}_D$ [30]. However, to avoid the computational burdensome SVD of the operator $\overline{\overline{G}}_D$ and further accelerate the process of optimization, the original current subspace spanned by the singular vector bases can be substituted by the discrete Fourier bases such that the FFT-TSOM was proposed in [30]. Thus,

$$\begin{aligned} \overline{I}_l^a &= \left(\overline{\overline{I}}_M - \overline{\overline{V}}_S^+ \cdot \overline{\overline{V}}_S^{+*}\right) \cdot \left[\overline{F}_1^D, \overline{F}_2^D, \ldots, \overline{F}_{M_0}^D\right] \cdot \overline{\beta}_l \\ &= \left(\overline{\overline{I}}_M - \overline{\overline{V}}_S^+ \cdot \overline{\overline{V}}_S^{+*}\right) \cdot \mathrm{vec}\{IDFT\{\overline{\overline{\gamma}}_l\}\}, \end{aligned} \tag{2.21}$$

where $\overline{F}_j, j=1, 2, \ldots, M_0$ is the vectorized discrete Fourier bases, and $\overline{\overline{\gamma}}_l$ is the 2-D Fourier coefficient tensor with nonzero elements corresponding to those low-frequency discrete Fourier bases (denoted as four blocks with size M_F in the four corners of the coefficient tensor in MATLAB®) and zero elements corresponding to the remaining high-frequency discrete Fourier bases. As mentioned in [30], low-frequency Fourier bases can be used to construct a current subspace as the approximation to the original current subspace spanned by the singular vectors with large singular values. The inverse discrete Fourier transform (IDFT) is performed by the 2-D FFT algorithm, and the computational complexity is $O(M\log_2 M)$, which is much smaller than the one of the direct multiplications in the TSOM. Detail of the FFT-TSOM could be found in [30].

After constructing the induced contrast source in the aforementioned way, the cost function is defined as follows. A residual error in the data (2.9) for lth incidence can be defined as

$$\Delta_l^{fie} = \left(\overline{\overline{G}}_S\left(\overline{I}_l^d + \overline{I}_l^a\right) - \overline{E}_l^{sca}\right). \tag{2.22}$$

And the relative residual error in the object function can be defined according to (2.8) under LSIE as

$$\Delta_l^{cur} = \left(\overline{L}(\overline{\overline{\gamma}}_l) - \overline{T}_l\right), \tag{2.23}$$

where $\overline{L}(\overline{\overline{\gamma}}_l) = \left(\overline{I}_l^a\right) - \chi \odot \overline{\overline{G}}_D\left(\overline{\overline{I}}_l^a\right)$ and $\overline{T}_l = \chi \odot \left[\overline{E}_l^{inc} + \overline{\overline{G}}_D\left(\overline{\overline{I}}_l^d\right)\right] - \overline{I}_l^d$. Consequently, the cost function is defined as follows:

$$f(\overline{\overline{\gamma}}_l, \chi) = \sum_{l=1}^{N_i} \left[\eta_l^S \|\Delta_l^{fie}\|_S^2 + \eta_l^D \|\Delta_l^{cur}\|_D^2\right], \tag{2.24}$$

where $\eta_l^S = 1/\|\overline{E}_l^{sca}\|_S^2$, and $\eta_l^D = 1/\|\overline{E}_l^{inc}\|_D^2$. The inversion is to minimize the objective function (2.24). This is a quadratic functional in $\overline{I}_l^a$, but nonlinear in χ. Different from the objective function (2.14), this objective function does not involve solving the forward problem by considering both the contrast and induced currents (or the coefficients) as unknowns. Doing so, the object equation acts no longer as a hard constraint but an objective to be satisfied. Such a type of objective function is usually less nonlinear compared with (2.14) and provides more freedoms in modeling. On the other hand, it requires more memory to store the physical states for every incidence.

In the inversion, the CSI/SOM-typed methods are used to minimize this cost function, in which two interlaced sequences updating $\overline{\overline{\gamma}}_l$ and χ via alternating application of the CG minimization method and least square (LS) method are constructed on the Fourier coefficients $\overline{\overline{\gamma}}_l$ and the updated contrast χ, respectively. As in [30], the FFT-TSOM is implemented as follows:

Step 1: Calculate $\overline{\overline{G}}_S$, $\overline{\overline{G}}_D$, and the thin SVD of $\overline{\overline{G}}_S$; obtain $\overline{I}_l^d$ by (2.17), $l = 1, 2, \ldots, N_i$.

Step 2: Initial step, $n = 0$: χ_0 is obtained from the back propagation [25,26]; select M_F, $\overline{\overline{\gamma}}_l = 0$; initialize the search direction $\overline{\rho}_{l,0} = 0$.

Step 3: $n = n+1$

Step 3.1: update $\overline{\overline{\gamma}}_{l,n}$: Calculate the gradient (Fréchet derivative) $\overline{g}_{l,n} = \nabla_{\overline{\overline{\gamma}}_l} f$ evaluated at $\overline{\overline{\gamma}}_{l,n-1}$ and $\overline{\overline{\chi}}_{n-1}$; determine the Polak–Ribière conjugate gradient search directions $\overline{\rho}_{\gamma;l,n} = \overline{g}_{l,n} + \left(Re\overline{g}_{l,n} - \overline{g}_{l,n-1}, \overline{g}_{l,n} / \| \overline{g}_{l,n}, \|^2 \right) \overline{\rho}_{\gamma;l,n-1}$ [25,26]. Define the scalar $d_{\gamma;l,n}$ by $\overline{\overline{\gamma}}_{l,n} = \overline{\overline{\gamma}}_{l,n-1} + d_{\gamma;l,n}\overline{\rho}_{\gamma;l,n}$. The objective function becomes quadratic in terms of the parameter $d_{\gamma;l,n}$, and it can be found from a line minimization as done in [25].

Step 3.2: Update $\overline{\overline{\chi}}_n$: For the mth cell, m=1, 2, …, M, update the induced contrast source $\overline{I}_{l,n} = \overline{I}_l^d + \left(\overline{\overline{I}}_M - \overline{\overline{V}}_S^+ \cdot \overline{\overline{V}}_S^{+*} \right) \cdot \mathrm{vec}\{IDFT\{\overline{\overline{\gamma}}_{l,n}\}\}$. Then update the total filed in the DoI, i.e., $\overline{E}_l^{tot} = \overline{E}_l^{inc} + \overline{\overline{G}}_D(\overline{I}_{l,n})$.

The objective function becomes quadratic in terms of $\overline{\overline{\chi}}_n$ and the solution is straightforwardly given by LS methods:

$$\left(\overline{\overline{\chi}}_n\right)_{m'n'} = \sum_{l=1}^{N_i} \frac{\left(\overline{E}_l^{tot}\right)^*_{m'n'}}{\|\overline{E}_l^{inc}\|} \cdot \frac{\left(\overline{I}_l^d\right)_{m'n'}}{\|\overline{E}_l^{inc}\|} \Big/ \sum_{l=1}^{N_i} \frac{\left(\overline{E}_l^{tot}\right)^*_{m'n'}}{\|\overline{E}_l^{inc}\|} \cdot \frac{\left(\overline{E}_l^{tot}\right)_{m'n'}}{\|\overline{E}_l^{inc}\|}. \tag{2.25}$$

Step 4: If the termination condition is satisfied, stop optimization. Otherwise, go to Step 3. Empirically, we stop the optimization when the values of the contrast do not noticeably change for successive three iterations.

It is obvious that the least-square update for the contrast is much more aggressive than the one-step CG update for the APIC. Therefore, one can attribute the main source of the nonlinearity onto the least-squares update of the contrast, which comes from the term $\overline{\overline{G}}_D(\overline{I}_l)$, especially when the scatterers are strong, those with large contrast and/or large dimensions in terms of wavelength, leading to much more significant contributions from $\overline{\overline{G}}_D(\overline{I}_l)$ than the ones from $\overline{E}_l^{inc}$.

To alleviate such a nonlinear effect, a family of CIE-I has been introduced in [33]. The discrete form of CIE-I could be given as

$$\beta\overline{\overline{I}}_l^d + \beta\overline{\overline{I}}_l^a = \overline{\overline{R}} \odot \left[\beta\overline{\overline{I}}_l^d + \beta\overline{\overline{I}}_l^a + \overline{\overline{E}}_l^{inc} + \overline{\overline{G}}_D\left(\overline{\overline{I}}_l^d\right) + \overline{\overline{G}}_D\left(\overline{\overline{I}}_l^a\right) \right], \tag{2.26}$$

where $\overline{\overline{R}} = \beta\overline{\overline{\chi}} / (\beta\overline{\overline{\chi}} + 1)$ is the modified contrast function, and β is a chosen auxiliary parameter to control the portion of the multiple scattering in estimating the contrast, which will be explained later in detail. Note that the CIE-I is mathematically equivalent to the LSIE, meaning that the former can be derived from the latter [33]. By properly choosing the β, (2.26) provides a new possibility to suppress the global nonlinearity embedded within the ISP that originates from the unknown multiple scattering effects with a new type of local nonlinearity. Such a transformation of nonlinearity can effectively constrain the error of estimations within a relatively small domain and thus increases the efficiency of handling highly nonlinear ISPs [33].

Given the object (2.26) and the two parts of induced current as earlier, the objective function of the TSOM-CIE-I scheme in [33] can also be defined as follows:

$$f\left(\bar{\bar{\gamma}}_l, \bar{\bar{R}}\right) = \sum_{l=1}^{N_i} \left[\eta_l^S \|\Delta_l^{fie}(\bar{\bar{\gamma}}_l)\|_S^2 + \eta_l^D \|\Delta_l^{cur}\left(\bar{\bar{\gamma}}_l, \bar{\bar{R}}\right)\|_D^2\right], \tag{2.27}$$

where the mismatch of the data equation is the same as (2.22), and $\Delta_l^{cur}\left(\bar{\bar{\gamma}}_l, \bar{\bar{R}}\right)$ measures the mismatch of the new object (2.26), defined as

$$\Delta_l^{cur}\left(\bar{\bar{\gamma}}_l, \bar{\bar{R}}\right) = \beta\left(\bar{\bar{I}}_l^d + \bar{\bar{I}}_l^a\right) - \bar{\bar{R}} \odot \left\{\beta\left(\bar{\bar{I}}_l^d + \bar{\bar{I}}_l^a\right) + \bar{\bar{G}}_D\left(\bar{\bar{I}}_l^d + \bar{\bar{I}}_l^a\right) + \bar{\bar{E}}_l^{inc}\right\}. \tag{2.28}$$

In the SOM or CSI, the contrast and the APIC (or the simply contrast sources in CSI) are updated alternatively. As mentioned in [33], the modified contrast for the nth iteration is estimated by the LS method,

$$\left(\bar{\bar{R}}_n\right)_{m'n'} = \sum_{l=1}^{N_i} \frac{\left(\Gamma_l^n\right)_{m'n'}^*}{\|\bar{\bar{E}}_l^{inc}\|} \cdot \frac{\left(\beta\bar{I}_l^d + \beta\bar{I}_l^a\right)_{m'n'}}{\|\bar{\bar{E}}_l^{inc}\|} \Bigg/ \sum_{l=1}^{N_i} \frac{\left(\Gamma_l^n\right)_m^*}{\|\bar{\bar{E}}_l^{inc}\|} \cdot \frac{\left(\Gamma_l^n\right)_{m'n'}}{\|\bar{\bar{E}}_l^{inc}\|}, \tag{2.29}$$

where

$$\left(\Gamma_l^n\right)_{m'n'} = \left[\bar{\bar{E}}_l^{inc} + \bar{\bar{G}}_D\left(\bar{\bar{I}}_l^d\right) + \bar{\bar{G}}_D\left(\bar{\bar{I}}_l^a\right)^n + \beta\bar{\bar{I}}_l^d + \beta\left(\bar{\bar{I}}_l^a\right)^n\right]_{m'n'}. \tag{2.30}$$

While the CIE-I can suppress the multiple scattering effects within the inversions, a proper regularization is needed to stabilize the inversions, since, as mentioned earlier, strong local wave effects have been introduced. In [33], the FFT-TSOM has been used to this end by constraining the induced current within a low-dimensional subspace. From numerical results therein, we clearly see that the FFT-TSOM effectively provides the regularization and effectively stabilizes the inversions with CIE-I model with large β. Nevertheless, such a low-dimensional subspace constraint might cause problems when tackling problems with even stronger nonlinearity where induced currents could have essential components outside the used subspace. To relax the subspace constraint onto the induced currents, a straightforward way is to put another regularization onto the contrast, leading to a hybrid regularization technique. We will discuss such a possible method in the next subsection.

2.3.2 Regularization with TSOM and MR

The TV technique is a useful approach to tackle ISPs, e.g., the multiplicative form in CSI method [26], where the TV introduces an extra constraint onto the reconstructed medium profile. Recently, it is shown that such an MR TV can work well with FFT-TSOM. And the numerical inversion results have shown that MR-TSOM provides convincing effects on inversions in terms of stability against noise [35], where we also notice that the subspace constraints within TSOM (or FFT-TSOM) have been relaxed with the MR.

For highly nonlinear ISP, as noticed in the previous section, the efficacy of using TSOM with the CIE-I to stabilize the inversions might still be good to some extent. When scatterers become even more strong, the low-dimensional subspace constraints onto the induced current could exclude some essential current components. Therefore, to further relax the TSOM subspace constraints, a possible way is to use the MR-TSOM, which is implemented as the following.

With the inclusion of the multiplicative TV regularizer, the object function at the nth iteration of the optimization can be further formulated in the generalized form,

$$H\left(\overline{\overline{\gamma}}_l, \overline{\overline{R}}\right) = f\left(\overline{\overline{\gamma}}_l, \overline{\overline{R}}\right) \cdot F_n^{TV}\left(\overline{\overline{R}}\right), \tag{2.31}$$

where $F_n^{TV}\left(\overline{\overline{R}}\right)$ is the MR factor. And it can be in the form of weighted L_1 and L_2 norms, which is represented by the following unified expression:

$$F_n^{TV}\left(\overline{\overline{R}}\right) = \frac{1}{A}\int_D \left(\frac{|\nabla R(r)|^2 + \delta_n^2}{|\nabla R_{n-1}(r)|^2 + \delta_n^2}\right)^{P/2} dV(r), \tag{2.32}$$

where A is the area of the test domain D and denotes the spatial differentiation with respect to r. If $P = 1$, the MR acts as a weighted L_1 norm TV-factor, and $P = 2$ as a weighted L_2 norm TV-factor. Both can recover smooth and "blocky" profiles.

The constant regularization parameter δ_n^2 is introduced for restoring differentiability of the TV regularizer in (2.31), and it plays a crucial role in the TV. The regularization parameter here is chosen as

$$\delta_n^2 = \frac{F_S\left(\overline{\overline{\gamma}}_l, \overline{\overline{R}}\right)}{\Delta^2} \times \Lambda(\beta, n), \tag{2.33}$$

where $F_S\left(\overline{\overline{\gamma}}_l, \overline{\overline{R}}\right) = \eta_l^D \Delta_l^{cur}\left(\overline{\overline{\gamma}}_l, \overline{\overline{R}}\right)_D^2$ is the right parts of (2.27). Δ is the mesh size of the discretized DoI D. Here, $\Lambda(\beta, n)$ is an auxiliary function of adaptive parameters relating to the CIE-I being used. The principles of choosing δ_n^2 include the following:

1. At the beginning, the optimization focuses on the update of the unknown contrast function $R(r)$.
2. The effect of MR should be increased as the iterative optimization proceeds by decreasing the value of δ_n^2.
3. The auxiliary function $\Lambda(\beta, n)$ should be well designed to guarantee that δ_n^2 is gradually reduced to a threshold [35].

Previously, the hybrid inversion method is named MR-TSOM-CIE-I, and the iterative algorithm can be referred to [36]. By setting TSOM as SOM (letting the

Fourier filter be an all-pass one [33]), only the MR works with the CIE-I, denoted as MR-SOM-CIE-I. TSOM provides the direct regularization effects onto the induced current, whereas there is only MR working with the CIE-I, the implication of the local wave effects by the induced current in (2.29) can only be indirectly remedied through the estimation of the contrast by the regularization of MR in the previous iteration. Thus, the TSOM should outperform the MR in this aspect. Nevertheless, MR is able to loosen the subspace constraints from TSOM, as indicated in [35,36]. We expect that they can help each other when working with CIE-I to increase the stability when handling the highly nonlinear ISPs.

2.3.3 Numerical Test I

In order to test the resolvability of the inversion algorithm MR-TSOM-CIE-I to tackle the scatterers with large contrasts and/or with electrically large dimensions, we present several inversion results from the synthetic data.

To evaluate the quality of the reconstructed images, the mean-square error of the estimation can be calculated as

$$ERR_{\varepsilon}^{tot} = \sqrt{\frac{1}{M}\sum_{n_1}\sum_{n_2}\frac{\left|\overline{\overline{\varepsilon}}_{r;n1,n2}^{inv}-\overline{\overline{\varepsilon}}_{r;n1,n2}^{true}\right|^2}{\left|\overline{\overline{\varepsilon}}_{r;n1,n2}^{true}\right|^2}}, \tag{2.34}$$

where the summation of indexes n_1 and n_2 are over the whole DoI. $\overline{\overline{\varepsilon_r}}^{inv}$ represents the relative permittivity of each iteration and $\overline{\overline{\varepsilon_r}}^{true}$ denotes the true relative permittivity of the DoI. To further evaluate the reconstruction qualities exactly on the unknown scatterers (apart from the background media), another type of inversion error ERR_{ε}^{sct} is defined with the summation of indexes m and n over only the domain where unknown scatterers distribute, and the corresponding total number of cells.

In all numerical tests, additive white Gaussian noise (AWGN) is added to the synthetic data and is quantified by $\|\overline{e}_l^{noise}\|_D^2/\|\overline{E}_{l;MoM}^{sca}\|_D^2 \times 100\%$, where $\|\cdot\|_D^2$ denotes the norm of the DoI D and $\overline{E}_{l;MoM}^{sca}$ is the numerical scattering data generated by MoM for lth incidence. The classic "Austria" profile is first considered, with different values of contrasts in different tests. "Austria" profile consists an annulus, two disks, and the background air [28–30]. The two disks are of the same 0.2-m radius and their centers are (−0.3, 0.6) m and (0.3, 0.6) m. The annual is centered at (0, −0.2) m with 0.3-m inner radius and 0.6-m outer radius. In all the simulations with "Austria" profile, the DoI D is a rectangular domain centered at the origin with 2 m×2 m. The DoI is illuminated by 16 plane wave incidences at $f = 400$ MHz (with the wavelength in the air being 0.75 m) from different angles evenly distributed in $[0, 2\pi)$ on a circle S with radius 3 m centered at the origin. For each incidence angle, $N_r = 32$ probes are evenly distributed along the same circle S with a radius 3 m to measure the scattered fields. In inversions, a 64×64-grid mesh of DoI D is used. On the other hand, in the forward problem, in order to avoid inverse crime, the scattering data are calculated with a finer 100×100-grid mesh.

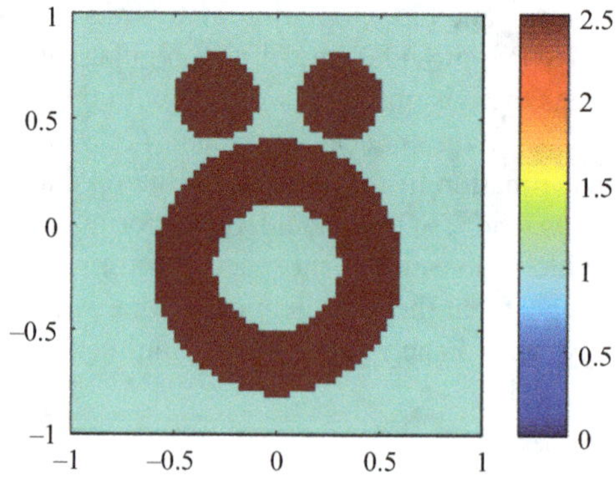

Figure 2.2 Exact "Austria" profile with $\varepsilon_r = 2.5$

Example 1: In the first example, all the three scatters (two disks and the annual) in "Austria" profile are lossless with the relative permittivity $\varepsilon_r = 2.5$, as shown in Figure 2.2. Due to the lossless scatterers, the null imaginary part of the profile is omitted here. 10% AWGN is added to the synthetic data unless otherwise stated. The value of L depends on the noise level and the singular values of the operator $\overline{\overline{G}}_S$. When given a measurement scheme and a DoI, $\overline{\overline{G}}_S$ is decided, so do its singular values. Then L is decided by the noise level, as mentioned in [28,30]. Here $L = 15$ is selected. And M_F determines how many low-frequency Fourier components are utilized to construct APIC [30].

Reconstructed results obtained by MR-TSOM-LSIE, SOM-CIE-I, and TSOM-CIE-I are depicted in Figure 2.3(a)–(c), respectively, where the reconstructed results by MR-TSOM-LSIE with $M_F = 12$ is not satisfactory, which shows that MR-TSOM-LSIE fails to locate the global solution when encountering highly nonlinear ISP. To alleviate the nonlinearity of ISP, the CIE-I is used to replace the LSIE. Following the principle in [36], $\beta = 3$ is used in CIE-I-based algorithms. One can see from Figure 2.3(b) that a rough "Austria" profile with some disturbances can be retrieved by SOM-CIE-I, which is certainly a substantial improvement compared to MR-TSOM-LSIE in Figure 2.3(a). In order to get better stability and better robustness against noise, TSOM with $M_F = 12$ is used to stabilize the inversion, the result of which is shown in Figure 2.3(c) with a further good improvement. The errors of reconstructions, ERR_ε^{tot}, in Figure 2.3(a)–(c) are 0.5205, 0.3283, and 0.2571, and ERR_ε^{sct} are 0.2522, 0.1010, and 0.0847. From the comparisons, we see that, as mentioned in [36], the TSOM-CIE-I algorithm can greatly improve the ability to resolve the strong nonlinearity in ISPs.

Example 2: To differentiate the TSOM-CIE-I and MR-TSOM-CIE-I in terms of the resolvability against the high nonlinearity. Thus, the relative permittivity of the "Austria" profile is increased to 4.5, which makes the ISP a highly nonlinear one. Here, we assume that the real and imaginary parts of the contrast are not smaller than 0 (by setting those elements smaller than 0 to be 0 after every iteration). The reconstructed results by the two methods are shown in Figure 2.4(a) and (b). In the first round, $M_F = 6$

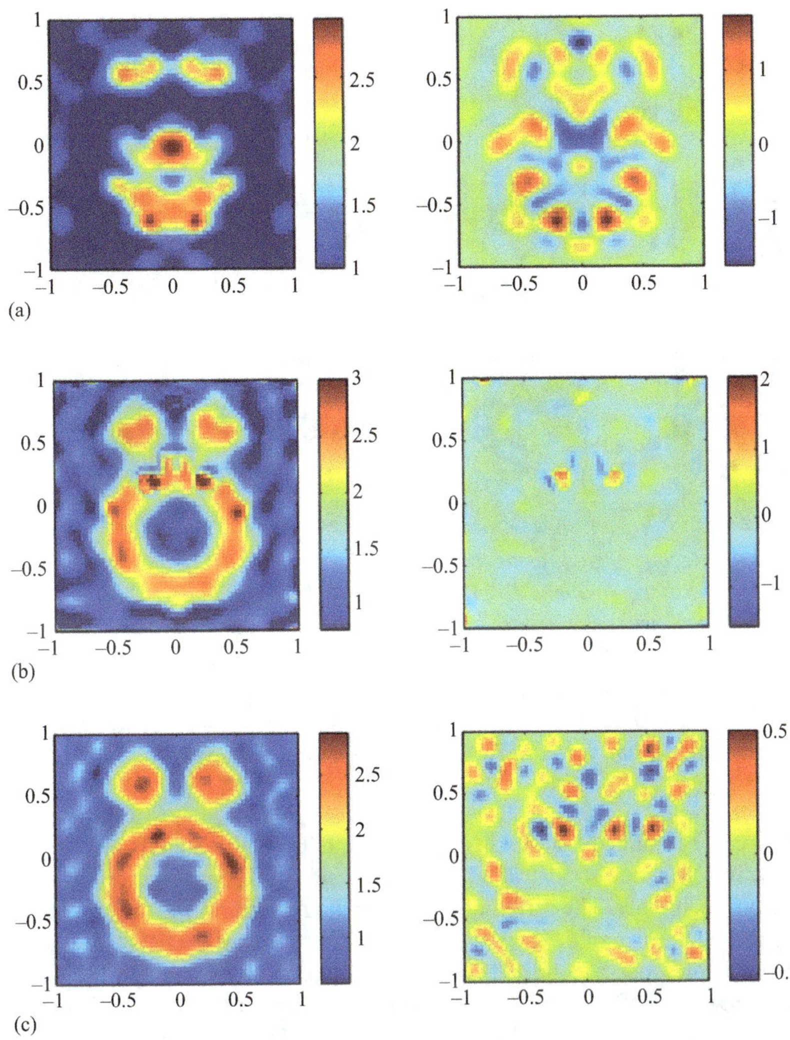

Figure 2.3 *Reconstructed results in Example 1 with 10% AWGN for "Austria" type scatterers with ε_r=2.5, the real (left) and imaginary (right) parts of the reconstruction relative permittivity ε_r when retrieved by (a) MR-TSOM-LSIE, (b) SOM-CIE-I, and (c) TSOM-CIE-I after 300 iterations*

and $\beta = 8$ are used in both methods and the reconstructed results after 100 iterations are given in the first row. In the second round, with $M_F = 12$ and $\beta = 0.5$ and results obtained in the first round as the starting points, the reconstructed profiles after 2,000 iterations are shown in the second row. After two rounds of optimization, the reconstructed result by MR-TSOM-CIE-I is quite satisfactory while the one obtained by TSOM-CIE-I is of far less quality, as indicated by the recorded errors in Figure 2.4.

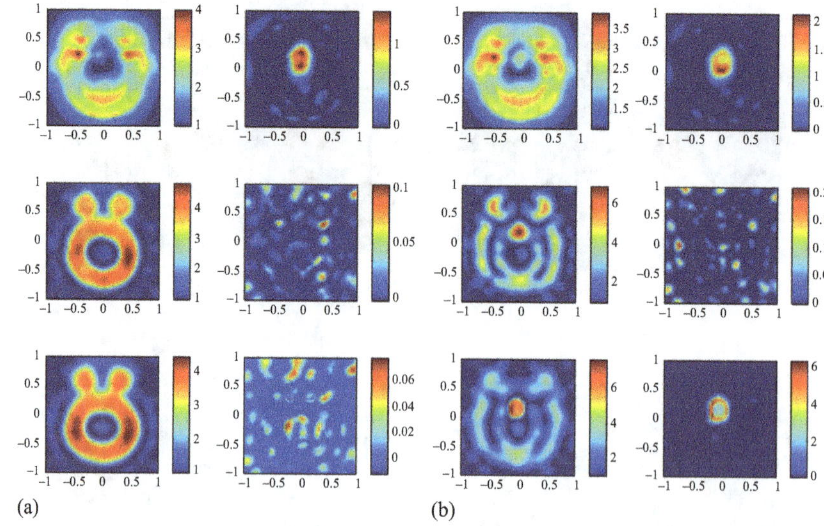

Figure 2.4 Reconstructed results in Example 2 with 10% AWGN for "Austria" type scatterers with $\varepsilon_r = 4.5$, the real (left) and imaginary (right) parts of the reconstruction relative permittivity ε_r using (a) weighted L_2 norm MR-TSOM-CIE-I and (b) TSOM-CIE-I, respectively. The first, second, and third rows correspond to M_F being 6, 12, and 10, and β_0 being 8, 0.5, and 0.5, respectively (with two kinds of two-rounds M_F iterated algorithm, including $\{M_F = 6, M_F = 12\}$ and $\{M_F = 6, M_F = 10\}$)

It is can be noticed that reconstructed results by both methods after the first-round optimization are similar, but after the second-round optimization, two results differ from each other. The difference between the first round and the second round mainly lies on the size of the current subspace. This comparison tells that when MR comes in, it provides a good extra regularization effect to stabilize the CIE-I in cases with relatively loosened TSOM subspace constraint (larger M_F). It is proved that the MR can loosen the subspace constraint in TSOM to provide more high-frequency current components that are needed to properly reconstruct the strong scatterers. To further confirm this, we set $M_F = 10$ and $\beta = 0.5$ for another trial of second round optimization, and the corresponding inversion results after 900 iterations are given in the third row. One can see that while very satisfactory results can be obtained by MR-TSOM-CIE-I, the TSOM-CIE-I still cannot provide good estimation on the profile.

In brief, two regularization methods (i.e., TSOM and MR) and their combination under the CIE-I model are studied. Numerical tests show that the MR can loosen the subspace constraint from TSOM and provides more high-frequency components of the induced sources for the CIE-I while keeping the inversions stable, which are vital for solving highly nonlinear ISPs. This tells that the hybrid regularization technique together with CIE-I or MR-TSOM-CIE-I, outperforms

TSOM-CIE-I, in terms of robustness against noise and resolvability against nonlinearity. This lays solid ground for tackling ISPs with strong scatterers, such as those appearing in the biomedical imaging.

On the other hand, due to the different tissues within the human body, the electrical properties vary largely from one tissue to another, such as those in the brain and breast. To handle such a complex background, a straightforward way is to use the associated Green's function, which, however, results in inefficient inversions due to the loss of the Toeplitz matrix structure of Green's function operator and thus the loss of the FFT type fast matrix–vector multiplication. To circumvent this drawback, in the next subsection, we will discuss the difference type IE model that is specifically designed for the ISPs with an inhomogeneous background.

2.4 Inversion with inhomogeneous background

2.4.1 Inversions with D-LSIE and with D-CIE-I

The previously mentioned methods are based on the problems with homogeneous background, in which closed-form Green's functions or semi-closed-form ones are available for simple media, like homogeneous or layered media. If we change our background medium from the homogeneous medium to another already known inhomogeneous medium, the object equation and the data equation are still valid if Green's functions are changed accordingly with inhomogeneous background. However, Green's function for inhomogeneous medium is usually not in a closed form, and the convolution type of the integration (the operator $\overline{\overline{G}}_D$) does not exist anymore. To deal with such a type of problem, a straightforward way is to use Green's function associated with the known inhomogeneous background, such as the DBIM [37], the finite-difference CSI method [38], and the SOM based on the finite-element method [39]. However, by involving Green's functions for inhomogeneous background media, the computational cost associated could be prohibitively large, especially when tackling large-scale problems. Here, the associated computations include those to generate these Green's functions and those to apply them into the calculation of fields. Most likely, fast algorithms, such as FFT [40] and fast multipole method (FMM) schemes [41], cannot be used in this case. If the modeling of ISPs based on the inhomogeneous background is directly used in the modeling equations, much more cumbersome inversions can be expected.

Recently, based on the LSIE and CIE-I, two types of difference IEs are proposed to study the difference-induced current within the DoI [42]. Referring them as difference LSIE (D-LSIE) and D-CIE-I, the closed-form Green's functions with homogeneous medium are used. In the inversion, the models of D-LSIE and D-CIE-I are applied in conjunction within the FFT-TSOM frame [30].

Without using Green's function with inhomogeneous background medium, this method is computationally more effective. And under the new CIE-I, the inversion methods based on the D-CIE-I model can handle ISPs with strong nonlinearity. In the following, the methods will be introduced. If the inhomogeneous background is known, then $\overline{\overline{\chi}}^{inh-b} = (\varepsilon_{inh-b} - \varepsilon_b)/\varepsilon_b$ is denoted as the contrast of known background inhomogeneous medium compared with the initial homogeneous background (e.g., air or coupling liquids used in biomedical imaging). And let the total contrast $\overline{\overline{\chi}}$ split into two parts $\overline{\overline{\chi}} = \overline{\overline{\chi}}^{inh-b} + \Delta\overline{\overline{\chi}}$, where $\Delta\overline{\overline{\chi}}$ is the unknown perturbation from the background inhomogeneous medium. The total internal electric field can also be split into two parts, $\overline{\overline{E}}_l = \overline{\overline{E}}_l^{inh-b} + \Delta\overline{\overline{E}}_l$, where $\overline{\overline{E}}_l^{inh-b}$ is the internal field when only the background inhomogeneous medium exists but not the unknown scatterers and can be obtained by solving the LSIE in advance,

$$\overline{\overline{E}}_l^{inh-b} = \overline{\overline{E}}_l^{inc} + \overline{\overline{G}}_D\left(\overline{\overline{I}}_l^{inh-b}\right), \tag{2.35}$$

where $\overline{\overline{I}}_l^{inh-b} = \overline{\overline{\chi}}^{inh-b} \odot \overline{\overline{E}}_l^{inh-b}$ being the contrast source generated by the inhomogeneous background medium $\overline{\overline{\chi}}^{inh-b}$. We denote the scattered fields generated by the inhomogeneous background medium as $\overline{\overline{E}}_l^{b;sca} = \overline{\overline{G}}_S\left(\text{vec}\left\{\overline{\overline{I}}_l^{inh-b}\right\}\right)$, the subtraction of which from (2.9) yields the difference data equation as

$$\Delta\overline{\overline{E}}_l^{sca} = \overline{\overline{E}}_l^{sca} - \overline{\overline{E}}_l^{b;sca} = \overline{\overline{G}}_S(\Delta\overline{I}_l), \tag{2.36}$$

where $\Delta\overline{I}_l = \text{vec}\{\Delta\overline{\overline{I}}_l\}$, and $\Delta\overline{\overline{I}}_l = \overline{\overline{I}}_l - \overline{\overline{I}}_l^{inh-b}$, $\overline{\overline{I}}_l$ is the contrast source generated by the inhomogeneous background medium $\overline{\overline{\chi}}^{inh-b}$ and unknown scatterers with the medium $\overline{\overline{\chi}}$. In virtue of (2.8), the formulation of $\overline{\overline{I}}_l$ and $\overline{\overline{I}}_l^{inh-b}$ can be achieved.

By the subtraction of one by another, we straightforwardly obtain a difference object equation based on LSIE as

$$\Delta\overline{\overline{I}}_l = \overline{\overline{\chi}}^{inh-b} \odot \overline{\overline{G}}_D(\Delta\overline{I}_l) + \overline{\overline{\chi}} \odot \left[\overline{\overline{E}}_l^{inh-b} + \overline{\overline{G}}_D(\Delta\overline{I}_l)\right], \tag{2.37}$$

which is referred to as D-LSIE.

Following the same procedure for the D-LSIE, we obtain the difference object equation based on the CIE-I as

$$\begin{aligned} \beta\Delta\overline{\overline{I}}_l = \overline{\overline{R}} \odot &\left[\overline{\overline{E}}_l^{inh-b} + \beta\overline{\overline{I}}_l^{inh-b} + \overline{\overline{G}}_D(\Delta\overline{I}_l) + \beta\Delta\overline{\overline{I}}_l\right] + \\ &\overline{\overline{R}}^{inh-b} \odot \left[\beta\Delta\overline{\overline{I}}_l + \overline{\overline{G}}_D(\Delta\overline{I}_l)\right], \end{aligned} \tag{2.38}$$

where $\overline{\overline{R}}^{inh-b} = \beta\overline{\overline{\chi}}^{inh-b} / \left(\beta\overline{\overline{\chi}}^{inh-b} + 1\right)$ is the modified contrast function for the inhomogeneous background medium and $\overline{\overline{R}} = \overline{\overline{R}} - \overline{\overline{R}}^{inh-b}$. We refer to this equation as the D-CIE-I.

From (2.36)–(2.38), we see that the new difference models (D-LSIE and D-CIE-I) focus on the perturbation of the contrast and the induced currents inside the DoI. And the new models still use Green's function for the homogeneous background, which therefore allows the fast computation of convolutional type multiplication of Green's function and the induced current through the FFT scheme or the FMM. This substantially saves cost from two aspects: (1) to avoid calculating the numerical Green's function for the inhomogeneous background and (2) to use the aforementioned fast algorithms instead of direct calculation of matrix–vector multiplication [from $O(M_2)$ to $O(M\log M)$]. Besides, the D-CIE-I can further improve the capability of solving the high nonlinear ISPs with inhomogeneous background.

2.4.2 FFT-TSOM-based inversions with D-LSIE and D-CIE-I

Different from the ISPs with homogeneous background, the unknown variables in the inversion, e.g., $\overline{\overline{I}}_l$ and $\overline{\overline{\chi}}$ (or $\overline{\overline{R}}$), are changed into the difference variables, e.g., $\Delta\overline{\overline{I}}_l$ and $\Delta\overline{\overline{\chi}}$ (or $\Delta\overline{\overline{R}}$). Therefore, as did in TSOM for homogeneous background [30], the unknown induced current $\Delta\overline{\overline{I}}_l$ in ISPs with inhomogeneous background is also split into two parts: a DPIC $\Delta\overline{I}_l^d$ and an APIC $\Delta\overline{I}_l^a$. Thus, based on (2.36) and similar to (2.17), the DPIC can be obtained as

$$\Delta\overline{I}_l^d = \sum_{j=1}^{L}\frac{\langle\Delta\overline{E}_l^{sca},\overline{u}_j^S\rangle}{\sigma_j^S}\overline{v}_j^S = \overline{\overline{V}}_j^S\cdot\overline{\alpha}_l^+. \tag{2.39}$$

On the other hand, as in [30], the APIC can either be expressed by

$$\Delta\overline{I}_l^a(\overline{\overline{\gamma}}_l) = \overline{I}_l^{tmp} - \overline{\overline{V}}_S^+\left(\overline{\overline{V}}_S^{+H}\cdot\overline{I}_l^{tmp}\right) = W_l(\overline{\overline{\gamma}}_l), \tag{2.40}$$

for FFT-TSOM, where $\overline{I}_l^{tmp} = \text{vec}\{IDFT\{\overline{\overline{\gamma}}_l\}\}$, and the operator $W_l(\overline{\overline{\gamma}}_l) = \left(\overline{\overline{I}}_M - \overline{\overline{V}}_S^+\cdot\overline{\overline{V}}_S^{+H}\right)\cdot\text{vec}\{IDFT\{\overline{\overline{\gamma}}_l\}\}$.

For the FFT-TSOM, the mismatch of the data (2.36) for lth incidence is given by

$$\Delta_l^{fie} = \left(\overline{\overline{G}}_S\left(\Delta\overline{I}_l^d + \Delta\overline{I}_l^a\right) - \Delta\overline{E}_l^{sca}\right), \tag{2.41}$$

where $\Delta\overline{I}_l^d$ and $\Delta\overline{I}_l^a$ are as in (2.39) and (2.40), respectively.

The object equation is another key equation to satisfy. Utilizing the current construction (2.36) and both objects (2.37) and (2.38), the operator corresponding with unknown APIC $\Delta\overline{I}_l^a$ a based on the D-LSIE and the D-CIE-I can be defined as, respectively,

$$L(\overline{\overline{\gamma}}_l)^{LSIE} = \Delta\overline{\overline{I}}_l^a - \chi^{inh-b}\odot\overline{\overline{G}}_D\left(\Delta\overline{\overline{I}}_l^a\right) - \Delta\chi\odot\overline{\overline{G}}_D\left(\Delta\overline{\overline{I}}_l^a\right), \tag{2.42}$$

$$L(\overline{\overline{\gamma}}_l)^{CIE-I} = \left(\beta - \beta R^{inh-b} - R^{inh-b}\odot\overline{\overline{G}}_D\right)\left(\Delta\overline{\overline{I}}_l^a\right) - \left(\beta\overline{\overline{R}} + \overline{\overline{R}}\odot\overline{\overline{G}}_D\right)\left(\Delta\overline{\overline{I}}_l^a\right), \tag{2.43}$$

where $\Delta\overline{\overline{I}}_l^a = \text{ten}\{\Delta\overline{I}_l^a(\overline{\overline{\gamma}}_l)\}$, and ten{} is the inverse operation of vec{}. Another operator related to DPIC $\Delta\overline{I}_l^d$ can be accordingly expressed as

$$\overline{\overline{T}}_l^{LSIE} = \Delta\chi\odot\left[\overline{E}_l^{inh-b} + \overline{\overline{G}}_D\left(\Delta\overline{\overline{I}}_l^d\right)\right] + \chi^{inh-b}\odot\overline{\overline{G}}_D\left(\Delta\overline{\overline{I}}_l^d\right) - \Delta\overline{\overline{I}}_l^d, \tag{2.44}$$

$$\begin{aligned}\overline{\overline{T}}_l^{CIE-I} &= -\left(\beta - \beta R^{inh-b} - R^{inh-b} \odot \overline{\overline{G}}_D\right)\left(\Delta \overline{\overline{I}}_l^d\right) \\ &+ \overline{\overline{R}} \odot \left[\overline{\overline{E}}_l^{inh-b} + \beta \Delta \overline{\overline{I}}_l^d + \beta \overline{\overline{I}}_l^{inh-b} + \overline{\overline{G}}_D\left(\Delta \overline{\overline{I}}_l^d\right)\right],\end{aligned} \tag{2.45}$$

where $\Delta \overline{\overline{I}}_l^d = \text{ten}\left\{\Delta \overline{I}_l^d\right\}$. With the abovementioned definitions, we can write the mismatch of the difference object functions (2.42), (2.44), and (2.43), (2.45) of LSIE and CIE-I uniformly as

$$\Delta_l^{cur} = \left(L(\overline{\overline{\gamma}}_l) - \overline{\overline{T}}_l^{LSIE/CIE-I}\right). \tag{2.46}$$

Finally, the cost function is constructed under the FFT-TSOM scheme:

$$f(\overline{\overline{\gamma}}_l, \chi \text{ or } R) = \sum_{l=1}^{N_i}\left[\eta_l^S \|\Delta_l^{fie}\|_S^2 + \eta_l^D \|\Delta_l^{cur}\|_D^2\right], \tag{2.47}$$

where $\eta_l^S = 1/\|\overline{\overline{E}}_l^{sca}\|_S^2$ and $\eta_l^D = 1/\|\overline{\overline{E}}_l^{inh-b}\|_D^2$. The optimization is to minimize the abovementioned objective function. In [25,28,30], the CG-type algorithm is adopted by alternatively updating the $\overline{\overline{\gamma}}_l$ and $\Delta\chi$ (or ΔR) at every iteration of the optimization. At last, the final dielectric profile can be obtained as $\overline{\overline{\varepsilon}}_r = \overline{\overline{\chi}}^{inh-b} + \Delta\overline{\overline{\chi}} + 1$.

We clearly see that, based on the D-LSIE and D-CIE-I, the bounded inhomogeneous background is fully considered, and the matrix–vector multiplicative computations associated with Green's function become much more efficient compared with the case of using the inhomogeneous background Green's function. Meanwhile, the inversions still focus onto the changes due to the unknown medium perturbations. This is achieved at the cost of including all the inhomogeneous background into the DoI. For biomedical imaging problems, such a modeling is proper since the concerned human body parts are not large in terms of the wavelength of the probing wave.

2.4.3 Numerical Test II

We perform several numerical experiments to test the inversion method. The synthetic data with inhomogeneous background, such as through-wall imaging, have been employed to validate the methods based on difference IEs (D-LSIE and D-CIE-I).

Example 3: Herein, through-wall imaging is selected as the testing scenario. A square wall with outer side length 1.6λ and inner side length 1.1λ is used as the inhomogeneous background, whose relative permittivity is 1.5, as shown in Figure 2.5. The unknown scatterer is an annulus with relative permittivity of 3, whose inner and outer radii are 0.25λ and 0.4λ, respectively. Both the wall and the annulus are centered at the origin. The null imaginary part of the profile is omitted here.

Real parts of the reconstructed profiles after 100 iterations obtained by DBIM, D-LSIE, and D-CIE-I are depicted in Figure 2.6(b)–(d), respectively. As shown in

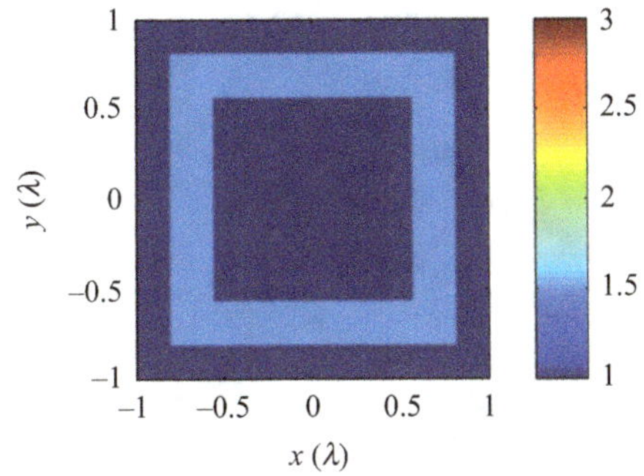

Figure 2.5 Exact configuration of the inhomogeneous background medium

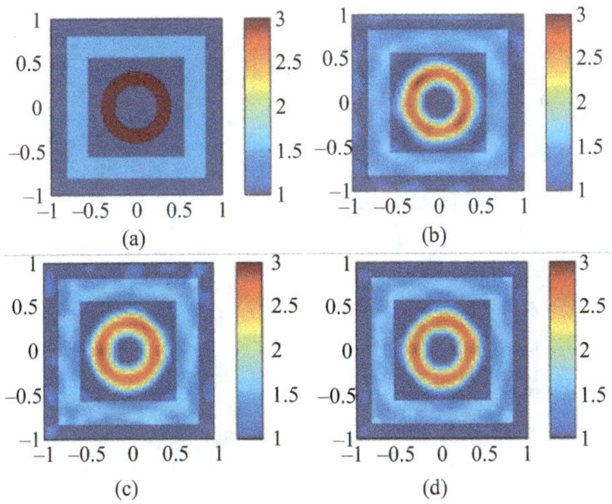

Figure 2.6 Reconstruction results in Example 3: (a) exact profile: real parts of reconstructed results after the 100 iterations with (b) DBIM, (c) D-LSIE, and (d) D-CIE-I

Figure 2.6, we can see that, although some small fluctuation (i.e., inside the square wall and the annulus) in the background exists, the annulus and the square inside the wall are obviously well reconstructed. Compared with the profile reconstructed by the DBIM, the results obtained by the D-LSIE and D-CIE-I are quite satisfactory. From the comparisons in this case, we see that, by virtue of D-LSIE and D-CIE-I and using Green's function for homogeneous medium, these new inversion methods can achieve similar reconstruction results compared with the methods based on the inhomogeneous Green's function, such as DBIM. However, in terms of efficiency, they are much faster compared with the DBIM.

Example 4: In order to further validate the effect, differentiate the two models (e.g., D-LSIE and D-CIE-I) in terms of the resolvability against highly

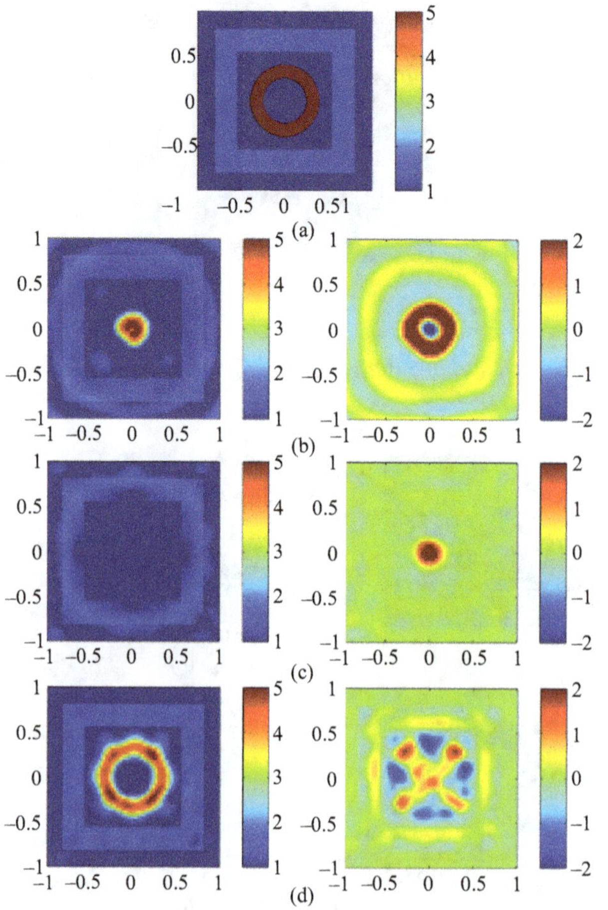

Figure 2.7 Reconstruction results in Example 4: (a) exact profile: real parts of reconstructed results after the 100 iterations with (b) DBIM, (c) D-LSIE, (d) D-CIE-I

nonlinear ISPs, the relative permittivity of the annulus inside is increased to 5. The reconstructed results by the DBIM, D-LSIE, and D-CIE-I methods after 200 iterations are shown in Figure 2.7(b)–(d). In order to highlight the difference among them, the imaginary parts of reconstructed results are also displayed. Both the DBIM and the D-LSIE cannot successfully reconstruct the profiles, as shown in Figure 2.7(b)–(c). On the contrary, the results reconstructed by D-CIE-I in Figure 2.7(d) are satisfactory, in which the annulus can be well recognized. These comparisons tell that the algorithms based on D-CIE-I are superior to the others, such as DBIM and the ones based on D-LSIE, in terms of the stability and the resolvability when tackling the highly nonlinear ISPs with inhomogeneous background.

2.4.4 Numerical test III for the biomedical microwave imaging

The previous discussions and experiment through numerical tests have validated that the D-CIE-I can significantly improve the capability of solving the highly nonlinear ISPs with the inhomogeneous background media. In the following, the D-CIE-I inversion method is used for the biomedical imaging for human tissues. In the following, three biomedical imaging cases are demonstrated for the effectiveness of the method, i.e., a human thorax, a human brain, and a human breast. These all have complex background media. The comparison of D-LSIE and D-CIE-I will be utilized to illustrate the effectiveness of the CIE-I model. And owing to the discussion with DBIM before, the comparison again to DBIM in biomedical imaging is not implemented.

Example 5: A simple human thorax model is used to validate the D-LSIE and D-CIE-I inversion methods. The exact profile is shown in Figure 2.8(a), in which the imaginary part of the complex permittivity is almost equal to zeros and is omitted here. The relative permittivity of the fat/skin, muscle, deflated lung, skull cancellous, heart muscle, and blood vessel wall are 5.57, 56.9, 54.2, 22.3, 65.3, and 46.7, respectively, which are slightly different from the permittivity distribution in [5]. The thorax is immersed in the glycerol medium with a relative permittivity of $\varepsilon_r = 45{:}8$. The DoI D is a square of side length 40 cm. The number of transmitters is 16 and the number of receivers is 32, and they are uniformly distributed on a circle S of radius 30 cm. The source operation frequency is 434 MHz. In inversions, a 64×64-grid mesh of the DoI D is used.

In this example, 10% AWGN is added to the synthetic data. The inhomogeneous background medium, as shown in Figure 2.8(b), includes the coupling

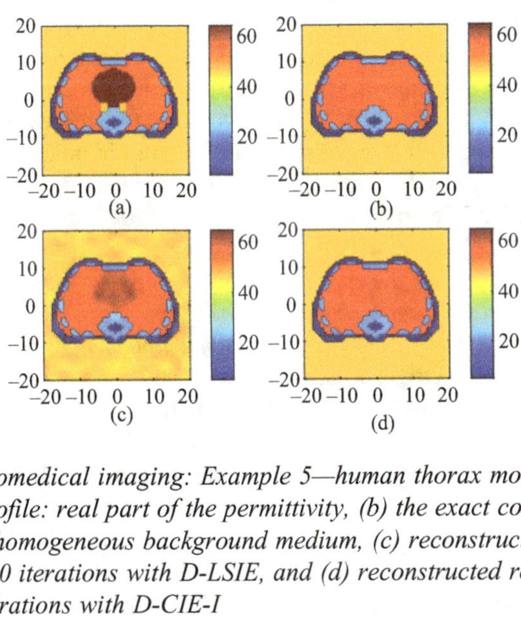

Figure 2.8 Biomedical imaging: Example 5—human thorax model: (a) exact profile: real part of the permittivity, (b) the exact configuration of the inhomogeneous background medium, (c) reconstructed result after 100 iterations with D-LSIE, and (d) reconstructed result after 100 iterations with D-CIE-I

glycerol liquid, skin layer, skull cancellous, and the muscle. So, the unknown tissues are the heart muscle inside and two blood vessels.

The value of L depends on the noise level and the singular values of operator G_S. Here $L=15$ is selected for the inversion. The reconstructed profiles after 100 iterations by D-LSIE and D-CIE-I are shown in Figure 2.8(c) and (d), respectively. As shown in Figure 2.8, one can see clearly that the unknown heart muscle inside could be obviously well reconstructed by both D-LSIE and D-CIE-I. The two blood vessels in front of the heart muscle cannot be recognized correctly since the permittivity is almost equal to that of background and in addition smaller than that of the lung. The errors of reconstructions ERR_{ε}^{tot} in Figure 2.8(c) and (d) are 0.0836 and 0.0809, respectively, which validate the better ability of the inversion under the D-CIE-I.

Example 6: A human brain tumor imaging is selected as the testing scenario. The exact profile is shown in Figure 2.9(a), the left profile is the real part of the model and the right part is the imaginary part of the model. The relative permittivity of the skin, skull, fat, meninges, gray matter, white matter, tumor, and environment are $39.0000-14.3801i$, $11.1000-2.5165i$, $4.9000-0.3595i$, $43.2000-17.2561i$, $50.7000-16.3573i$, $37.5000-10.4256i$, $61.2000+22.5573i$ and 34, respectively. A square with side length 24 cm is used as DoI D. In inversions, the DoI is discretized into 96×96-grid meshes. A total of 16 incidences uniformly distributed on the 2π angle are employed, while 32 receivers evenly located on a circle (with radius 30 cm) centered at the origin of the DoI measure the scattering data for each incidence. The source operation frequency is 400 MHz. This example is more complicated compared to the previous one.

In this example, 10% AWGN is added into the synthetic data. The imaging profiles in Figure 2.9(b) are used as the inhomogeneous background, including the skin, skull, and other environment. In the inversions, the unknown parts are the rest tissues. The noise level and the singular values of G_S determine the value of L. The value of L is chosen as 15 here. The reconstructed results after 100 iterations by D-LSIE and D-CIE-I are shown in Figure 2.9(c) and (d), respectively. From those results, we can see that both methods can successfully identify tumors. However, the retrieval results by D-CIE-I can more accurately detect the tumor compared to the one with D-LSIE. The errors of reconstructions ERR_{ε}^{tot} in Figure 2.9(c) and (d) are 0.02 and 0.016, respectively. Both the imaging results and reconstructed errors validate the better ability for the inversion of high nonlinear ISPs under the D-CIE-I method.

Example 7: To further validate the inversion methods, in this example, a human breast tumor model is selected. The exact profile is shown in Figure 2.10(a); similarly, the left profile is the real part of the model and the right one is the imaginary part of the model. The breast model is developed using MRI images from Wisconsin University repository (heterogeneously dense breast, ID: 07194) [14]. The relative permittivity of the skin, muscle, interstitial fluid, and immersion medium are $20.0932+0.7440i$, $27.2768+0.7785i$, $12.4283+0.0022i$, and 14, and three fibro-connective glandular are $26.5261+0.4722i$, $19.2627+0.7210i$, and $24.3507+0.8214i$, and three fatty tissues are $14.0980+0.0214i$, $14.8373+0.0377i$, and $17.6651+0.0864i$,

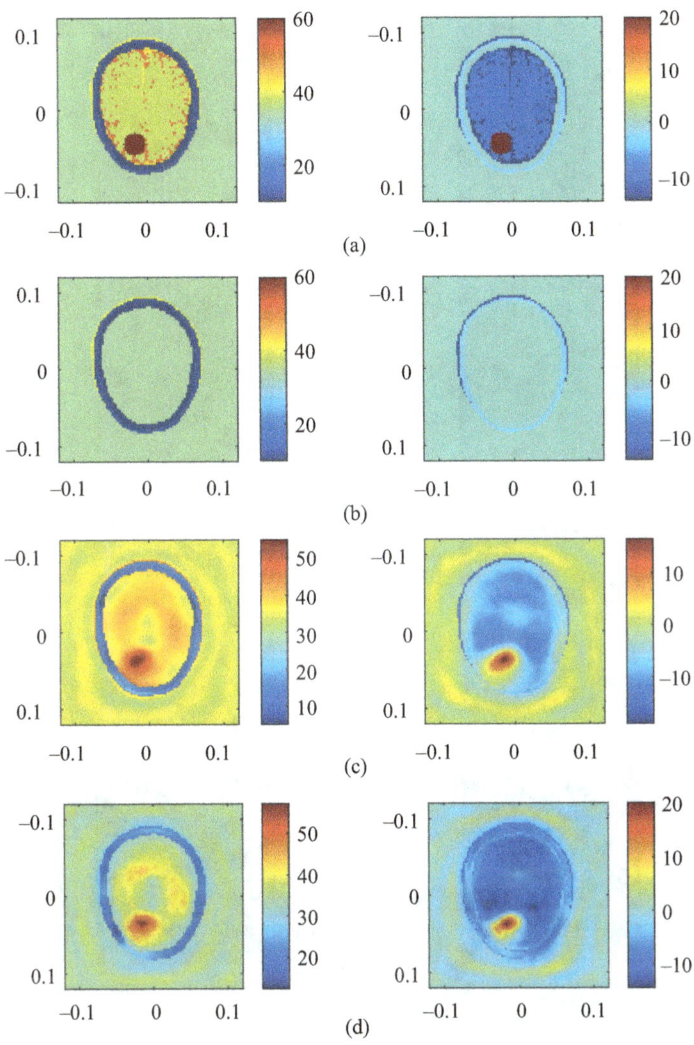

Figure 2.9 Biomedical imaging: Example 6—human brain tumor model: (a) exact profile: real part and imaginary part of the permittivity, (b) the exact configuration of the inhomogeneous background medium, (c) reconstructed result after 100 iterations with D-LSIE, and (d) reconstructed result after 100 iterations with D-NIE

respectively. In the inversion, DoI (with a length of 15 cm) is calculated using an 84×84-grid mesh. The DoI is illuminated with 16 plane waves from different angles evenly distributed in [0, 2 π) and scattered fields are collected by 40 receivers uniformly distributed along a circle centered at the origin of coordinates with a radius 20 cm. The operating electromagnetic waves frequency is 2.4 GHz.

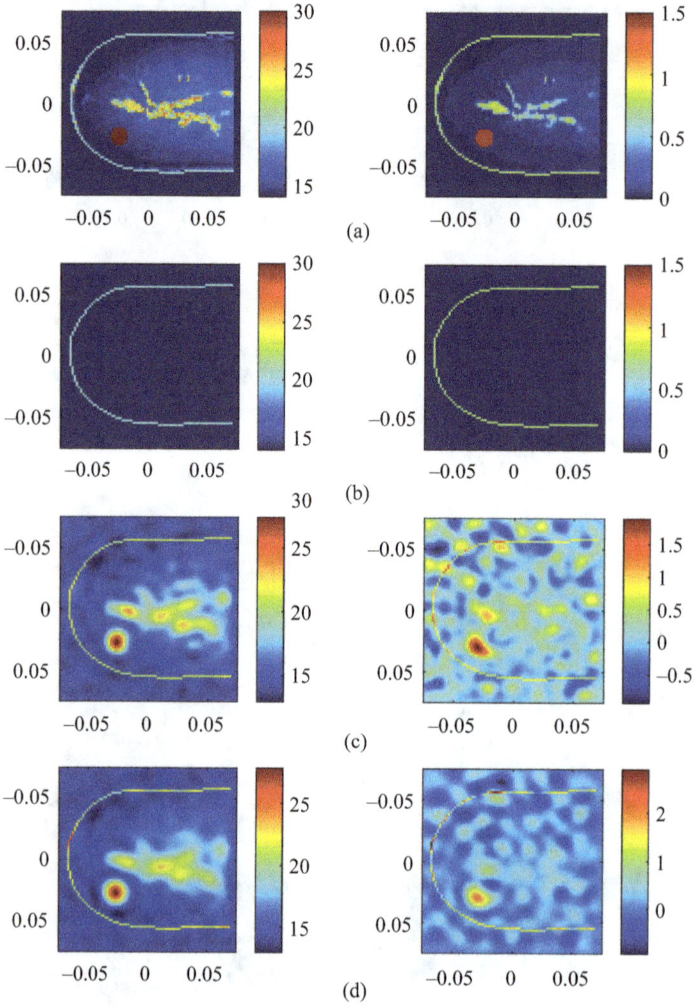

Figure 2.10 Biomedical imaging: Example 7—human breast tumor model: (a) exact profile: real part and imaginary part of the permittivity, (b) the exact configuration of the inhomogeneous background medium, (c) reconstructed result after 100 iterations with D-LSIE, and (d) reconstructed result after 100 iterations with D-CIE-I

In this example, 10% AWGN is added into the synthetic data. The profiles in Figure 2.10(b) are used as the inhomogeneous background, including the skin and immersion medium. Here L is chosen as 10 and other configurations are similar to *Example 2*. The reconstructed results after 100 iterations are shown in Figure 2.10 (c) and (d) generated by D-LSIE and D-CIE-I, respectively. From the retrieval profiles, the imaging results by the D-CIE-I are clearer and more distinguishable compared to the ones by D-LSIE. And the errors of reconstructions ERR_{ε}^{tot} by D-LSIE and D-CIE-I are 0.001 and 0.00098, and as can be seen from Figure 2.10, the background noise of the image retrieved by D-CIE-I is even less. Therefore, compared to the D-LSIE, both the reconstructed profiles and quantitative errors prove that D-CIE-I has the better performance and stability.

The previous microwave imaging tests validate the capability of the D-CIE-I when dealing with the biomedical imaging with high nonlinearity under complicated inhomogeneous background media. All the numerical examples show that the D-CIE-I under new IE have better inversion ability and robustness compared with the D-LSIE based on the traditional LSIE.

By taking the full advantage of the models based on difference IEs, the closed form Green's function with homogeneous background is used such that the burdensome uses of the numerical Green's function for the inhomogeneous background medium are avoided via fast algorithms, such as FFT or FMM, that can efficiently handle the multiplication of Green's function and the induced currents. Within the frame of FFT-TSOM, both D-LSIE and D-CIE-I are able to efficiently tackle the concerned ISPs. Especially, the D-CIE-I is designed to handle the highly nonlinear ISPs with bounded inhomogeneous background medium.

2.5 Conclusion

In order to alleviate the two challenges in the microwave biomedical imaging, i.e., strong nonlinearity and complicated inhomogeneous background media, a new type of modeling, CIE-I, has been implemented. First, in the frame of the CIE-I, MR-TSOM-CIE-I is discussed for solving the highly nonlinear ISPs, i.e., those scatterers with high contrast or electrically large dimension. The MR-TSOM-CIE-I shows much better inversion capability than the traditional methods based on LSIE. Further, D-CIE-I is applied to solve the ISPs with high contrasts under the inhomogeneous background media. Both the MR-TSOM-CIE-I and D-CIE-I have been numerically validated with the tests against synthetic data. At last, several biomedical imaging cases have been studied. Numerical results show that the D-CIE-I can well resolve the microwave biomedical imaging problem and has better performance and better stability than the D-LSIE. Besides the biomedical imaging, many practical applications involving inhomogeneous backgrounds, such as through-wall imaging, and geophysical survey, can find good interest in the inversion methods discussed in this chapter.

References

[1] D. Colton and R. Kress, *Inverse Acoustic and Electromagnetic Scattering Theory*. Berlin: Springer, The 2nd edition, 1998.

[2] T. Ueda and M. S. Zhdanov, "Fast numerical modeling of multi-transmitter electromagnetic data using multigrid quasi-linear approximation," *IEEE Trans. Geosci. Remote Sens.*, vol. 44, no. 6, pp. 1428–1434, 2006.

[3] P. M. Meaney, M. W. Fanning, D. Li, S. P. Poplack, and K. D. Paulsen, "A clinical prototype for active microwave imaging of the breast," *IEEE Trans. Microwave Theory Tech.*, vol. 48, no. 11, pp. 1841–1853, 2000.

[4] Q. H. Liu, Z. Q. Zhang, T. T. Wang *et al.*, "Active microwave imaging. I. 2-D forward and inverse scattering methods," *IEEE Trans. Microwave Theory Tech.*, vol. 50, no. 1, pp. 123–133, 2002.

[5] S. Caorsi, A. Massa, M. Pastorino, and M. Donelli, "Improved microwave imaging procedure for nondestructive evaluations of two-dimensional structures," *IEEE Trans. Antennas Propag.*, vol. 52, no. 6, pp. 1386–1397, 2004.

[6] L.-P. Song, C. Yu, and Q. H. Liu, "Through-wall imaging (TWI) by radar: 2-D tomographic results and analyses," *IEEE Trans. Geosci. Remote Sens.*, vol. 43, no. 12, pp. 2793–2798, 2005.

[7] F. Xu and Y. Q. Jin, "Imaging simulation of bistatic synthetic aperture radar and its polarimetric analysis," *IEEE Trans. Geosci. Remote Sens.*, vol. 46, no. 8, pp. 2233–2248, 2008.

[8] M. Bertero, "Linear inverse and III-posed problems," *Adv. Electron. Electron Phys.*, vol. 75, pp. 1–120, 1989.

[9] X. Chen, *Computational Methods for Electromagnetic Inverse Scattering*. Hoboken, NJ, USA: Wiley, 2018.

[10] Y. Zhong, "Subspace-based inversion methods for solving electromagnetic inverse scattering problems," Ph.D. dissertation, Nat. Univ. Singapore, Singapore, 2010.

[11] M. S. Zhdanov, *Geophysical Inverse Theory and Regularization Problems*. Amsterdam: Elsevier, 2002.

[12] S. Caorsi, A. Massa, M. Pastorino, and M. Donelli, "Improved microwave imaging procedure for nondestructive evaluations of two-dimensional structures," *IEEE Trans. Antennas Propag.*, vol. 52, no. 6, pp. 1386–1397, 2004.

[13] L. Song, C. Yu, and Q. Liu, "Through-wall imaging (TWI) by radar: 2-D tomographic results and analyses," *IEEE Trans. Antennas Propag.*, vol. 43, no. 12, pp. 2793–2798, 2005.

[14] A. Abubakar, P. M. van den Berg, and J. Mallorqui, "Imaging of biomedical data using a multiplicative regularized contrast source inversion method," *IEEE Trans. Microwave Theory Tech.*, vol. 50, no. 7, pp. 1761–1771, 2002.

[15] P. M. Meaney, M. W. Fanning, D. Li, S. P. Poplack, and K. D. Paulsen, "A clinical prototype for active microwave imaging of the breast," *IEEE Trans. Microwave Theory Tech.*, vol. 48, no. 11, pp. 1841–1853, 2000.

[16] T. Cui, W. C. Chew, A. A. Aydiner, and S. Chen "Inverse scattering of two-dimensional dielectric objects buried in a lossy earth using the distorted Born iterative method," *IEEE Trans. Geosci. Remote Sens.*, vol. 39, no. 2, pp. 339–346, 2001.

[17] Y. M. Wang and W. C. Chew, "An iterative solution of the two-dimensional electromagnetic inverse scattering problem," *Int. J. Imaging Syst. Technol.*, vol. 1, no. 1, pp. 100–108, 1989.

[18] L. Li, W. Zhang, and F. Li, "Tomographic reconstruction using the distorted Rytov iterative method with phaseless data," *IEEE Geosci. Remote Sens. Lett.*, vol. 5, no. 3, pp. 479–483, 2008.

[19] R. Palmeri, M. T. Bevacqua, L. Crocco, T. Isernia, and L. Di Donato, "Microwave imaging via distorted iterated virtual experiments," *IEEE Trans. Antennas Propag.*, vol. 65, no. 2, pp. 829–838, 2017.

[20] T. Habashy, R. Groom, W. Ross, and B. Spies, "Beyond the born and Rytov approximations: A nonlinear approach to electromagnetic scattering," *J. Geophys. Res.*, vol. 98, no. B2, pp. 1759–1775, 1993.

[21] W. C. Chew and Y. M. Wang, "Reconstruction of two-dimensional permittivity distribution using the distorted born iterative method," *IEEE Trans. Med. Imaging*, vol. 9, no. 2, pp. 218–225, 1990.

[22] Y. Wang and W. Chew, "An iterative solution of the two-dimensional electromagnetic inverse scattering problem," *J. Imaging Syst. Technol.*, vol. 1, no. 1, pp. 100–108, 1989.

[23] L. Li, W. Zhang, and F. Li, "Tomographic reconstruction using the distorted Rytov iterative method with phaseless data," *IEEE Geosci. Remote Sens. Lett.*, vol. 5, no. 3, pp. 479–483, 2008.

[24] T. Habashy, R. Groom, W. Ross, and B. Spies, "Beyond the born and Rytov approximations: A nonlinear approach to electromagnetic scattering," *J. Geophys. Res.*, vol. 98, no. B2, pp. 1759–1775, 1993.

[25] P. M. van den Berg and R. E. Kleinman, "A contrast source inversion method," *Inverse Prob.*, vol. 13, no. 6, pp. 1607–1620, 1997.

[26] P. M. van den Berg, A. Abubakar, and J. T. Fokkema, "Multiplicative regularization for contrast profile inversion," *Radio Sci.*, vol. 38, no. 2, pp. 1–10, 2003.

[27] P. Mojabi and J. LoVetri, "Overview and classification of some regularization techniques for the Gauss-Newton inversion method applied to inverse scattering problems," *IEEE Trans. Antennas Propag.*, vol. 57, no. 9, pp. 2658–2665, 2009.

[28] X. Chen, "Subspace-based optimization method for solving inverse-scattering problems," *IEEE Trans. Geosci. Remote Sens.*, vol. 48, no. 1, pp. 42–49, 2010.

[29] Y. Zhong and X. Chen, "Twofold subspace-based optimization method for solving inverse scattering problems," *Inverse Prob.*, vol. 25, no. 8, p. 085003, 2009.

[30] Y. Zhong and X. Chen, "An FFT twofold subspace-based optimization method for solving electromagnetic inverse scattering problems," *IEEE Trans. Antennas Propag.*, vol. 59, no. 3, pp. 914–927, 2011.

[31] P. Rocca, M. Benedetti, M. Donelli, D. Franceschini, and A. Massa, "Evolutionary optimization as applied to inverse scattering problems," *Inverse Prob.*, vol. 25, no. 12, p. 123003, 2009.

[32] C.-C. Chiu, C.-H. Sun, C.-L. Li, and C.-H. Huang, "Comparative study of some population-based optimization algorithms on inverse scattering of a two-dimensional perfectly conducting cylinder in dielectric slab medium," *IEEE Trans. Geosci. Remote Sens.*, vol. 51, no. 4, pp. 2302–2315, 2013.

[33] Y. Zhong, M. Lambert, D. Lesselier, and X. Chen, "A new integral equation method to solve highly nonlinear inverse scattering problems," *IEEE Trans. Antennas Propag.*, vol. 64, no. 5, pp. 1788–1799, 2016.

[34] A. F. Peterson, S. L. Ray, and R. Mittra, *Computational Methods for Electromagnetics*. Piscataway, NJ, USA: IEEE Press, 1998.

[35] K. Xu, Y. Zhong, R. Song, X. Chen, and L. Ran, "Multiplicative regularized FFT twofold subspace-based optimization method for inverse scattering problems," *IEEE Trans. Geosci. Remote Sens.*, vol. 53, no. 2, pp. 841–850, 2015.

[36] K. Xu, Y. Zhong, and G. Wang, "A hybrid regularization technique for solving highly nonlinear inverse scattering problems," *IEEE Trans. Microwave Theory Tech.*, vol. 66, no. 1, pp. 11–21, 2018.

[37] C. Yu, M. Yuan, and Q. H. Liu, "Reconstruction of 3D objects from multi-frequency experimental data with a fast DBIM-BCGS method," *Inverse Prob.*, vol. 25, no. 2, p. 024007, 2009.

[38] X. Chen, "Subspace-based optimization method for inverse scattering problems with an inhomogeneous background medium," *Inverse Prob.*, vol. 26, no. 7, p. 074007, 2010.

[39] A. Abubakar, W. Hu, P. M. van den Berg, and T. M. Habashy, "A finite-difference contrast source inversion method," *Inverse Prob.*, vol. 24, no. 6, p. 065004, 2008.

[40] M. F. Catedra, R. F. Torres, J. Basterrechea, and E. Gago, *The CG-FFT Method: Application of Signal Processing Techniques to Electromagnetics*. Boston, MA, USA: Artech House, 1995.

[41] W. C. Chew, J.-M. Jin, E. Michielssen, and J. Song, *Fast and Efficient Algorithms in Computational Electromagnetics*. Norwood, MA, USA: Artech House, 2001.

[42] K. Xu, Y. Zhong, X. Chen and D. Lesselie, "A fast integral equation-based method for solving electromagnetic inverse scattering problems with inhomogeneous background," *IEEE Trans. Antennas Propag.*, vol. 66, no. 8, pp. 4228–4239, 2018.

Chapter 3

Electromagnetic sources for THz imaging and DNP NMR spectroscopy

Sergey Ponomarenko[1], Sergey Kishko[1], Alexander Likhachev[1], Eduard Khutoryan[2] and Alexei Kuleshov[1]

Application of THz radiation is attractive and promising in biology and medicine, in particular, in order to remove ionizing X-rays in imaging test and to enhance the nuclear magnetic resonance (NMR) signal. At present the problem of lack of powerful and compact-style sources of THz radiation in the frequency range from 300 GHz to 1 THz still exists. Especially for high sensitive and high-resolution dynamic nuclear polarization (DNP) NMR spectroscopy, the increase of the operating frequency and output power of THz sources is a key issue. In this chapter, we will analyze the physical principles of classical electromagnetic (EM) sources of THz radiation those are widely applied in THz imaging systems and in DNP-enhanced NMR Spectroscopy. The advantages of solid-state oscillators (Gunn, impact ionization avalanche transit-time (IMPATT) and TUNNET diodes together with multipliers), vacuum electron devices (VEDs) (backward wave oscillators (BWOs), clinotrons, diffraction radiation oscillators (DROs), orotrons, extended interaction klystrons and oscillators (EIKs and EIOs), gyrotrons), and combined systems for different THz applications have been discussed. State-of-the-art of compact frequency-tunable sources and up-to-date research and development activities on high-frequency medium power VEDs have been presented. Special attention is paid to THz-imaging and spectroscopy schemes and modules based on existing sources. The examples of THz-image processing of the biological objects and its application in medical diagnostics are presented.

[1]Department of Vacuum Electronics, O.Ya. Usikov Institute for Radiophysics and Electronics of the National Academy of Sciences of Ukraine, Kharkiv, Ukraine
[2]Department of Theory of Difraction and Difraction Electronics, O.Ya. Usikov Institute for Radiophysics and Electronics of the National Academy of Sciences of Ukraine, Kharkiv, Ukraine

3.1 Introduction

The terahertz radiation (100 GHz–10 THz) has a set of advantages that make it outstanding compared to conventional microwave radiation and photonics. The THz waves provide a nonionizing effect on the penetrated objects due to very low energy of photon compared to the X-rays. Since rotational, vibration, and translation energy levels in molecules appear in the THz range, the additional information about a substance can be obtained by THz waves, and it cannot be reached by traditional techniques of microwave and X-rays. The THz radiation is sensitive to dielectric material, and especially to the quantity of water in it.

Nowadays the problem of "THz gap" still exists and many researches are being conducted to develop the powerful, frequency-tunable, efficient, and compact-style THz oscillators for a big number of practical applications. At present the solid-state THz sources are being actively developed to increase their levels of the output power and, thus, to provide more advantages in comparison with VEDs. The main advantage of the THz solid-state sources is their real compact style since in the operation they do not require a high-magnetic field as in the case of VEDs of cyclotron resonance masers (CRMs) type or in the case of traditional compact style VEDs (BWO, traveling wave tube (TWT), orotron, clinotron, etc.) in order to focus the electron beams (EBs). Also, the compact air cooling systems are applied in THz solid-state oscillators while a big number of powerful VEDs require water cooling systems with rather big chillers (refrigerators). Lastly, THz solid-state devices operate at low voltages while VEDs operation requires accelerating voltages usually from several kV up to several dozens of kV.

The numbers of papers and reviews on the state-of-the-art of the THz solid-state devices are increasing every year that shows the big potentials of such devices to cover the whole frequency range from the millimeter range up to the infrared region [1,2]. However, nowadays the frequency tuning range of any THz solid-state oscillator is rather narrow and customers are required to purchase the series of the sources operating in some separate parts of the THz range. Moreover, it is still required for customers to make a choice of the oscillator, which can fit for not a wide range of tasks but only for the specific ones. Indeed, the solid-state sources capable of generating very short pulses of the THz radiation are unable to operate in continuous-wave mode.

Powerful compact-style VEDs such as BWOs, clinotrons, orotrons, DROs, and EIOs are commonly used as tunable sources in mm-wave range and there are attempts to use them in sub-THz and THz ranges (0.3–1.2 THz). EIOs have a Watt level of output power at sub-THz, but they have a very narrow frequency tuning range and they are very expensive. BWOs have the widest tuning frequency range; however, its typical levels of output power are about several mW. Clinotron is a powerful modification of BWO comprising advantages of frequency tuning in wide range with the output power up to 1.5 W at 200 GHz and 100 mW at 0.4 THz. In Section 3.2, the state-of-the-art of existing THz oscillators is discussed, Section 3.3 discusses the frequency-tunable powerful BWO–clinotron tubes in greater detail. Finally, Sections 3.4 and 3.5 separately discuss the benefits of the applications of powerful THz sources in DNP NMR spectroscopy and THz imaging.

3.2 Sources of THz radiation: vacuum electron devices and solid-state oscillators

There is a big family of the THz solid-state sources, such as THz quantum cascade lasers (QCLs), resonant tunneling-diodes (RTDs), injection-seeded THz-wave parametric generators [3], optical photoconductive materials (OPMs) and photomixers, complementary metal–oxide–semiconductor (CMOS) [4], and heterojunction bipolar transistor (HBT). In the sub-THz range, the Schottky diode-based multipliers are a key technology for high-power terahertz solid-state sources [5]. Schottky diode-based THz sources rely on the nonlinearities of the Schottky diode to produce harmonics of an input signal, thus generating power at integer multiples of the drive frequency. In THz oscillators, the Schottky diodes are typically applied with lower frequency active devices such as Gunn or IMPATT oscillators [6]. Current levels of the output power of the 264-GHz source developed at Virginia Diodes using Schottky diode technology reach more than 100 mW [7] that is higher than the output power of BWO. Such VDI THz systems are based on the oscillator at 11 GHz, which is fed into an MMIC (monolithic microwave integrated circuit) premultiplier and amplifier, with an output frequency of 33 GHz and a saturated output power of 3 W. This MMIC is the final active stage in the chain, and after this there are only Schottky diode multiplication stages. For this system, there are three high-efficiency Schottky varactor multipliers with outputs at 66, 132, and 264 GHz, producing a peak output power higher than 100 mW [6].

THz oscillators based on CMOS technology provide the output power from 22 μW to 2.6 mW in the frequency bands between 0.288 and 0.498 THz [1]. Different triplers are applied to multiply the frequency from X-band to sub-THz with the help of nm-CMOS technology, which results in the output power 2.6 mW at 0.498 THz. THz sources based on HBT technology showed higher output powers from 10 mW at 0.215 THz to 12 μW at 0.92 THz with the efficiency up to 3.2% in comparison with CMOS oscillators [8].

At present, the OPM method of the generation of the short pulses of the THz radiation together with the femtosecond laser technique as the pumping system are utilized in laboratories [1]. The OPM is based on semiconductors such as low-temperature grown GaAs with the carrier lifetime of hundreds femtoseconds. An OPM emitter is composed of an ultrafast photoconductor connected to a terahertz antenna and driven by an external optical pump [9]. Femtosecond laser pulses generate carriers on the semiconductor surface, which are further accelerated by DC voltage. Application of the three-dimensional plasmonic contact electrodes allows photocarriers to be generated within nanoscale distances from the photoconductor contact electrodes and drifted to the terahertz-radiating antenna in a sub-picosecond timescale to efficiently contribute to terahertz radiation [9]. Broadband terahertz radiation with an output power level of 0.1 mW and an optical-to-terahertz power conversion efficiency of 7.5% in the 0.1–2-THz frequency range was demonstrated [9].

It should be mentioned that the OPM method can be applied for the case of continuous wave (CW) or quasi-CW THz radiation excitation when the periodic generation of electrons and holes in semiconductors occurs as the result of the absorption of two interfering laser beams [10]. The interference results in intensity modulation of the laser beams and, hence, the THz-periodic carrier generation. The emission of THz radiation originates either directly from the (phase-coherent) acceleration of the individual photocarriers, or it originates from the collective current of these carriers, generated within a very small area and being fed into an antenna [10]. Highly efficient continuous-wave terahertz emission using nanogap electrodes in a photoconductive antenna-based photomixer showed the maximal level of output power about 0.1 mW at 0.4 THz [11].

In the frequency range from 1 up to 10 THz the QCLs are the most powerful solid-state sources of terahertz radiation that are uniquely poised to target a range of potential applications in fields as diverse as astronomy, atmospheric science, biology, medicine, and chemical analysis. Terahertz QCLs could be designed to emit output power in the range tens of mW at cryogenic temperatures [12]. In contrast to the conventional semiconductor lasers where light is generated by the electron–hole-radiative recombination across the bandgap of the active material, in a quantum-cascade laser the electrons propagate through a potential staircase of coupled quantum wells, where the conduction band is split by quantum confinement into a number of distinct sub-bands [13]. The layer thickness, applied electric field, carrier lifetimes, and tunneling probabilities of each level determine the conditions of the population inversion between two sub-bands in a series. The radiation frequency corresponds to the energy spacing of the lasing sub-bands, allowing in principle operation at arbitrarily long wavelengths [14].

In contrast to QCL, the RTDs have two barriers and the energy levels are quantized; thus, only one type of carrier (electron) has the energy for tunneling. The tunneling process is rather fast to excite the radiation of THz range. The output power level of 0.61 mW at 0.62 THz was reported in [15].

Another promising solid-state oscillators in the frequency range from 0.4 to 1.5 THz are the THz emitters, which are based on the Josephson effect. The THz emitters are based on the high critical temperature (T_c) superconductor $Bi_2Sr_2CaCu_2O_{8+\delta}$ (Bi-2212) [16]. The best devices reach an output power of around 100 μW. It was already possible to give some demonstrations of potential applications, e.g., in THz imaging or in THz spectroscopy, further showing that Bi-2212-based emitters are highly interesting both for science and for technology.

Also, we should mention about the THz gas lasers [17], which still have very narrow frequency bands, and free-electron lasers (FELs) [18], which are the specific installations at the International Research Centers.

THz VEDs mainly operate at frequencies lower than 1.2 THz and they are devices in which EB moves in a vacuum and interacts with EM fields [19,20]. An EB is generated by an electron gun, which consists of an emitter of electrons and electron-optic system (EOS) providing a motion of electrons with desired velocity and shape. During EB–wave interaction, the EB kinetic energy is transferred into the energy of an EM field. Spent electrons fall on a beam collector and the excited EM wave is radiated into a load through an output port and vacuum window that separates vacuumed volume of VED with the space.

For efficient exchange between EB and EM energies, the EB and EM wave phase should be close since the interaction power P has a maximum at the vicinity of $v_{el} = v_{em}$ [21,22]. The interaction power is defined as follows:

$$P = \frac{1}{2}\int_V \vec{j}\vec{E}^{*} dV. \tag{3.1}$$

The resonant condition of phase equality is known as synchronism between EB and EM wave. There are several ways to classify VEDs. One way is based on the mechanism that provides synchronism. The first mechanism that we consider here is the Cherenkov radiation [23–26]. In this case to synchronize EB with EM wave, the EM wave velocity should be slowed down to be equal to that of an EB. It can be realized by inserting the material with dielectric permittivity ε_{so} that $v_{em} = c/\sqrt{\varepsilon}$. Namely, the effect of Vavilov–Cherenkov was revealed when fast electrons moved through liquids. Also, periodic circuit named as slow-wave structure (SWS) causes enlarging the EM wave path with respect to this of an EB one along the EB trajectory and hence causes slowing down an EM wave (or its space harmonic). THz VED based on Cerenkov mechanism containing SWS are TWT [27–29], BWO [19,30–32], clinotrons [33], orotrons [34–37], DRO [38–40], EIKs and EIOs [41–43], etc. Sketches of TWT/BWO, DRO–orotron based on the grating type SWS, EIO are shown in Figure 3.1.

In all these VEDs, a linear sheet or pencil-like EB moves along SWS. Due to SWS periodicity, an EM field can be represented as a series of the space harmonics:

$$E_z = \sum_{n=-\infty}^{\infty} A_n e^{-\alpha_n x} e^{i(k_{zn}z-\omega t)}, \tag{3.2}$$

where $k_{zn} = k_{z0} + 2\pi n/l$, $\alpha_n = \sqrt{k_{zn}{}^2 - (\omega/c)^2}$. Velocity of nth harmonic is $v_{phn} = \omega/k_{zn}$ and for a given beam voltage, the SWS period should be decreased with a frequency increase that requires special technology for an SWS fabrication at THz range, especially for nonrelativistic devices. Since the velocity of the synchronous with EB harmonic is less than c (speed of light), the transverse wavenumber of the harmonic $\alpha_n \approx \omega/v_{phn}$ is real that means that the EM field decays in the transverse direction

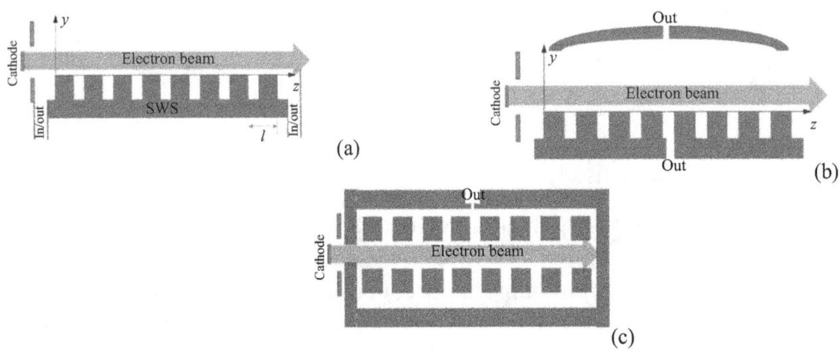

Figure 3.1 Principles of TWT/BWO (a), DRO–orotron based on the grating type SWS (b), and EIO tube (c)

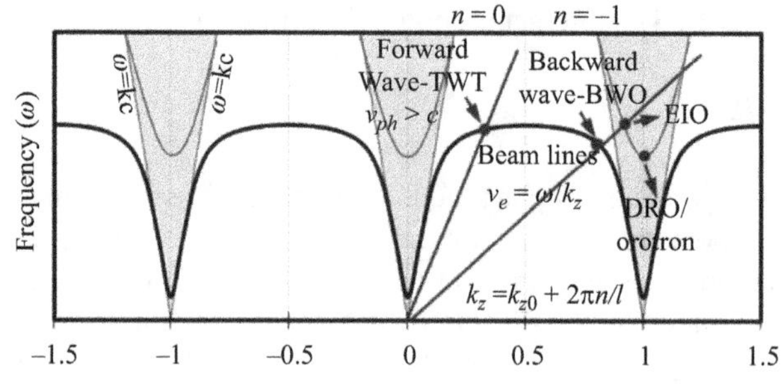

Figure 3.2 Operation of VEDs at dispersion diagram

from a grating and hence such field is called surface one. And this is one of the main reasons why the efficiency of Cherenkov VED drops at THz range—the interaction space in the transverse direction $\Delta x \cong 1/\alpha_n$ becomes very thin that necessities very thin and intense EB that is quite difficult to attain. Also, a common feature of this type of device is that they are placed in a magnetic focusing system to provide an efficient transportation of an EB.

The main difference between VEDs shown in Figure 3.2 is the mode type of an EM wave interacting with an EB that is defined by the dispersion curve.

In the case of the surface wave Cherenkov VEDs such as TWT and BWO, all space harmonics are surface (Figure 3.2). TWT is an amplifier and the group velocity of the wave is of the same direction as of an EB motion. The signal to be amplified is input through a waveguide from the cathode side and an output signal is radiated into a waveguide from the SWS end. BWO is an oscillator and the group velocity is the opposite to the EB velocity to provide a feedback (beam line intersects dispersion curve in the point corresponding to the negative derivative is $v_{gr} = \partial\omega/\partial k_z < 0$). Therefore, the output signal propagates through a waveguide placed at the cathode side. However, in THz range, because of high ohmic loss and oversized cavity dimensions, the efficiency of such radiation output is usually low.

In contrast to BWO, in orotron, DRO, EIO one harmonic (usually 0th) is radiating, i.e., α_0 is an imagine value and the dispersion curve of such wave corresponds to the volume mode. In this case, additionally to an SWS, several reflectors are applied to return radiating harmonic back to the interaction space and, therefore, to provide feedback. Output waveguide in such devices can be located far from SWS (Figure 3.1).

The activities for an increase of Cherenkov VED performances are mainly going in several directions:

- to generate and to transport thin intense EB with defined profile and velocity spread providing maximal EB–wave interaction;
- to develop the SWS providing high coupling impedance and low loss (e.g., ohmic loss in metal), mechanically and thermally robust and technological;
- to reduce diffraction losses, including not desired mode transformation in oversized cavities, to develop a radiation output with high efficiency;
- to find cavity/SWS modes that provide wide frequency operation.

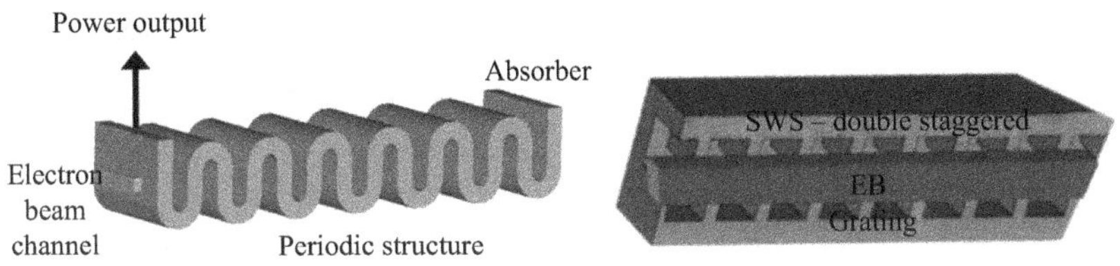

Figure 3.3 Interaction structures of THz BWO and TWT tubes

Let us discuss some recent achievements regarding those activities. For example, last one relating to the requirement of broadband operation is different for amplifiers and oscillators. The amplifiers are designed in such a way that for a given EB voltage, an EB is synchronous with a wave in a wide frequency band with close coupling impedance. Use of SWS as double staggered grating [44–48], folded waveguide [49–51] (see Figure 3.3) may provide an amplification of 25±2 dB at bandwidth wider than 10% for 0.2-, 0.3-THz TWTs and is promising for the design of even higher frequencies TWT, especially by use of the LIGA technology [19,52].

Usually, oscillators are designed to generate single-frequency radiation unless special options of multifrequency and noise oscillators. Frequency-tuning range in single-frequency oscillators is provided by the change of some beam or circuit parameter, mostly of EB voltage. This so-called electron frequency tuning allows fast frequency switch, fast frequency modulation, etc. Widest frequency-tuning range is in nonresonant BWO and, for example, it is about 200 GHz for 0.5 THz as one can see in Table 3.1 [19,32,53]. Due to this fact, BWOs with relatively low power (see Table 3.1) have strong demand in applications where wide frequency-tuning range is important. Frequency tuning of resonant BWO and clinotron is not so smooth and may contain gaps, but the total range may be the same as in non-resonant BWO (see Table 3.1) with much higher output power [33,54–57]. In contrast to this, the resonant VEDs with volume waves have a quite narrow electron frequency-tuning range. In DRO and orotrons instead of electron frequency tuning, the additional mechanical tuning may be applied by changing the distance between mirrors that affects the resonant frequency [34–38]. However, it is very slow and cannot be applied when fast frequency modulation is needed. Also, the frequency step is relatively big, especially in THz range and devices with movable mirrors are not robust for mechanical vibrations.

The second mechanism that we consider here, which provides synchronism between EB and EM wave, is the cyclotron radiation [58,59]. VEDs based on this principle are called CRM. The most famous and widely used CRM is a gyrotron (gyromonotron, Gyro-TWT, gyro-BWO, gyro-klystron) that is being developed at Russia, EU, USA, Japan, China, etc. [59–61]. Compared to the tubes based on Cherenkov radiation, they are bulkier, but at the same time, they are much more compact than the accelerator-based sources and FELs.

Electrons placed in a strong magnetic field B are gyrating with cyclotron frequency $\omega_{cyc} = eB/\gamma m$ where e and m are electron's charge and mass and $\gamma = (1 - \beta^2)^{-1/2}$ is the Lorentz factor appearing due to relativistic mass

Table 3.1 Performance of resonant and nonresonant BWOs and clinotrons

Type, model	Frequency (GHz)	Max power (mW)	Max voltage (kV)	Max current (mA)
BWO OV-24	163–263	40	3.8	25
BWO OV-30	203–377	20	4	40
BWO OV-32	370–547	15	4.5	40
BWO OV-80	438–711	10	6	45
BWO OV-81	690–850	5	6	45
BWO OV-83	910–1,100	5	5.5	45
BWO OV-84	1,070–1,250	2	6	45
BWO OV-85	1,150–1,420	1.5	6	45
Carcinotron CO.20A	152–158	1,500	6	60
Carcinotron CO.10	285–310	60	6	60
Carcinotron CO.10.1	275–290	1,000	11	30
Clinotron C200	166–231	500–1,000	5	150
Clinotron C260	250–263	300–800	5	200
Clinotron C315	272–334	50–120	5.5	150
Clinotron C352	315–362	30–100	5.5	150
Clinotron C400	345–410	30–50	4.5	170
Clinotron C485	460–510	50–95	5.6	170

dependence on the velocity that is responsible to the negative mass instability in a gyrotron. The resonance condition for the EB–wave interaction is met when the wave frequency equals the cyclotron frequency or its harmonic s:

$$\omega = s\omega_{cyc} + k_z v_z, \tag{3.3}$$

where $k_z v_z$ is the Doppler shift term appearing when gyrating electron moves in longitudinal direction z with velocity v_z. The wave interacting with an EB in gyrotron is usually TE_{mn} mode of circular hollow waveguide of the z direction with following dispersion:

$$\frac{\omega^2}{c^2} = k^2 = {k_\perp}^2 + {k_z}^2, \tag{3.4}$$

where $k_\perp = \chi_{m,n}/R$ is transverse wavenumber determined by nth zero of derivative of the Bessel function $J_m(x)$ and by the waveguide radius. The gyrotron operation occurs near the intersection of the beam-wave resonance line and the TE_{mn} mode dispersion (Figure 3.4). Circular waveguide with down-taper and up-taper sections at its ends forms a gyrotron cavity. These sections provide reflections that in its turn provide resonance properties of a gyrotron, diffraction output, and cut the radiation propagation to the cathode. Especially high Q-factor providing strong feedback occurs near regular waveguide cutoff frequency. The schematic drawing of a gyrotron (Figure 3.5) shows its key elements: magnetron injection gun (MIG)

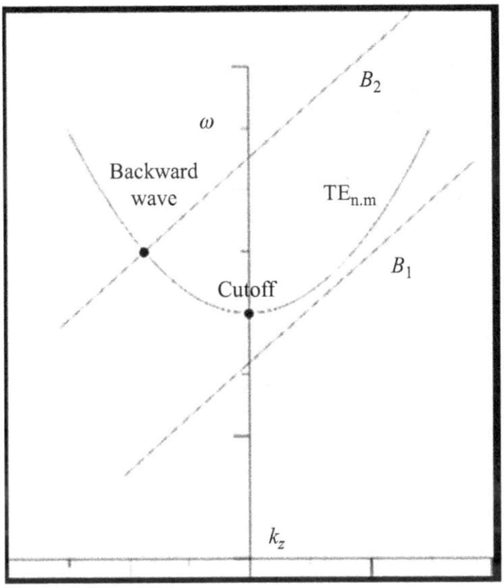

Figure 3.4 Operation regime of gyrotron oscillator

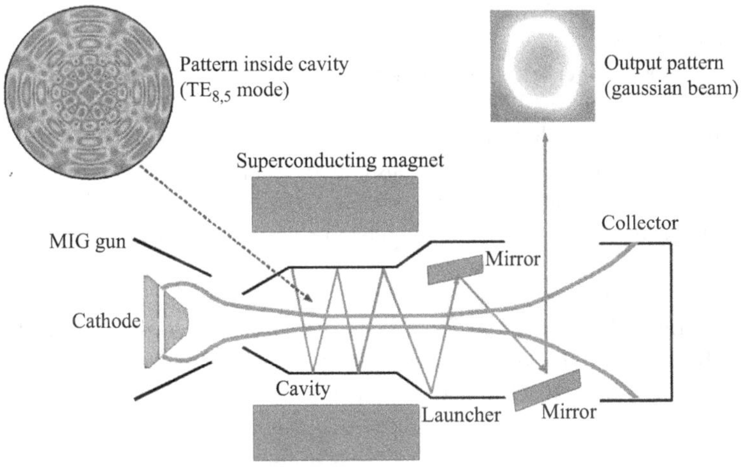

Figure 3.5 Schematic drawing of a gyrotron

generating electrons and providing the required ratio of transverse to longitudinal velocity $g = v_{\perp}/v_z$ in the cavity region; superconducting magnet (SCM) providing gyration of electrons with a certain frequency; a cavity where EB–wave interaction occurs; electron collector; a radiation output. In most gyrotrons, the radiation of TE_{mn} mode is converted into much suitable for transmission and focusing Gaussian-like TEM_{00} radiation (Figure 3.5) by a special quasioptical system with efficiency more than 90% [62–64].

Table 3.2 Performance of gyrotrons operating at the second harmonic

Gyrotron	Frequency (GHz)	Max power (W)	Max B (T)
FU CW CI	395	120	8
FU CW G0	460	40	10
FU CW C	780	15	15

As one can see one of the most bulk and expensive part and frequency-limiting reasons in gyrotron is an SCM. Modern cryogen-free continuously operating SCM produces a maximum 15–20 T of magnetic field [65] that approximately corresponds to 400–560 GHz of the cyclotron frequency. To generate radiation above 1 THz at the first cyclotron harmonic, a pulsed solenoidal magnet producing up to 40 T was utilized [66,67]. However, the radiation pulse was very short and the repetition rate was very low. One way to reduce the magnetic field for the given frequency is an operation at harmonics of cyclotron resonance. Gyrotrons operating on first cyclotron harmonic may generate output power up to several MW, for example, at frequencies 110–170 GHz [68,69] and achieve more than 50% efficiency. High-power levels are needed for such applications as plasma heating, plasma diagnostics, material processing, radar, and communication. For medical and biological applications, the required level of output power is several dozen W for some spectroscopy techniques (e.g., DNP NMR, emission spectroscopy) [70] and is less than 1 W for medical THz imaging, treatments requiring low tissue heating or even below heating effect [71,72]. Such medium and low power gyrotrons usually operate at the second cyclotron harmonic. This fact allows a double decrease of the magnetic field and hence makes the source more compact and cheaper. In addition, the operation at the second cyclotron harmonic allows CW operation at frequencies that are not achievable at the fundamental harmonic operation. For example, a series of gyrotrons operating at the second harmonic was designed in FIR UF (Table 3.2) for operation frequencies 0.395, 0.46, 0.78 THz, including achieving the breakthrough threshold of 1-THz CW operation [73]. Let us note that the main obstacle for the output power increase when operating at the second cyclotron harmonic is a mode competition with fundamental harmonic [74–76]. The same valid for the attempts of the further decrease of the magnetic field when operate at third cyclotron harmonic. The activities to solve this problem include the development of the special cavities design providing advantage (Q-factor, interaction length, etc.) for certain modes [77–81] and the creation of the special EBs effectively exciting certain modes (large-orbit gyrotrons, double beam gyrotron, etc.) [82–85].

Next gyrotron research activity is the extension of the frequency tenability that is going in three different ways. The first one is stepwise frequency change by switching between different modes when varying the cyclotron frequency (by change of the magnetic field or the accelerating voltage). Such method may be appropriate at the fundamental harmonic operation with oversized cavity because the frequency steps are small in this case. In the medium power gyrotron, the magnetic field sweeping causes switching between modes with big frequency step (Figure 3.6 shows this for

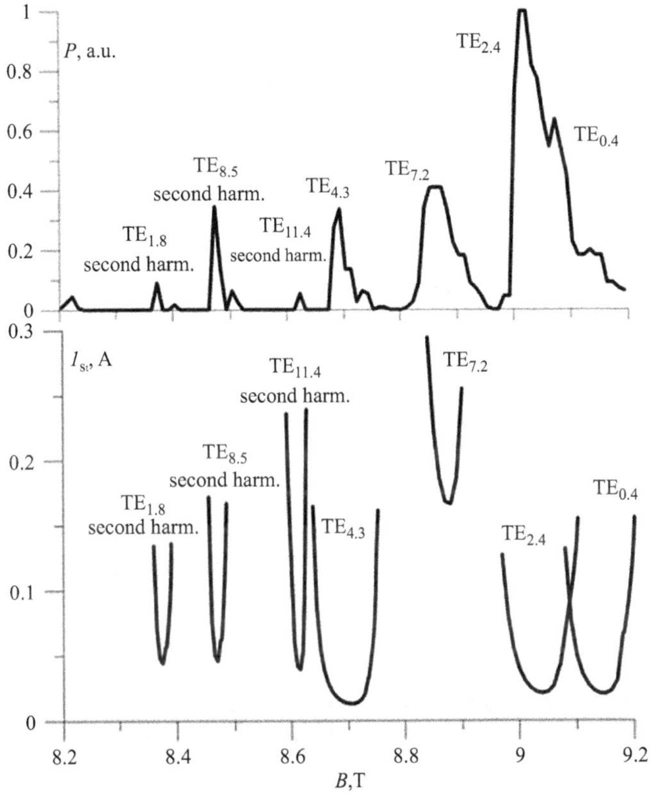

Figure 3.6 Modes excitation at magnetic field sweep

FU-GO-II gyrotron [86,87]), especially in the case of the second harmonic operation. The second way of frequency tuning is the excitation of the sequence of high-order axial modes (HOAM) [88] that allows continuous frequency tuning by varying the cyclotron frequency. However, because of differences of Q-factors, RF field profile, and especially because of the high sensitivity of HOAM to the EB velocity spread, the output power corresponding to fundamental axial mode is usually much higher of this corresponding to HOAM (Figure 3.7, [86,87]). The third way is the creation of cavities in which the changeable shape (mechanically, thermally, or by another way) resulting in the resonant frequency change. However, this way is slow and severe additional technical complications are introduced with such a method.

Demand of compact THz sources resulted in the activity to design a compact gyrotron. On one hand, the availability of compact cryo-free SCM [65] has made it possible to develop much more compact gyrotrons. For example, the compact gyrotrons FU CW CI and FU CW CII designed in FIR FU have smaller overall volume, mass, and dimensions and are more suitable for table-top laboratory applications [59,89,90]. Their EOSs have specially designed MIGs with minimized

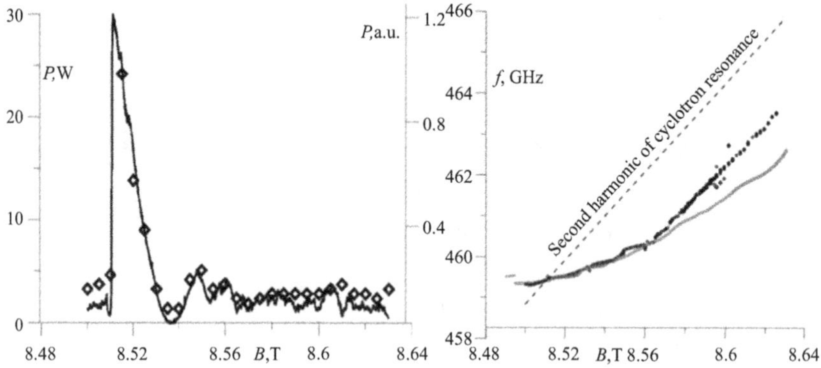

Figure 3.7 Frequency tuning during excitation of HOAM at magnetic field sweep

radial dimensions in order to accommodate them to the reduced diameter of the inner bore of the most compact magnets. On the other hand, recent activities on low-voltage gyrotron operation [91–94] (from 1.5 to 5 kV) are also promising for more the compact style of a gyrotron and high voltage power supply.

3.3 Compact frequency-tunable THz oscillators: backward-wave oscillator and a clinotron

3.3.1 Operating principles

In Section 3.2, we have briefly described VEDs based on Cherenkov radiation such as BWO and a clinotron, which have broadband electronic frequency tuning and the compact style that made them attractive for application in THz imaging and spectroscopy. In this section, we discuss them in more detail.

The type of a SWS applied in BWO depends on the operating parameters such as frequency range and output power. For instance, helical and coupled-cavity structures are used in centimeter and millimeter wavelength ranges. The helical BWOs provide low-power broadband operation, while coupled-cavity BWOs demonstrate output power up to kilowatt with relatively low-frequency tuning.

In submillimeter-wave range, the application of such structure has no advantages due to a bunch of physical effects and technological limitations [20,29,32]. As was shown in Section 3.2, SWS dimensions in THz frequency range become too small and issues of manufacture and heat transfer emerge. In this connection, SWSs of a comb type are more suitable for submillimeter-wavelength operation. In Particularity, there are several micro-fabrication methods such as wire electrical discharge machining, deep reactive ion etching, LIGA technology based on ultraviolet radiation or X-ray and computer numerical control milling (CNC-milling). Recently CNC-milling method had become widely spread for manufacturing both double corrugated and double staggered grating structures [19,48,52].

The decrease of the RF field localization of the synchronous harmonic becomes the key physical limitation in the THz frequency range. Another obstacle is high-frequency ohmic losses that cause the attenuation of EM wave. The additional reasons of such losses are thermal heating due to the EB interception and surface roughness that become comparable with the skin depth in the THz range.

The beam–wave interaction process can also be improved by the modification of a periodic structure, such as double-grating and multi-row SWS [34,44–48,95]. A similar approach was implemented in BWOs of the OV series, which covered a frequency range up to 1.5 THz. Typical operation parameters of these tubes are listed in Table 3.1. In contrast to conventional BWO operating with a thin EB, clinotron oscillators employ thick sheet EB tilted to the surface of a periodic structure. Therefore, clinotron oscillator does not suffer from the requirement of the application of the intense EB in comparison with BWO.

Clinotron oscillators were proposed as a modification of a resonant BWO, in which improved beam–wave interaction is realized by an inclination of the intense EB to the SWS and by providing resonant conditions.

All these modifications provide a significant improvement of the beam–wave interaction efficiency resulting in an increase of output power compared to conventional THz BWO [54–57]. Because of the high output power of a clinotron, there is an attractive opportunity to use clinotron together with frequency multipliers in order to obtain reasonable output power at higher frequencies.

In the oversized system of THz clinotrons, structural inhomogeneities such as the radiation output, electron gun cause both reflection of the surface (interacting with EB) wave and transformation of the surface mode into a higher waveguide modes and vice versa (Figure 3.8). Evidently the resonant property of THz clinotron would be determined not only by surface mode resonances but also by resonances of higher modes and their mutual transformations.

Hence, the theory of THz clinotron was extended by applying the consideration of scattering matrices of an oversized EM system, which includes T-junctions and structural peculiarities at the ends of a periodic structure for that reason [96]. This approach provides frequency-dependent coefficients for reflection and transformation of almost all modes that propagate in the interaction system in operating frequency range. Particularly, the elements can display the transformation of slow grating modes into fast ones and vice versa as well as the reflection of EM energy back into the interaction region or it is propagation to the output waveguide.

To solve the scattering problem, it is required to find the scattered EM field and its decomposition by eigenmodes of the interaction system. To overcome the difficulty of the scattering problem, the entire design of the interaction system is separated by individual parts connected by the short sections of rectangular waveguide. For instance, the power output unit has been presented by three-port junction, which contains port of an output waveguide, port of an anode slot, and port of an interaction region as well. EM fields in the first two ports are represented as a superposition of the modes of the rectangular waveguides. The main feature of the last one port is the consideration of semi-infinite SWS. The mode basis of the SWS contains only propagating eigenmodes those were found by using the solution

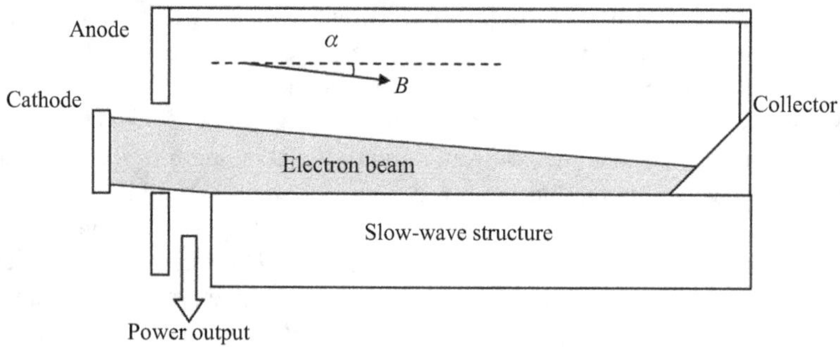

Figure 3.8 Principles of clinotron tube

of dispersion equation providing both slow and fast modes. The chamfer transitions related to the original design have been considered by the use of a stepwise approximation.

The calculation of scattering problem is carried out by the mode-matching technique and the method of generalized scattering matrices. Let us notice that this approach can be applied to consider 2D design as well as 3D. Finally, the coefficients of the matrix $S_{km}(i,j)$ that display the jth mode transformation of the mth port into ith mode of the kth port are used to define boundary conditions at the ends of the periodic structure during the solution of the beam–wave interaction problem. The system of nonstationary equations describes the propagation of surface and space waves inside the interaction region and the beam–wave interaction that occurs only with the backward surface wave as well. This assumption is valid while the coupling impedance for the highest modes is low compared to the surface mode that is actually observed in the THz frequency range.

Finally, the calculation of the beam–wave interaction problem provides the amplitudes of the EM waves propagating in the system at a given frequency. The EM power propagating in a certain port (particularly to the output waveguide) can be evaluated as a sum of powers of all modes propagating there. In Figure 3.9, the results of simulation together with the experimental data have been shown for 300-GHz clinotron and good agreement was obtained. Therefore, to increase clinotron output power, based on this theory, the optimization of the radiation output and plunger section is currently being carried out. This will allow minimize the radiation into the cathode area to minimize the reflection coefficient of the surface mode back into interaction space, etc.

The quality of EB in BWO and clinotrons plays an important role in the beam–wave interaction process. One of the factors affecting on the tubes operation is the quality of EB which is formed by an EOS. Designers of EOS try to form a sheet EB with minimal velocity spread for application in THz tubes since the velocity spread usually results in a decrease of the efficiency.

However, several effects such as space charge, thermal velocities, and lens effect result in velocity spread of electrons. Diocotron oscillations are additional effect provided by significant space charge that causes the dependence of

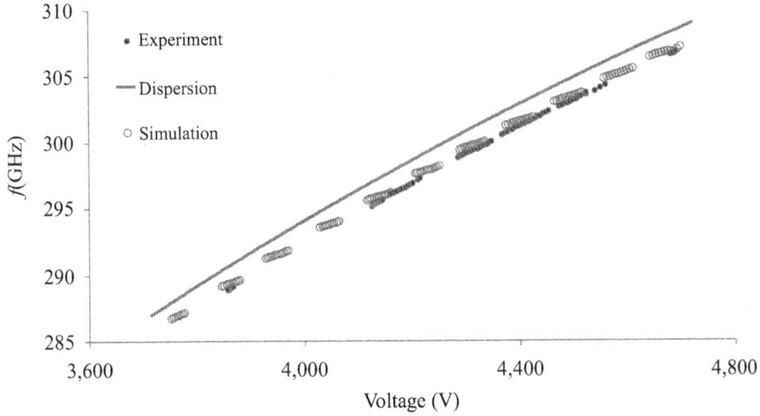

Figure 3.9 Simulation results for 300-GHz CW clinotron compared with the experimental data

longitudinal velocity on the transversal coordinates. The velocity spread usually results in a decrease of the beam–wave interaction efficiency and broadening of the spectrum linewidth. In this connection, the main aim of the design of an EOS is forming of EB with minimal distortions of the beam shape, and minimal velocity spread. Nowadays, the development of both electron-optic and transporting system is carried out through the numerical simulations with the use of professional software packages [96–98].

EB enters the interaction space after the EOS, where it is transported with minimal deformation by means of a magnetic focusing system. In THz clinotrons and BWOs, the permanent magnetic focusing systems based on Nd–Fe–B or Sm–Co alloys are utilized. In clinotrons, EOS produces sheet EB without compression. Oscillators of THz frequency range have a cross-section of an emitting area within 0.1–0.15 mm×2–2.5 mm while EB current reaches up to 200 mA. The electron gun operates in the mode of temperature limited emission.

The velocity spread is a negative effect from the traditional point of view of beam–wave interaction principles of BWO. However, in the case of a clinotron, special velocity distribution over the cross-section of the EB may provide additional features during the beam–wave interaction [99]. The analysis of the particle tracking in clinotron has shown several cases of velocity distribution. Mainly, those cases are result of lens and space charge effects. For instance, the lens effect arises due to displacement of the cathode relatively to the anode lens. Together with the inclination of an EB, these factors provide appearance of beam fractions having different velocities in different longitudinal positions along the periodic structure of a clinotron. As a result, the interaction of different velocity fractions with EM field of different amplitudes is occurring in the interaction region.

The theoretical investigation of this effect in clinotron had shown that the increase of output power occurs in the case of linear velocity distribution over the beam thickness while the lower layer of the beam has increased velocity compared to the upper layer. In the opposite case, the beam–wave interaction becomes less effective. The change of output power has been referred to the case of uniform velocity distribution corresponding to the case of a single-velocity beam. The variation of interaction efficiency is explained by velocity mismatch between electrons and wave. This parameter has different optimal values for different amplitudes of synchronous EM field. The optimal mismatch shifts to the higher values when the amplitude of the EM field increases. If the velocity mismatch of lower electron layers is high enough, the nonlinear beam–wave interaction occurs with a high efficiency. Because of the principles of backward wave operation, the upper electrons impose the oscillation frequency on the lower particles inside the beam. Therefore, the interaction efficiency decreases if the mismatch parameter is negative corresponding to the case of faster lower electrons and slower upper ones.

A specific case is observed when the mismatch parameter shifts to acceleration phase of the wave showing the energy absorption by electrons and resulting in sufficient decrease of the output power. Additional peculiarity can occur if the operation beam current exceeds the start current of oscillations; thus the independent oscillations could excite by lower and upper layers with frequencies corresponding to their velocities showing the multifrequency operation.

3.3.2 *Excitation of hybrid space-surface waves in a clinotron and BWO*

The increase of operation frequency toward THz values results in the enhancement of high-frequency ohmic loses. Consequently, the dissipation of EM energy of the surface wave is occurring in the periodic structure. This is the main reason of the output power decrease in VEDs based on Cherenkov radiation. Besides, in resonance devices, the reflected surface wave is strongly attenuated causing a reduction of resonant properties for an extensive EM system. The last one feature is important for THz clinotron oscillators that contain several hundreds of periods in their interaction system.

Space waves of interaction system have a fast zero spatial harmonic that is also transit EM energy, but it has low sensitivity to the ohmic losses compared to slow harmonics. The operation at the space waves occurs in oscillators based on diffraction radiation such as orotron, DRO, and ledatron. However, the interaction efficiency of such oscillators operated in a nonrelativistic regime is compatible to clinotron. This fact is explained by low coupling impedance of the synchronous slow harmonic of the fast wave compared to the operating harmonic of the surface wave.

The key benefits of operation at both surface and slow waves can be combined by using a complex periodic structure that has additional periodicity [100,101]. The dispersion of such periodic structure contains natural leaky waves that propagate along the structure and radiate energy by means of the fast spatial harmonic at the same time [102–110]. In antenna technology, such periodic structure is called leaky-wave antenna.

In clinotron, nonuniform grating with periodically modified grooves has been proposed to optimize the power output unit. The principles of beam–wave interaction in this system are exactly the same as for conventional clinotron. The main difference is the operation point that is chosen at the dispersion curves in order to ensure the phase velocity greater than c for the zero spatial harmonic.

Total EM field near the periodic structure can be represented with Floquet series by space harmonics, while the field inside the grooves is decomposed by waveguide modes. In the long wavelength approximation, where wavelength is greater than structural period, the dispersion relation is obtained by using the technique of field matching and decomposition. The final dispersion relation of unbounded nonuniform grating can be presented as following [102]:

$$\sum_{p_0=1}^{N} D_{p_0}\left[\delta_p^{p_0}\cos\left(kh_p\right)+i\frac{kd}{L}\sin\left(kh_{p_0}\right)\sum_{r=-\infty}^{\infty}\left(\frac{\sin(k_r d/2)}{k_r d/2}\right)^2\frac{e^{ik_r(p-p_0)l}}{q_r}\right]$$
$$=0,\quad p=1,N \tag{3.5}$$

The example of dispersion diagram of nonuniform structure is presented in Figure 3.10. The dispersion curve of nonuniform grating contains several branches that quantity is defined by large period L. The wavenumber of the highest branches has a complex value in the region that corresponds to the space wave operation ($k_0<k$). This feature of nonuniform structure ensures the power loss of the traveling wave via outgoing radiation. The intensity of outgoing radiation can be studied by simulating the scattering EM field of bunched EB traveled near the periodic structure.

A typical radiation pattern simulated by such method is shown in Figure 3.11. The angle of the main lobe strictly depends on the synchronism conditions, which is related to both wavenumber and phase velocity. These conditions define the operation regime and therefore restrict the broadband operation for such method of output power extraction. Nevertheless the main advantage of unbounded

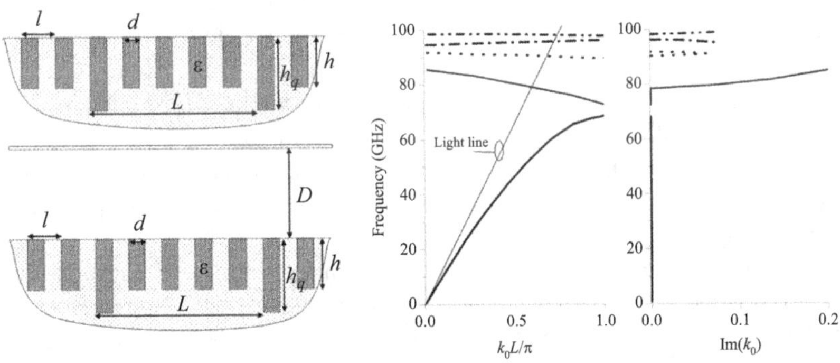

Figure 3.10 Dispersion diagram of W-band nonuniform grating structure with period L=5l: period is l=0.28 mm, groove depth h=0.66 mm, grove depth h_q=1.4h

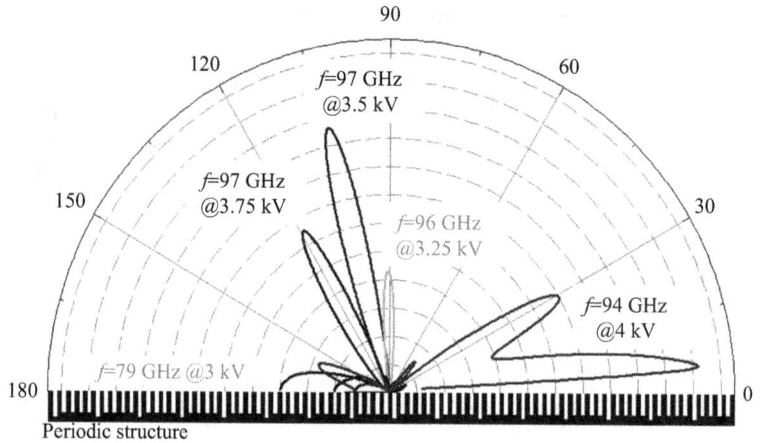

Figure 3.11 Radiation pattern of unbounded nonuniform grating structure that has dispersion presented in Figure 3.10

nonuniform periodic structure is forming of radiation pattern that can be compatible with quasioptic transmission lines. The design of clinotron with modified quasioptic power output may contain a correction dielectric lens placed on the way of outgoing radiation to extend the operation frequency range and make the radiation beam straighter.

Another configuration of the beam–wave interaction system, which utilizes the principle of leaky-waves, has been proposed to provide a reduction of ohmic losses in THz frequency range [102,103]. For that reason, a nonuniform grating is placed in a cavity resonator ensuring a feedback loop by fast harmonics. The EM radiation reflected from the opposite cavity mirror diffracts on the periodic structure. It results in energy exchange between the space component which propagates inside the volume of a cavity and the surface component that propagates near the structure. This effect has resonant nature and occurs under the certain incident angle or frequency. For instance, the variation of the reflection coefficient of the plane wave diffracted on nonuniform grating is shown in Figure 3.12. The reflection coefficient takes minimal values in the case of sufficient transformation of the plane wave into the natural modes of nonuniform periodic structure. In order to adjust the feedback at a given frequency range, the design of such EM system contains a movable cavity mirror. The design of clinotron employed this operation is presented in Figure 3.13 [103].

In contract to unbounded nonuniform interaction structure, the nonuniform periodic structure placed in a cavity resonator has additional operation modes related to the space modes of such complex EM structure. The low cutoff frequency of these modes depends on distance D between the periodic structure and opposite cavity mirror. These modes may overlap the natural modes of nonuniform system causing the regions of so-called mode interaction at certain values of D. Such points denote the resonant transformation of the space wave into the surface one

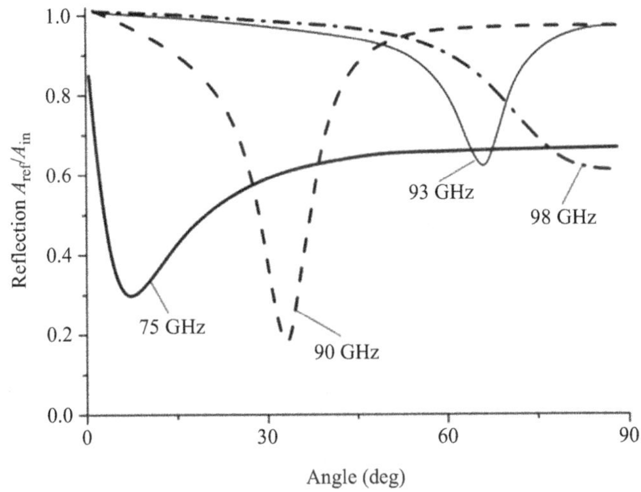

Figure 3.12 Reflection coefficients of the plane waves diffracted on the nonuniform grating at different incidence angles and frequencies

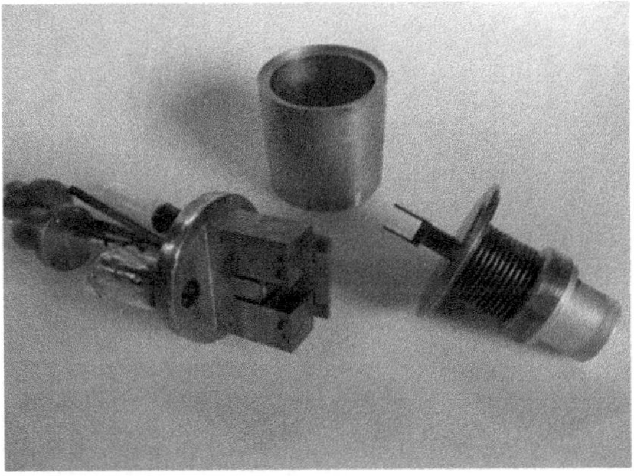

Figure 3.13 Parts of experimental clinotron with three-stage grating structure designed for operation in the frequency range from 70 to 105 GHz. The oscillator is equipped with movable cavity mirror that provided the adjustment of feedback loop

and vice versa [104]. The main conditions of intermode interaction for two specified modes are equality of wavenumbers at the same frequency, equality of diffraction Q-factor, and being the same class of symmetry. The demonstration of this effect is shown in Figure 3.14 that shows the pattern of EM field of eigen-modes for different points at the dispersion curves.

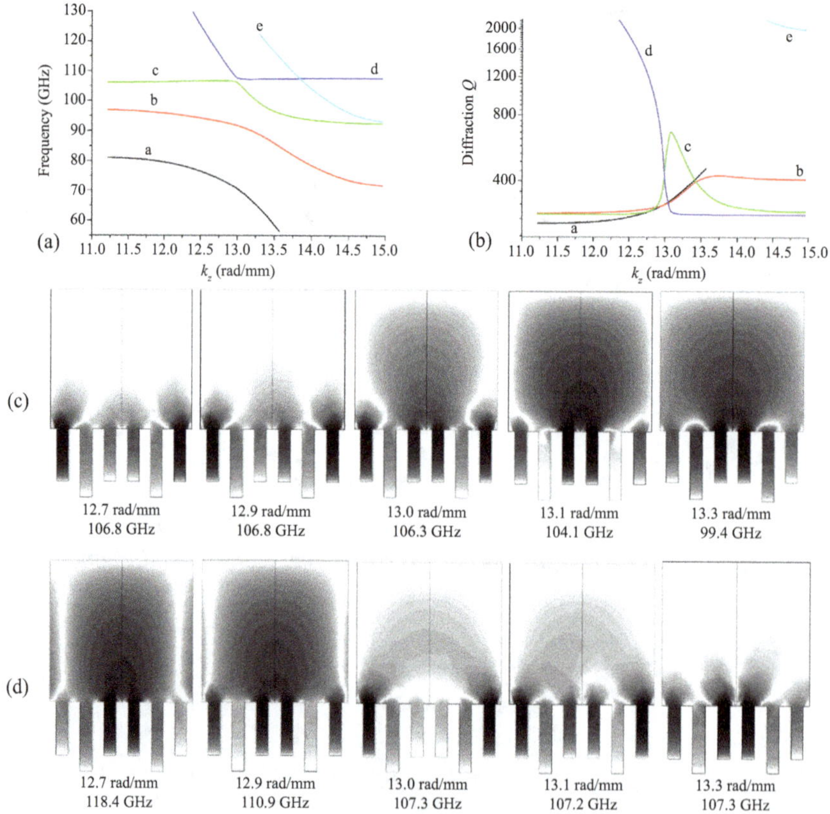

Figure 3.14 Dispersion curves and corresponding diffraction Q-factor showing the regions of intermode interaction (top (a) and (b)). The evolution of patterns for electromagnetic field near the region of intermode interaction (bottom (c) and (d))

Synchronism condition of EB with the part of dispersion curve which ensures that the excitation mechanism of leaky waves results in oscillations of the EM field with a complex structure. Because of localization of EM field occurring near the periodic structure as well as inside the volume of resonator, this kind of EM wave is called as hybrid surface-space wave highlighting the difference between DRO–orotron and clinotron.

Both increased Q-factor compared to the pure surface wave operation and the presence of additional feedback loop make the beam–wave interaction at a surface-space wave less susceptible to high-frequency ohmic losses. Consequently, in THz frequency range, the efficiency of the beam–wave interaction and output power can be improved in such way. In Table 3.3, the operating parameters of clinotrons are shown for different types of interaction systems based on nonuniform grating [105,106].

Table 3.3 Performance of clinotrons with nonuniform periodic structures

Frequency (GHz)	Output power (W)	Voltage (kV)	Current (mA)	Type of grating
		Nonuniform grating in cavity resonator		
70–105	1–2	2–4	20–150	3-Stage
120–145	1–2	2–5	20–150	4-Stage
		Unbounded grating		
125–132	1–5	3.2–3.8	200	5-Stage
375	0.7	4.3	165	5-Stage

3.4 Application of THz oscillators in DNP NMR spectroscopy

Nowadays, there is a strong demand on THz radiation sources to increase the sensitivity of NMR spectroscopy that is a powerful tool for diagnostics in medicine and biology [107–109]. The sensitivity increase is due to so-called DNP effect [70,110–115]. The main principles of the idea are as follows.

There are a large number of nuclei, such as ^{1}H, ^{13}C, and ^{15}N that comprise biological molecules and have a nonzero spin angular momentum I. In the presence of an external magnetic field B_0, the energy levels split into $(2I+1)$ sublevels (Zeeman energy levels). Energy difference between neighboring Zeeman levels

$$\Delta E = \frac{\gamma h B_0}{2\pi}, \tag{3.6}$$

where γ is the gyromagnetic ratio of the nucleus. Therefore, EM oscillation with so-called Larmor frequency $f{=}\Delta E/h$ can cause transfer between those energy levels. In the thermal equilibrium state, the number of nucleus with lower energy level is bigger than those in the higher level that means that EM wave propagating through the substance is absorbed. This absorption (intensity of NMR signal) increases with the difference of population between energy levels and the number of nuclei. In accordance with the Boltzmann distribution, the difference of population between energy levels increases with ΔE (correspondingly with B and γ) and decreases with the sample temperature T. Since different nuclei differ by gyromagnetic ratio γ and hence by Larmor frequency, the NMR spectral lines corresponding to different nuclei are quite far from each other that allows easily to recognize the type of nucleus and study of different nuclei independently.

When a nucleus is a part of a molecule, it is surrounded by its atom electrons and by the neighboring nuclei, which slightly disturb the effect of the external magnetic field for an isolated nucleus. They are the origin of several interaction types such as spin–spin coupling (interaction of adjacent nuclei spins through the bonding electrons), and dipole–dipole coupling (coupling of spins through the space). They also cause appearing of spin–lattice and spin–spin relaxation times that are related to the structure and mobility of the molecule. In addition, it slightly changes resonant frequency from the Larmor one; such change is called as chemical shift and is expressed in ppm. Since those interactions depend on the distance and angle between nuclei, the peaks in the NMR signal provide important molecular three-dimensional structure information such as torsion angles, anomerization, internuclear distances with high precision. Multidimensional NMR technique even enriches information about molecular structure with respect to 1D NMR one [116–120] and may provide the information that is not available by any other method.

This information about biological molecules is very important for the understanding of their functioning, interaction with drugs to identify groups of diseases and to determine a comprehensive mechanism of the pathology. Thus, the NMR spectroscopy is a powerful tool in the biological study, medical diagnostics (especially in early detection of various diseases), pharmacy, etc. Furthermore, NMR is nondestructive; thereby the further analysis of the same sample is allowed.

For example, NMR spectroscopy was applied for the study of dynamics of membrane protein acting as H^+ pump [121] (Bacteriorhodopsin), detection of the misfold of proteins since it may cause numerous diseases such as Alzheimer's, pathogenic aggregates [122–125], sometimes referred to as amyloid fibrils or prions.

NMR spectroscopy is a suitable technique for metabolomics [126–129]. Several studies have utilized ^{1}H NMR spectroscopy to analyze various body fluids such as plasma, blood, and urine. Advancement in metabolomics has included biomarker determination indicative of disease and clinical diagnostics. Metabolic changes due to certain diseases can be detected in biological fluids before the clinical symptoms develop, generating useful fingerprints. Further along, these characteristic fingerprints of the pathology may then serve as metabolic biomarkers, in which various diseases can be detected through the analysis of tissues or biofluids [130–132]. This lends way to the importance of biomarkers in medicine. It should be noted that the analysis has high reproducibility, confirming that the metabolic effects detected by the instrument are much higher than the analytical variability.

The information gathered via NMR lends insight to the mechanisms of biochemical disease processes and drug metabolism [133]. NMR-based metabolite profiling allows a "snapshot" of the metabolite's molecular dynamics and mobility, simultaneously detecting the wide range of metabolites in the sample [134]. Therefore, ^{1}H NMR-based metabolomics has also shown the potential for monitoring the progression of toxicological effects and the identification of biomarkers of toxicity [133], as a potential diagnostic tool for inborn errors of metabolism. Pioneer biomarkers such as creatinine, glucose, and cholesterol have been utilized to detect organ rejection (kidney transplant rejection), diabetes, and lipid metabolism [133,134]. At studies of diabetes type 2 and type 1, the urine sample ^{1}H NMR spectroscopy showed much more informative data for early diagnostics, monitoring inpatients and for creating new treatment and medicine. Recently ^{1}H NMR-based urinary metabolomics have been applied as a powerful early diagnostic tool to lung, gastric adenocarcinoma, prostate, and bladder cancer [135].

In multiple studies in [136], ^{1}H NMR spectroscopy has been utilized for identifying and quantifying the common uropathogens of urinary tract infections.

Despite the above mentioned numerous advantage of NMR spectroscopy, the main obstacle to its wide implementation is very low sensitivity since the difference of population between energy levels is low. To increase SNR (signal-to-noise ratio) of NMR signal the acquisition time in an experiment should be increased [107–109,137]. Some investigations requiring high sensitivity and resolution, especially utilizing the multidimensional technique, are almost impossible or require quite extremely long time of an experiment even at high magnetic fields. One of the most present powerful methods of enhancing NMR signals in solid state and solution is microwave-driven DNP method. It is based on the transfer of polarization from electrons (of some agent) to the nuclei. The theoretical maximum enhancement for 1D DNP-NMR k_{1D} in the case of ^{1}H nucleus is determined by the difference of population between energy levels for electrons and protons and hence by the ratio of electron and proton gyromagnetic ratios γ and is about 660. Correspondingly, the enhancement of 2D DNP-NMR is $k_{2D} = k_{1D}{}^2$ and hence it allows several hours of diagnostics instead of several months without the DNP technique. To stimulate the transfer of polarization from electrons (of a radical) to the studied nuclei, microwave with the frequency close to this of electron spin resonance (ESR) should irradiate a sample. The transfer occurs due to several mechanisms such as solid effect (SE) and the cross effect (CE).

The SE is a two-spin process when both nucleus and electron spin flip under irradiation frequency $f = f_{ESR} \pm f_{NMR}$ where both signs "+" and "−" correspond to enhancement minima and maxima correspondingly. The CE is a three-spin effect, involving flipping of the two electron one nuclear spins in the case when inhomogeneous breadth is wider than NMR frequency $\Delta > f_{NMR}$. In this case, the ESR frequencies of two electrons are related with NMR frequency as follows $f_{ESR1} - f_{ESR2} = f_{NMR}$ and irradiation frequency is close either to $f_{ESR\ 1}$ or $f_{ESR\ 2}$.

For high resolution and sensitive NMR, a higher magnetic field is to be applied. Since the ratio of electron and proton gyromagnetic ratios γ and is about 660, the radiation source frequency for ESP pumping should be about 660 times higher of NMR frequency. This provides THz radiation sources with frequencies of 132, 264, 395, 460 GHz for 200, 400, 600, 700-MHz NMR correspondingly. Further increase of NMR frequency is limited by available magnetic fields. Now projects of 28 and 40-T NMR experiments are under development. As a result, sources with an output frequencies of 780 GHz and 1.1 THz are also being developed [85]. Therefore, nowadays the DNP frequency of most interesting applications lies in the range from 130 GHz to 1.1 THz known as THz gap and it is important motivation to develop Watt level THz oscillators. In 1992, the first use of a gyrotron for a DNP NMR experiment was reported in [138,139]. Signal enhancements for polystyrene doped with BDPA of 10 for ^{1}H and 40 for ^{13}C were reported when comparing NMR spectra recorded with and without microwave power. Frequency and CW output power were 140 GHz and 20 W, respectively. Further advance in DNP-NMR scheme led to an enhancement increase. For example, a 250-GHz DNP NMR system [140,141] was commissioned at MIT in 2000 with a design that improved upon the 140-GHz spectrometer. This gyrotron produced 15 W, and ^{1}H enhancements of up to 170 have been observed for ^{1}C-glycine at temperatures of 20K using a MAS probe.

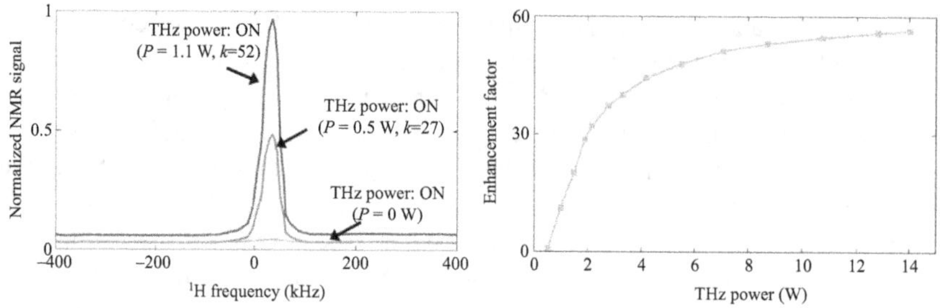

Figure 3.15 NMR signal recorded for various THz power levels (left) and typical dependence of enhancement factor on irradiation power (right)

The requirement on the power level is determined by the dependence of DNP enhancement factor on microwave/THz irradiation power [70] and this dependence in turn is determined by sample volume, temperature, radical type, concentration, type of NMR (static, MAS), etc.

Typical dependence is shown in Figure 3.15. One can see that the DNP enhancement is usually significantly lower than the maximal theoretical value discussed before. However, the enhancement is still high enough to improve the sensitivity in NMR experiments by factors of 20–400 (corresponding to 400–160,000 in acquisition time) [70]. The increased signal intensity shortens the acquisition time, reduces the amount of sample required, and allows the acquisition of multidimensional spectra with high SNR.

In majority of DNP-NMR schemes, the minimal required output is 50 mW, whereas optimal power is several tens of W. As was discussed before, nowadays, solid-state oscillators cannot provide such levels of output power in the THz range that imposes mainly use of VEDs as irradiation sources.

Up to now, Watt output power level laboratory sources at frequencies higher than 0.5 THz are gyrotron and its use for DNP-NMR provided main progress. The activity of development EIO, clinotron, orotron, DRO makes them also candidates for use at DNP-NMR at high frequencies [56,70]. Their advantage at gyrotrons is compact size and possibility to be installed quite close to NMR probe that may significantly simplify transmission lines and decrease transmission losses.

Requirements for long-term (NMR signal acquisition may take several days to increase sensitivity) stable output power and frequency ($\Delta P/P<1\%$, $\Delta f<1$ MHz) have caused development of various schemes for gyrotron and clinotron output parameters stabilization, including PID schemes and frequency locking [142–148]. In addition, there are new methods of increasing the DNP NMR sensitivity [70] requiring sources with options of fast frequency modulation and tuning. Rapid frequency modulation is reported to improve the DNP enhancement when nitroxide radicals are used as the polarizing agent, especially for static samples [149]. This can be understood as an increased number of saturated electron spins participating the DNP process. Two 0.46-THz gyrotrons FU-CW-GO-I and FU-CW-GO-II

[86,87] have been designed to meet these requirements for 700-MHz NMR ^{13}C experiments in Osaka University, Institute for Protein Research [70].

3.5 THz-imaging systems: schemes and achievements

3.5.1 Imaging technologies in medicine

The application of THz radiation is attractive not only for scientific research, but also for imaging techniques in security, industry, medical diagnostic, etc. Because of shorter wavelength, THz waves provide better resolution compared to microwaves. For instance, the resolution of several hundreds of μm can be achieved.

Available medical diagnostics include modern technologies such as X-ray, ultrasound, optics, and magnetic resonance. Besides the known advantages, these methods have some specific weakness those may restrict the area of possible application. For instance, the conventional X-ray computed tomography (CT) requires additional securing due to the ionizing effect. Since that such medical research cannot be carried out frequently. Also, such method provides low contrast for the soft tissues and typical resolution lies within 1–2-mm range. For that reason, a contrast material can be applied in some cases. Positron emission tomography (PET) is a variation of computer tomography in sense of using the ionizing radiation and it is also known as nuclear magnetic imaging. The mechanism of PET is based on the detection of low ionizing radiation that is produced by a small amount of radioactive materials that have been injected into a patient before the PET investigation. The kind of radioactive materials depends on the studied disease, and particularly the ability of some organs to accumulate the material during a short period of time. The material is accumulated in regions of inflammation and can be detected during PET session [150].

At the present time, magnetic resonance imaging may be the most frequently used method for medical diagnostics. This method employs strong magnetic fields and radio waves to obtain the image of the internal organs of a patient. The typical image resolution in mm fraction strongly depends on magnetic field induction that can exceed several Tesla. This feature defines the main drawback of MRI system related with expensive magnets. Besides, the method is time-consuming, especially when the additional spatial resolution is required [151].

The real-time imaging without ionizing radiation can be provided with use of ultrasound diagnostics. However, the method requires the object under study to be immersed in a liquid medium. Also, the ultrasound waves strongly attenuate in the inhomogeneous medium and provide poor resolution.

Another real-time technology applied in a medical study is optical coherence tomography (OCT). This method captures an image by analyzing the backscattered optical radiation at tissues under study. Because of nanometers wavelengths, the spatial resolution of 10 μm can be demonstrated easily. However, the penetration depth of optical radiation strictly depends on the tissue properties. Since that OCT technology has become widely used in ophthalmology and applied for the investigation of skin diseases [152].

Summarizing the properties of the presented methods, one can see that neither method of medical imaging is excellent. At the same time, the advantages of THz radiation make the imaging technique suitable in some cases and it can provide additional medical information. Also, it is attractive to combine THz radiation with other available technologies to provide more accurate diagnoses.

The key technology limitation for THz imaging is the low power of radiation that penetrates an object with significant EM loss. Therefore, the lack of compact radiation sources with reasonable output power and efficient detectors operated at room-temperature cause the limitation in wide THz radiation utilizing. The variation of instrumentation methods and principal approaches are developed to overcome such obstacles and improve the reconstruction. Here and after, we consider an active THz imaging technology, since passive technology is akin to infrared imaging and has low resolution due to a heat diffusion nature. Thus, the active imaging shows appropriate resolution and robust results in parcel inspection [153]. The recent achievements of THz technology were obtained in research of proteins and acids as well as in medical diagnostics of tissues, teeth, and oncological diseases [154,155].

3.5.2 Principles of an interaction of THz waves with biological tissues

THz imaging provides an attractive opportunity to define the structural peculiarities of an internal body in a noninvasive and nonionizing manner. The main mechanism of THz imaging is different absorption of THz radiation by substances differing in their dielectric properties, so the quality of the restored image depends on the dielectric contrast of a sample. For instance, soft tissues contain a significant amount of water while bones contain different minerals.

In the loss medium, the propagation of EM wave is defined by complex propagation constant $k^*=\omega\varepsilon^{*1/2}\ \mu^{*1/2}$, where complex permittivity is $\varepsilon^*=\varepsilon'-j\varepsilon''$ and complex permeability is $\mu^*=\mu'-j\mu''$. The relative permeability of human tissues is very close to 1. The deviations from unity appear due to perfusion of tissues, since iron presence in blood. However, such influence is very small, so the magnetic properties of tissues can be neglected. Since that, the attenuation of EM radiation in human tissues can be defined by dielectric loss tangent $\tan\delta=(\omega\varepsilon''+\sigma)/\omega\varepsilon'$.

The complex permittivity of biological tissues can be simulated by using the properties of water. For that reason, the effective permittivity is introduced as a function of the water content for a certain kind of tissue. Particularly, two mathematical models may be applied in the simulation of dielectric properties of biological tissues at different frequencies. There are Cole–Cole model and the Debye model. Also, several empirical models such as Havriliak–Negami are used for simulations as well. In the sub-THz range, the complex permittivity depends on frequency because of a sufficient polarization of water molecules. Besides, the permittivity varies with the temperature. In the MHz range, the attenuation is relatively low; however, it increases toward the THz frequencies. Finally, the skin-depth d becomes narrower because it inversely proportional to the attenuation coefficient Imk*. Typically the skin-depth varies from several hundred μm to several mm in sub-THz and THz frequency ranges [156]. Consequently, the direct imaging of the internal body with THz waves is limited.

Since the small penetrating depth, available THz imaging techniques are capable of investigating only a thin layer of tissue, which is specially prepared for the study (in vitro). At the same time, the investigation of human skin peculiarities can be realized "in vivo." The insured regions can be detected by measuring the permittivity, absorption, transmission, and reflections of THz signal. For instance, the regions of burned skin have water content different from the normal skin that results in a reduction of effective dielectric constant. Therefore, injured regions provide the contrast of reflectivity and they can be detected with THz radiation [157]. The same technique is used to investigate the tissues affected by a neoplasm. In such case, the imaging of water concentration gradient provides the information that cannot be obtained by optical and infrared tools. Another possible medical application of THz waves is dental diagnostics. In the case of caries, the attenuation of EM wave becomes higher in the tooth because of higher water content than healthy enamel and dentil have [158,159].

The level of exposure is important safety parameter that has to be defined in the case on "in vivo" study. The relevant researches have been carried out in the frequency range up to 3 THz to define the mechanism of interaction of THz waves with biological objects [160–163]. There are several effects of THz radiation have been defined. On the one hand, the irradiation at 120 and 130 GHz cannot induce either genotoxicity or alteration of cell cycle kinetics in human blood cells within 20 min [161]. Besides, the study of keratinocytes showed neither specific inhibition, nor stimulation of cell activity, while the exposure not exceeds 0.45 J/cm^2 [160]. However, the cytotoxic effect of EM radiation on a rat glial cell line has been demonstrated in the frequency range from 120 to 180 GHz and power density of 3.2 mW/cm^2 [164]. The investigation of a long-term impact of continuous-wave radiation with relatively low-power density has also showed the genomic instabilities of human lymphocytes at 100 GHz [165].

The parameters of EM radiation such as frequency, pulse duration, exposure, and incident power should be selected for the certain individual cases since biological tissues are heterogeneous and have a complex structure.

3.5.3 Pulsed and continuous-wave mode of THz imaging

For the last years, the number of researchers involved in THz imaging has sufficiently increased. Since the recent progress in compact sources of THz radiation and detectors, the bunch of THz systems had become commercially available [166,167]. At the present time, there are two possible solutions for THz imaging: pulsed and CW.

Generic pulsed THz-imaging system is based on laser, which has an average power of hundreds of mW and pulse duration of several hundred fs [168–170]. Such pulse duration corresponds to extremely wide distribution of spectral density providing simultaneously analysis at different frequencies. The average output power of laser beam is up to several hundred mW [168–170]. The beam is guided by the optical system containing off-axis parabolic mirrors, beam splitters, and time delay system; and it is used for the generation and detection of coherent THz pulse. According to design of the imaging system, the guiding system may include dielectric lenses, such as Fresnel lenses and axicon lenses to collimate and focus the THz radiation at a sample.

The pumping beam provided by the beam splitter is transformed to THz radiation by a photoconductive antenna. After the THz beam interacted with the sample, it is received by detection system. To increase the magnitude of detected signal, the THz beam can be focused onto a detector. The application of time-delay system provides the detection of different parts of THz pulse, so the complete form of the THz pulse can be obtained in the time domain by changing the delay time. Such scanning approach is quite time-consuming; however, it deals with the time-domain signals and, hence, provides the time-of-flight information. The information is required to restore the configuration of the object in depth. The additional spectrum information about scattering objects can be collected as well.

The photoconductive module consists of a microstrip dipole antenna fabricated on a semiconductor substrate that serves as a photoconductor. The dipole has a gap of several μm that is supplied with a bias voltage. The pulse of THz radiation is generated by the antenna when the gap is irradiated by pulsed laser radiation and sort pulse of current passes across the bias. Modern photoconductive antennas are capable of providing the THz radiation with maximal power up to several hundreds of μW and the bandwidth that exceeds 400 GHz [171].

The antenna can be used for the detection of THz radiation as well. For that purpose, additional photoconductive module should be included in the system. The detection is performed when the antenna is irradiated by both THz beam and laser "probe" beam additionally provided by the splitter. The signal is measured at the moment, when both THz and probe beams arrive at the detection device.

Otherwise, the THz radiation can be detected directly by using either compact Schottky diode [172] or pyroelectric sensor [173] or Golay cell [174] those have sufficient sensitivity and can operate at room temperature. An array of sensors can be applied to reduce the scanning time [175]. In some cases, the low-frequency modulation of the THz beam is applied; in particular, when a pyroelectric sensor is used.

In contrast to the pulsed approach, the CW-based system employs THz radiation directly, without photoconductive modules. The radiation can be generated by a huge variety of solid-state and VEDs, so the optimal operation characteristics of imaging system can be provided for each individual case. The imaging system based on CW technique may be operated either in a single frequency or frequency-modulated mode. The single-frequency CW imaging provides the distribution of transmitted/reflected energy as a projection at the sample plane during the short period of time. In contrast to that, the use of frequency-modulated mode allows to define the time-of-flight and phase information about the object under study. In the frequency-modulated mode, a voltage-controlled oscillator such as BWO or Schottky diode should be applied. The frequency stabilization is provided by using the phase-locked loops or PID-control in wide operating range [176,177]. The application of BWO is attractive for THz-imaging systems due to the advantages of high output power, compact style, and ease of operation. Besides, it is possible to extend the operation frequency range with use of frequency multipliers to provide reasonable output power at frequencies above 1 THz because of sufficient output power at basics frequencies.

Other possible ways of CW THz generation are photomixing technique and application of QCLs. The photomixing approach has advantage of extremely broadband operation that can be up to several THz [178]. This feature is provided by the generation of THz radiation at a photomixing device from the beat-frequency of two frequency separated laser beams.

Both pulsed and CW THz-imaging systems have been compared in [179] considering the problem of the detection of flaws in a space shuttle insulating foam. Particularly, investigating the voids and delimitations in the sample, it was concluded that CW imaging approach provides more useful results and less resource consuming compared to pulse imaging.

3.5.4 Reflective and transmission configuration of THz imaging systems

Both pulsed and CW THz-imaging systems can be realized in two different ways, either reflective or transmission configuration. The reflective configuration is preferable in the applications related to highly attenuated substances. Such imaging systems have been applied in dental healthcare, recognition of skin cancer, breast cancer, lung neoplasm, and uterine cervical neoplasm up to the present moment [180,181]. In Figure 3.16(a), the principal scheme of reflective THz-imaging system is presented for the case of pulsed operation. Reflective configuration is often applied with CW radiation sources; however, the output information is a power distribution only. Basics scheme of THz imaging setup is presented for transmission configuration in Figure 3.16(b). The application of transmission configuration is suitable for the samples that demonstrate reasonable contrast in dielectric

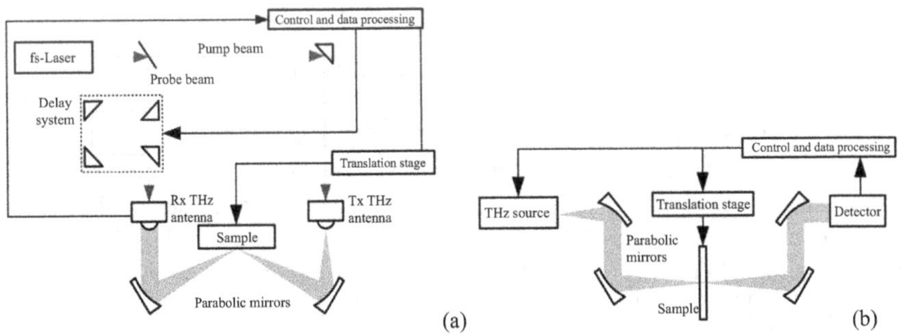

Figure 3.16 The principal schemes of THz imaging systems designed for reflection configuration (a) and transmission configuration (b)

properties and low attenuation. For instance, the THz-imaging investigations of paraffin-embedded biological objects have been previously reported [182,183]. The scheme can be extended to measure the phase shift of radiation transmitted across the sample by using the interferometer method.

Both configurations assume that the output data are obtained by raster scanning of the sample across the THz beam by using a displacement stage. The beam is focused in a small spot at the sample plane by using the focusing system, so the spot size often relates to the image pixel. The focusing system can contain off-axis parabolic mirrors and dielectric lenses. The spatial resolution of THz-imaging system also depends on factors related to numerous parameters such as operation frequency, aperture, and focal length of focusing device and scan step. In the case of 3D imaging with frequency-modulated method, the numbers of frequency samples and total frequency range are becoming additional critical parameters. The spatial resolution can be theoretically evaluated by using the Rayleigh criterion that demonstrates the improvement of the resolution while the frequency of incident THz beam and focal length decrease, and the aperture for focusing element increases. However, the spatial resolution of a real system is several times worse than it has been predicted, because of the combination of effects mentioned before [184]. The spot size of the beam and the tolerance of sample displacement at the scan plane can be evaluated from the Rayleigh length. The parameter relates to the depth of focus that shows the region of incident beam where the EM field corresponds to the plane wave. Besides, the depth of focus limits the thickness of a sample. If the sample thickness is less than the focus depth, the image blurring can be observed.

In the case of Gaussian distribution, the spot size decreases while the wavelength and focal length reduce. The beam pattern essentially depends on the bunch of parameters such as waveform at the output of THz radiation source, aberration, misalignment, and diffraction in transmission line. The actual spot size of THz beam can be measured by using the knife-edge technique. The experimental researches demonstrate that the spot size can be achieved near the diffraction limit in THz range [185].

Another effect that can be observed during the scan is interference that occurs due to reflections of EM wave between the focusing elements of transmission system. Also, the Fabry–Pérot effect can be observed during reflection measurements as well [184]. In this case, the quality of image can be improved by applying the slope of sample [184,185].

The experimental testing of spatial resolution for THz-imaging system is carried out by scanning the various resolution targets either custom or industrial, such as USAF resolution target [172,184,186].

Because of sufficient attenuation of THz EM wave inside the biological objects, the target signal should have a reasonable SNR to be detected and processed. A high SNR can be obtained by applying the integration procedure at each pixel by using either synchronous detection or gated integration. In the case of CW imaging, the THz radiation is additionally modulated with an optical chopper placed in the front of the output port of the radiation source, and synchronized with a lock-in amplifier. Besides, a high SNR is provided in a system equipped with a powerful THz radiation source having low noise and good stability. For instance,

THz-imaging system equipped with BWO demonstrates a 40-dB SNR [185]. Consequently, the target signal is processed by a computer providing output data.

Generally, the displacement stage contains linear 2D displacement providing the scanning of sliced samples. However, in the case of THz tomography method, the stage is equipped with an additional rotation stage [187]. The various designs of THz-imaging system have been presented in [168,170,172].

3.5.5 Basics of data-processing methods

The final image can be obtained with an appropriate processing of collected data depending on the configuration of the THz-imaging system. In the case of pulsed THz imaging, a probe pulse interacts with a sample and generates the output signal that contains a sequence of pulses contained information about various interfaces inside the sample. The output temporal waveform of THz pulse is detected by a photoconductive device with changing arriving time of a probe laser pulse that depends on the optical delay. The output pulse may include echoes that correspond to the reflection of the THz pulse from the elements of the sample holder. Often the sample is mounted on a quartz plate; therefore, the parasitic reflections can excite at the quartz–air interface [168,170]. Therefore, the signal-processing steps are plied to extract the target signal [188,189]. The presence of atmospheric water vapor provides additional fluctuation in the signal. The noise can be filtered by applying the deconvolution of the raw signal with the reference pulse, obtained in the absence of a sample. A band-pass filter is applied further to filter the frequency components falling outside the operation frequency range.

Typical waveform of collected THz pulse is shown in Figure 3.17. By using the waveform, the THz image can be generated in two different ways. One approach assumes processing of maximal amplitude of a waveform at a given scanning position to render the 2D surface image of the sample. Another approach provides the 3D image providing in-depth visualization. This approach is based on the "time-post-pulse" (TPP) technique [189]. Another name is the "time-of-flight." The depth information of the internal structure of the sample is obtained from the time that is required for the pulse to travel over a certain distance. The THz pulse width depends on the absorption properties of the sample. The higher absorption in the sample the greater the broadening of the pulse is. The pulse boarding refers to a TPP value, which refers to the waveform amplitude A_t normalized by the minimal amplitude A_{min}.

The 2D THz image is produced by plotting the TPP value at a particular time for each pixel over the sample. In the case of 3D visualization, a depth value can be calculated from the reference time by assuming a certain refractive index for the each layer inside the object. For instance, the refractive index of skin is assuming to be as 2 in THz frequency range [168,169]. Let us notice, the depth value can be calculated approximately because of unknown dispersion and diffraction properties of real biological object. In practice, reference time is chosen to provide the best contrast between the injured and normal tissue.

Generic design of pulsed THz-imaging system can be modified to provide a real-time imaging. The main idea is to use the THz pulse with an enhanced diameter together with charge-coupled device (CCD). The probe THz beam penetrates

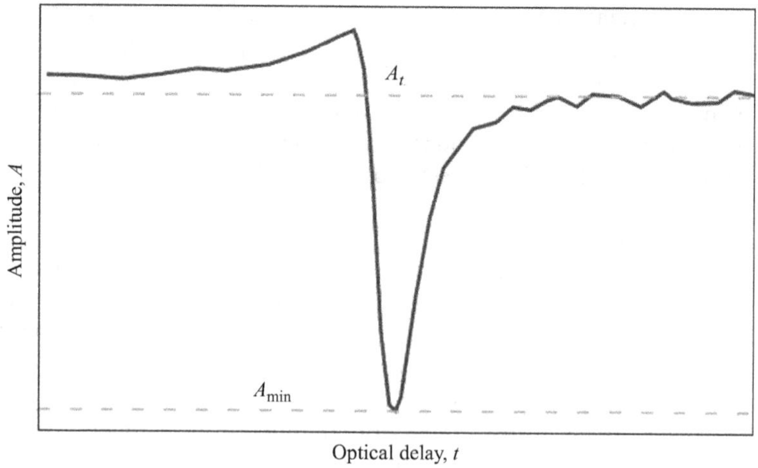

Figure 3.17 Typical waveform of target time-domain THz pulse

the sample and interacts with the preliminary polarized reference optical beam at the electro-optical crystal, such as ZnTe. Finally, the combination of CCD and analyzer of polarization provides the detection of polarization changes that occur on a large area of the crystal [188].

In the case of continuous-wave operation of THz imaging system, output 2D image of a sample is reconstructed by processing the amplitude of detected THz radiation at a given frequency [185]. Consequently, CW THz imaging is less time-consuming in contrast to pulsed configuration that is especially important for real-time medical imaging. Both large-aperture antenna systems and sensor array are often used instead of the beam focusing systems to improve the data acquisition time. Besides, the application of frequency-modulated method provides the 3D visualization. However, broadband THz radiation source with electronically controlled frequency is required for that purpose to provide reasonable spatial resolution in depth.

The THz holography method is often applied for the frequency-modulated continuous wave imaging. The hologram is produced by moving the object within the radiation pattern of the antenna. The reference signal is mixed with the probe signal to extract the difference signal that contains information about the amplitude and phase. Consequently, the distribution of complex amplitude is defined at the scanning plane. This distribution corresponds to the set of secondary radiation sources that reproduces the structure of the object. The final 2D image can be reconstructed by using the methods based on deconvolution algorithms [186]. The 3D image is reconstructed by applying the "time-of-flight" technique.

The THz diffraction method is applied to measure the scattered THz field from the object, including both amplitude and phase distribution. The projection image of the sample is provided by using the reconstruction algorithm based on the Fourier transform. The example of 2D image reconstruction of the composite sample is shown in Figure 3.18.

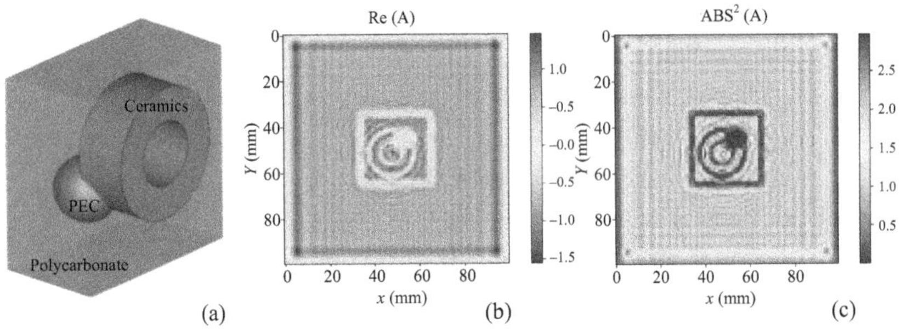

Figure 3.18 Composite object (a) and its 2D images (b, c) reconstructed by using the Rayleigh–Sommerfeld diffraction method

Eventually, basic THz-imaging methods listed before can be extended by applying the tomographic data processing [187,190]. The THz CT provides sectional images of the object. Besides, the spectroscopic information about internal structure can be collected in the case of pulsed configuration [190]. According to the applied configuration of imaging setup, the amplitude and phase of detected THz wave are measured at multiple projection angles [191]. The number of projections can be sufficiently reduced by using the tomosynthesis methods [190]. The image reconstruction procedure employs mathematical algorithms, such as inverse Radon transform or iterative reconstruction [192,193]. Moreover, several methods have been proposed to decrease the data acquisition time for pulsed 3D THz imaging such as diffraction tomography and coherent lens less imaging [194].

Generally, in the case of pulsed configuration, data processing is more complex than for the case of continuous-wave approach. Nevertheless, pulsed systems can provide additional spectroscopic information about the sample under study by applying Fourier transform to the waveforms collected during measurements. Taking into the consideration the frequency response of imaging system without the sample, the THz spectra of the sample can be extracted. Numerous researches demonstrate absorption lines for water vapor at the frequency domain power spectra in such way. Consequently, the contrast image of the sample can be obtained at the different THz frequencies. One of the attractive applications is the identification of different compounds such as concealed explosives and medicines. Since the resolution of frequency-domain power spectrum depends on both the range of temporal scan and the number of temporal samples, the delay system with large displacement range is required for the imaging system.

Glossary

BWO	backward wave oscillator
CCD	charge-coupled device
CMOS	complementary metal–oxide–semiconductor
CW	continuous wave regime

CT	computed tomography
CE	cross effect
CNC	computer numerical control
CRM	cyclotron resonance maser
DNP	dynamic nuclear polarization
DRO	diffraction radiation oscillator
EIO	extended interaction oscillator
EB	electron beam
EM	electromagnetic (wave)
EOS	electron-optic system
FEL	free-electron laser
HBT	heterojunction bipolar transistor
HOAM	high-order axial modes
IMPATT	impact ionization avalanche transit-time diode
MMIC	monolithic microwave integrated circuit
NMR	nuclear magnetic resonance
OPM	optical photoconductive material
OCT	optical coherence tomography
PET	positron emission tomography
QCL	quantum cascade laser
RTD	resonant tunneling-diode
SNR	signal-to-noise ratio
SWS	slow-wave structure
SCM	superconducting magnet
SE	solid effect
TWT	traveling wave tube
VED	vacuum electron device

References

[1] Yazgan A., Jofre L., and Romeu J. (eds.). 'The state of art of terahertz sources: A communication perspective at a glance'. *Proceedings of the 40th International Conference on Telecommunications and Signal Processing (TSP)*; Barcelona, Spain, July 2017. Brno: Brno University of Technology; 2017. pp. 810–816.

[2] Park G.-S., Kim Y.H., Han H. *et al.* (eds.). *Convergence of Terahertz Sciences in Biomedical Systems*. The Netherlands: Springer; 2012. p. 435.

[3] Murate K. and Kawase K. 'Perspective: Terahertz wave parametric generator and its applications'. *Journal of Applied Physics*. 2018; **124**: 160901. DOI: 10.1063/1.5050079.

[4] Fujishima M. 'Key technologies for THz wireless link by silicon CMOS integrated circuits'. *Photonics*. 2018; **5**: 50. DOI: 10.3390/photonics5040050.

[5] Hesler J. L. and Crowe T. *High-Power Solid-State Terahertz Sources* [online]. 2015. Available from https://spie.org/news/5859-high-power-solid-state-terahertz-sources?SSO=1 [Accessed 1 July 2020].

[6] Hesler J., Prasankumar R., and Tignon J. 'Advances in terahertz solid-state physics and devices'. *Journal of Applied Physics*. 2019; **126**: 110401. DOI: 10.1063/1.5122975.

[7] Virginia D. Custom Transmitters [online]. 2020. Available from https://vadiodes.com/en/products/custom-transmitters [Accessed 1 July 2020].

[8] Yun J., Yoon D., Kim H., and Rieh J.S. '300-GHz InP HBT oscillators based on common-base cross-coupled topology'. *IEEE Transactions on Microwave Theory and Techniques*. 2014; **62**(12): 3053–3064.

[9] Yang S.-H., Hashemi M. R., Berry C. W., and Jarrahi M. '7.5% optical-to-terahertz conversion efficiency offered by photoconductive emitters with three-dimensional plasmonic contact electrodes'. *IEEE Transactions on Terahertz Science and Technology*. 2014; **4**(5): 575–581.

[10] Preu S., Dohler G. H., Malzer S., Wang L. J., and Gossard A.C. 'Tunable, continuous-wave Terahertz photomixer sources and applications'. *Journal of Applied Physics*. 2011; **109**: 061301.

[11] Tanoto H., Teng J. H., Wu Q. Y. *et al.* 'Greatly enhanced continuous-wave terahertz emission by nano-electrodes in a photoconductive photomixer'. *Nature Photonics*. 2012; **6**: 121–126.

[12] Khanal S., Gao L., Zhao L., Reno J. L., and Kumar S. 'High-temperature operation of broadband bidirectional terahertz quantum-cascade lasers'. *Scientific Reports*. 2016; **6**: 32978. DOI: 10.1038/srep32978.

[13] Faist J., Capasso F., Sivco D. L., Sirtori C., Hutchinson A. L., and Cho A.Y. 'Quantum cascade laser'. *Science*. 1994; **264**: 553–556.

[14] Köhler R., Tredicucci A., Beltram F. *et al.* 'Terahertz semiconductor-heterostructure laser'. *Nature*. 2002; **417**: 156–159.

[15] Asada M. and Suzuki S. 'Room-temperature oscillation of resonant tunneling diodes close to 2 THz and their functions for various applications'. *Journal of Infrared, Millimeter, and Terahertz Waves*. 2016; **37**(12): 1185–1198.

[16] Kleiner R. and Wang H. 'Terahertz emission from $Bi_2Sr_2CaCu_2O_{8+x}$ intrinsic Josephson junction stacks'. *Journal of Applied Physics*. 2019; **126**: 171101. DOI: 10.1063/1.5116660.

[17] Chevalier P., Armizhan A., Wang F. *et al.* 'Widely tunable compact terahertz gas lasers'. *Science*. 2019; **366**: 856–860.

[18] O'Shea P. G. and Freund H.P. 'Free-electron lasers: Status and applications'. *Science*. 2001; **292**: 1853–1858.

[19] Barker R.J., Booske J.H., Luhmann N.C. Jr., and Nusinovich G.S. (eds.). *Modern Microwave and Millimeter-Wave Power Electronics*. Hoboken, New Jersey: Wiley-IEEE Press; 2005.

[20] Booske J.H., Dobbs R.J., Joye C.D. *et al.* 'Vacuum electronic high power terahertz sources'. *IEEE Transactions on Terahertz Science and Technology*. 2012; **1**(1): 54–75.
[21] Gewartowski J.W. and Watson H.A. *Principles of Electron Tubes*. Princeton, New Jersey: D. Van Nostrand Company, Inc.; 1965.
[22] Tsimring S.E. *Electron Beams and Microwave Vacuum Electronics*. Hoboken, NJ: John Wiley and Sons; 2007.
[23] Jelle J.V. 'Cerenkov radiation and its applications'. *British Journal of Applied Physics*. 1955; **6**: 277.
[24] Cherenkov P.A. 'Visible emission of clean liquids by action of γ radiation'. *Doklady Akademii Nauk SSSR*. 1934; **2**: 451.
[25] Tamm I.E. and Frank I.M. 'Coherent radiation of fast electrons in a medium'. *Doklady Akademii Nauk SSSR*. 1937; **14**: 107.
[26] Luo C., Ibanescu M., Johnson S.G., and Joannopoulos J.D. 'Cerenkov radiation in photonic crystals'. *Science*. 2003; **299**(5605): 368–371.
[27] Pierce J.R. 'Traveling wave tubes'. In: *Bell Lab Series*. Princeton, New Jersey: D Van Nostrand; 1950.
[28] Antonsen T.M. and Levush B. 'Traveling-wave tube devices with nonlinear dielectric elements'. *IEEE Transactions on Plasma Science*. 1998; **26**(3): 774–786.
[29] Gilmour A.S. Jr. *Klystrons, Traveling Wave Tubes, Magnetrons, Crossed-Field Amplifiers, and Gyrotrons*. Norwood, MA: Artech House; 2011.
[30] Johnson H.R. 'Backward-wave oscillators'. *Proceedings of the IRE*. 1955; **43**(6): 684–697.
[31] Kantorowicz G. and Palluel P. 'Backward wave oscillators' in Button K. (ed.). *Infrared and Millimeter Waves*, **Vol. 1**, Chap. 4, New York: Academic Press; 1979.
[32] Korolev A.N., Zaitsev S.A., Golenitskij I.I. *et al.* 'Traditional and novel vacuum electron devices'. *IEEE Transactions on Electron Devices*. 2001; **48**(12): 2929–2937.
[33] Usikov A.Ya. (eds.). *The Clinotron*. Kiev: Naukova Dumka; 1992 (in Russian).
[34] Bratman V.L., Ginsburg V.A., Grishin Yu.A., Dumesh V.S., Rusin F.S., and Fedotov A.E. 'Pulse wideband orotrons of MM and SUBMM waves'. *Radiophysics and Quantum Electronics*. 2006; **49**(11): 866–871.
[35] Myasin E.A., Evdokimov V.V., and Il'yin A.Yu. 'Experimental study of the possibility to generate radiation at a frequency of up to 400 GHz in an orotron with a double-row periodic structure'. *Radiophysics and Quantum Electronics*. 2016; **9**(5): 409–422.
[36] Rusin F. and Bogomolov G. 'Orotron – An electronic oscillator with open resonator and reflecting grating'. *Proceeding of IEEE*. 1969; **57**: 720.
[37] Bratman V.L., Dumesh B.S., Fedotov A.E., Makhalov P.B., Movshevich B. Z., and Rusin F.S. 'Terahertz orotrons and oromultipliers'. *IEEE Transactions on Plasma Science*. 2010; **38**(6): 1466–1471.

[38] Shestopalov V.P. (eds.). *Diffraction Radiation Generators*. Kiev: Naukova Dumka; 1991 (in Russian).

[39] Kucherenko S.N., Lukin K.A., Skrynnik B.K., Khlopov G.I., and Shestopalov V.P. 'A study of transient processes in diffraction radiation oscillators'. *Radiophysics and Quantum Electronics*. 1988; **31**: 64–69.

[40] Lukin K., Khutoryan E., and Tsvyk A. 'Mode self-synchronization in diffraction radiation oscillator'. *Proceedings of the IEEE International Vacuum Electronics Conference*; Monterey, CA, 2008. pp. 62–63.

[41] Steer B., Roitman A., Horoyski P., Hyttinen M., Dobbs R., and Berry D. 'Advantages of extended interaction klystron technology at millimeter and sub-millimeter frequencies'. *Proceedings of the 16th IEEE International Pulsed Power Conference*, 2007. **2**. pp. 1049–1053.

[42] Roitman A., Berry D., and Steer B. 'State-of-the-art W-band extended interaction klystron for the Cloud Sat program'. *IEEE Transactions on Electron Devices*. 2005; **52**(5): 895–898.

[43] Roitman A., Horoyski P., Steer B., and Berry D. 'High power CW 264 GHz tunable extended interaction oscillator'. *Proceedings of the 14th International Vacuum Electronics Conference*; Paris, France, 2013. pp. 1–2.

[44] Shin Y.-M., Baig A., Barnett L.R., Tsai W.-C., and Luhmann N.C. 'System design analysis of a 0.22-THz sheet-beam traveling-wave tube amplifier'. *IEEE Transactions on Electron Devices*. 2015; **59**(1): 234–240.

[45] Baig A., Gamzina D., Kimura T. *et al.* 'Performance of a nano CNC machined 220-GHz traveling wave tube amplifier'. *IEEE Transactions on Electron Devices*. 2017; **64**(5): 2390–2397.

[46] Rozhnev A.G., Ryskin N.M., Karetnikova T.A. *et al.* 'Studying characteristics of the slow-wave system of the traveling-wave tube with a sheet electron beam'. *Radiophysics and Quantum Electronics*. 2014; **56**(8–9): 542–553.

[47] Karetnikova T.A., Rozhnev A.G., Ryskin N.M., Fedotov A.E., Mishakin S. V., and Ginzburg N.S. 'Gain analysis of a 0.2-THz traveling-wave tube with sheet electron beam and staggered grating slow wave structure'. *IEEE Transactions on Electron Devices*. 2018; **65**(6): 2129–2134.

[48] Ploskih A.E., Ryskin N.M., Burtsev A.A., Danilushkin A.V., and Navrotsky I.A. 'Performance improvement of a sub-THz traveling-wave tube by using an electron optic system with a converging sheet electron beam'. *Results in Physics*. 2019; **12**: 799–803.

[49] Bhattacharjee S., Booske J.H., Kory C.L. *et al.* 'Folded waveguide traveling-wave tube sources for terahertz radiation'. *IEEE Transactions on Plasma Science*. 2004; **32**(3): 1002–1014.

[50] Tsutaki K., Neo Y., Mimura H., Masuda N., and Yoshida M. 'Design of a 300 GHz band TWT with a folded waveguide fabricated by microelectromechanical systems'. *Journal of Infrared, Millimeter, and Terahertz Waves*. 2016; **37**(12): 1166–1172.

[51] Zhang X., Cao L., Li F., He J., and Huang M. 'Design and study of slow wave structure of the THz folded waveguide TWT over 60W'. *Journal of Physics: Conference Series*. 2020; **1486**: 062026.

[52] Shin Y.-M., So J.-K., Han S.-T., Jang K.-H., and Park G.-S. 'Microfabrication of millimeter wave vacuum electron devices by two-step deep-etch X-ray lithography'. *Applied Physics Letters*. 2006; **88**(9): 2006. 10.1063/1.2178770.
[53] Thompson-CSF. *Microwave Tubes and Devices*. Vol. 3, 1977.
[54] Ponomarenko S.S., Kishko S.A., Zavertanniy V.V., *et al.* '400-GHz continuous-wave clinotron oscillator'. *IEEE Transactions on Plasma Science*. 2013; **41**(1): 82–86.
[55] Lysenko Ye.Ye., Pankov S.V., Pishko O.F., Chumak V.G., and Churilova S. A. 'Problems and the status of engineering of CW clinotrons for the frequency range from 400 GHz to 500 GHz'. *Electromagnetic Waves and Electromagnetic System*. 2010; **15**(112): 63–71 (in Russian).
[56] Likhachev A., Danik A., Kovshov Yu. *et al.* 'Compact radiation module for THz spectroscopy using 300 GHz continuous-wave clinotron'. *Review of Scientific Instruments*. 2019; **90**(3): 034703.
[57] Kovshov Y.S., Ponomarenko S.S., Kishko S.A., Khutoryan E.M., and Kuleshov A.N. 'Numerical simulation and experimental study of sub-THz and THz CW clinotron oscillators'. *IEEE Transactions on Electron Devices*. 2018; **65**(6): 2177–2182.
[58] Monreal B. 'Single-electron cyclotron radiation'. *Physics Today*. 2016; **69** (1): 70.
[59] Nusinovich G. *Introduction to the Physics of Gyrotrons*. Baltimore, Maryland: The Johns Hopkins University Press; 2004.
[60] Nusinovich G.S., Thumm M., and Petelin M.I. 'The gyrotron at 50: Historical overview'. *Journal of Infrared, Millimeter, and Terahertz Waves*. 2014; **35**: 325–381.
[61] Idehara T. and Sabchevski S.P. 'Gyrotrons for high-power terahertz science and technology at FIR UF'. *Journal of Infrared, Millimeter, and Terahertz Waves*. 2016; **38**(1): 62–86.
[62] Denisov G.G., Kuftin A.N., Malygin V.I., Venediktov N.P., Vinogradov D. V., and Zapevalov V.E. '110 GHz gyrotron with a built-in high-efficiency converter'. *International Journal of Electronics*. 1992; **72**(5–6): 1079–1091.
[63] Vlasov S.N., Zagryadskaya L.I., and Petelin M.I. 'Transformation of a whispering gallery mode, propagating in a circular waveguide into the beam of waves'. *Radio Engineering & Electronic Physics*. 1975; **20**: 14–17.
[64] Bogdashov A.A., Chirkov A.V., Denisov G.G. *et al.* 'Mirror synthesis for gyrotron quasi-optical mode converters'. *International Journal of Infrared and Millimeter Waves*. 1995; **16**(4): 735–744.
[65] Japan Superconductor Technology, Inc. (JASTEC). *Pioneer in Superconductor Technology* [online]. 2020. Available from https://www.jastec-inc.com [Accessed 15 Jun 2020].
[66] Glyavin M.Yu., Denisov G.G., Zapevalov V.E. *et al.* 'Terahertz gyrotrons: State of the art and prospects'. *Journal of Communications Technology and Electronics*. 2014; **59**: 792–797.

[67] Glyavin M.Yu., Luchinin A.G., and Golubiatnikov G.Yu. 'Generation of 1.5-kW, 1-THz coherent radiation from a gyrotron with a pulsed magnetic field'. *Physical Review Letters*. 2008; **100**: 015101.

[68] Thumm M. 'Recent advances in the world wide fusion gyrotron development'. *IEEE Transactions on Plasma Science*. 2014; **42**(3): 590–599.

[69] Thumm M. 'MW gyrotron development for fusion plasma applications'. *Plasma Physics and Controlled Fusion*. 2003; **45**: A143–161.

[70] Matsuki Y., Idehara T., Fukazawa J., and Fujiwara T. 'Advanced instrumentation for DNP-enhanced MAS NMR for higher magnetic fields and lower temperatures'. *Journal of Magnetic Resonance*. 2016; **264**: 107–115.

[71] Miyoshi N., Idehara T., Khutoryan E. *et al.* 'Combined hyperthermia and photodynamic therapy using a sub-THz gyrotron as a radiation source'. *Journal of Infrared, Millimeter and Terahertz Waves*. 2016; **37**: 805–814.

[72] Sabchevski S.P., Idehara T., Ishiyama S., Miyoshi N., and Tatsukawa T. 'A dual-beam irradiation facility for a novel hybrid cancer therapy'. *Journal of Infrared, Millimeter and Terahertz Waves*. 2013; **34**(1): 71–87.

[73] Idehara T., Ogawa I., Mori H., Kobayashi S., Mitsudo S., and Saito T. 'A THz gyrotron FU CW III with a 20T superconducting magnet'. *Journal of Plasma and Fusion Research Series*. 2009; **8**: 1508–1511.

[74] Levush B. and Antonsen T.M. 'Mode competition and control in higher-power gyrotron oscillators'. *IEEE Transactions on Plasma Science*. 1990; **18**(3): 260–272.

[75] Saito T., Tatematsu Y., Yamaguchi Y., *et al.* 'Observation of dynamic interactions between fundamental and second-harmonic modes in a high-power sub-terahertz gyrotron operating in regimes of soft and hard self-excitation'. *Physical Review Letters*. 2012; **109**(15): 155001.

[76] Zapevalov V.E., Zarnitsyna I.G., and Nusinovich G.S. 'Excitation of parasitic modes that resonate with the first harmonic of the cyclotron frequency in a gyrotron operating on a mode that resonates with the second harmonic'. *Radiophysics and Quantum Electronics*. 1979; **22**(3): 254–259.

[77] Melnikova M.M., Rozhnev A.G., Ryskin N.M. *et al.* 'Electromagnetic modeling of a complex-cavity resonator for the 0.4-THz second-harmonic frequency-tunable gyrotron'. *IEEE Transactions on Electron Devices*. 2017; **64**(12): 5141–5146.

[78] Zapevalov V.E., Malygin S.A., Pavel'ev V.G., and Tsimring S.E. 'Coupled-resonator gyrotrons with mode conversion'. *Radiophysics and Quantum Electronics*. 1984; **27**(9): 846–852.

[79] Dumbrajs O. and Borie E. 'A complex cavity with mode conversion for gyrotrons'. *International Journal of Electronics*. 1988; **65**(3): 285–295.

[80] Huang Y., Li H., Yang S., and Liu S. 'Study of a 35-GHz third-harmonic low-voltage complex cavity gyrotron'. *IEEE Transactions on Plasma Science*. 1999; **27**(2): 368–373.

[81] Tatematsu Y., Saito T., Fukunari M. *et al.* 'Experimental and numerical study of the 0.4-THz second-harmonic gyrotron with a complex-cavity

resonator'. *Proceedings of the 44th International Conference on Infrared, Millimeter, and Terahertz Waves*; Paris, France, 2019. pp. 1–2.
[82] Bratman V.L., Kalynov Y.K., and Manuilov V.N. 'Large-orbit gyrotron operation in the terahertz frequency range'. *Physical Review Letters*. 2009; **102**(24): 245101.
[83] Idehara T., Manuilov V.N., Watanabe O. *et al.* 'Electron gun for powerful large orbit gyrotron'. *International Journal of Infrared and Millimeter Waves*. 2004; **25**(1): 3–14.
[84] Zapevalov V., Idehara T., Sabchevski S. *et al.* 'Design of a large orbit gyrotron with a permanent magnet system'. *International Journal of Infrared and Millimeter Waves*. 2003; **24**(3): 253–260.
[85] Mitsudo S., Glyavin M., Khutoryan E. *et al.* 'An experimental investigation of a 0.8 THz double-beam gyrotron'. *Journal of Infrared, Millimeter, and Terahertz Waves*. 2019; **40**: 1114–1128.
[86] Idehara T., Khutoryan E.M., Tatematsu Y. *et al.* 'High-speed frequency modulation of a 460-GHz gyrotron for enhancement of 700-MHz DNP-NMR spectroscopy'. *Journal of Infrared, Millimeter, and Terahertz Waves*. 2015; **36**(9): 819–829.
[87] Idehara T., Tatematsu Y., Yamaguchi Y. *et al.* 'The development of 460 GHz gyrotrons for 700 MHz DNP-NMR spectroscopy'. *Journal of Infrared, Millimeter, and Terahertz Waves*. 2015; **36**(7): 613–627.
[88] Chang T.H., Idehara T., Ogawa I., Agusu L., and Kobayashi S. 'Frequency tunable gyrotron using backward-wave components'. *Journal of Applied Physics*. 2009; **105**: 063304.
[89] Sabchevski S. and Idehara T. 'Design of a compact sub-terahertz gyrotron for spectroscopic applications'. *Journal of Infrared, Millimeter, and Terahertz Waves*. 2010; **31**: 934–948.
[90] Mudiganti J., Idehara T., Tatematsu Y. *et al.* 'Design of a 394.6 GHz compact gyrotron FU CW CI for 600 MHz DNP-NMR spectroscopy'. *Proceedings of the 36th Int. Conf. Infrared, Millimeter THz Waves*; Houston, USA, 2011. pp. 1–2.
[91] Kuleshov A., Ishikawa Y., Tatematsu Y. *et al.* 'Low-voltage operation of the double-beam gyrotron at 400 GHz'. *IEEE Transactions on Electron Devices*. 2019; **67**(2): 673–676.
[92] Bratman V., Fedotov A., and Kalynov Y. 'Numerical study of a low-voltage gyrotron ('gyrotrino') for DNP/NMR spectroscopy'. *IEEE Transactions on Plasma Science*. 2017; **45**(4): 644–648.
[93] Sirigiri J.R. and Maly T. *Integrated high-frequency generator system utilizing the magnetic field of the target application*. U.S. Patent 8 786 284, 2014.
[94] Bratman V.L., Fedotov A.E., Kalynov Y.K., Osharin I.V., and Zavolsky N. A. 'Smooth wideband frequency tuning in low-voltage gyrotron with cathode-end power output'. *IEEE Transactions on Electron Devices*. 2017; **64**(12): 5147–5150.
[95] Yefimov B.P. and Levin G.Ya. 'Multiwave resonance BWT of clinotron type MM-radio waveband'. *International Journal of Infrared and Millimeter Waves*. 1997; **18**(11): 31–39.

[96] Kovshov Y.S., Ponomarenko S.S., Kishko S.S. *et al.* 'Effect of mode transformation in THz clinotron'. *Journal of Infrared, Millimeter, and Terahertz Waves*. 2018; **39**: 1055–1064.

[97] Xie W., Wang Z.-C., Luo J., and Zhao D. 'Three dimensional nonlinear analysis of a single-grating rectangular waveguide Cerenkov maser'. *Physics of Plasmas*. 2015; **22**(4): 042307.

[98] Kovshov Yu., Ponomarenko S., Kishko S., *et al.* 'Tracking analysis of a sheet electron beam for clinotron tube'. *Proceedings of the 17th International Conference on Mathematical Methods in Electromagnetic Theory*; Kiev, 2018. pp. 330–333.

[99] Likhachev A.A., Danik A.A., Kovshov Yu.S., *et al.* 'Effect of electron beam velocity spread in a clinotron'. *IEEE Transactions on Electron Devices*. 2019; **66**(3): 1540–1544.

[100] Buzik L.M. 'Application of the open multi-step slow-wave structures in millimeter and submillimeter wave oscillators'. *Proceedings of International Conference on Millimeter and Submillimeter Waves and Applications*; San Diego, CA, Jan 1994. SPIE; 1994. p. 225032.

[101] Buzik L.M., Pishko O.F., Churilova S.A., and Sheremet O.I. 'Dispersion characteristics of multi-step open slow-wave systems of finite width: Analysis'. *Telecommunications and Radio Engineering*. 1997; **51**(8): 77–84.

[102] Khutoryan E.M., Kovshov Y.S., Likhachev A.S. *et al.* 'Excitation of hybrid space-surface waves in clinotrons with non-uniform grating'. *Journal of Infrared, Millimeter, and Terahertz Waves*. 2018; **39**: 236–249.

[103] Ponomarenko S.S., Kishko S.A., Khutoryan E.M., Kuleshov A.N., and Yefimov B.P. 'Development of 94 GHz BWO-klynotron with 3-stage grating'. *Telecommunications and Radio Engineering*. 2014; **73**(3): 271–281.

[104] Wood R.W. 'Anomalous diffraction gratings'. *Physical Review*. 1935; **48** (12): 928–936.

[105] Lusenko E.E., Pishko O.F., Chumak V.G., and Churilova S.A. 'Current tendencies in the development of millimeter wavelength clinotrons'. *Radiofizika i Elektronika*. 2008; **13**: 315–320 (in Russian).

[106] Lysenko E.E., Pishko O.F., Chumak V.G., and Churilova S.A. 'Experimental research of clinotron with distributed quasioptical power output'. *Radio Physics and Radio Astronomy*. 1999; **4**(1): 13–19 (in Russian).

[107] Ionin B.I. and Ershov B.A. 'The fundamentals of NMR spectroscopy'. In: *NMR Spectroscopy in Organic Chemistry. Physical Methods in Organic Chemistry*. Boston, MA: Springer;1970.

[108] AIn R. *Vivo NMR Spectroscopy: Principles and Techniques*. 2nd edn. Hoboken, New Jersey: John Wiley & Sons, Ltd; 2007.

[109] Maly T., Debelouchina G.T., Bajaj V.S. *et al.* 'Dynamic nuclear polarization at high magnetic fields'. *The Journal of Chemical Physics*. 2008; **128** (5): 052211.

[110] Abragam A. and Goldman M. 'Principles of dynamic nuclear polarization'. *Reports on Progress in Physics*. 1976; **41**(3): 395–467.

[111] Akbey U., Linden A.H., and Oschkinat H. 'High-temperature dynamic nuclear polarization enhanced magic-angle-spinning NMR'. *Applied Magnetic Resonance*. 2012; **43**(1–2): 81–90.

[112] Barnes A.B., Paëpe G.D., Van Der Wel P.C.A. *et al.* 'High-field dynamic nuclear polarization for solid and solution biological NMR'. *Applied Magnetic Resonance*. 2008; **34**(3–4): 237–263.

[113] Ni Q.Z., Daviso E., Can T.V. *et al.* 'High frequency dynamic nuclear polarization'. *Accounts of Chemical Research*. 2013; **46**(9): 1933–41.

[114] Wind R.A., Duijvestijn M.J., Van Der Lugt C., Manenschijn A., and Vriend J. 'Applications of dynamic nuclear polarization in ^{13}C NMR in solids'. *Progress in Nuclear Magnetic Resonance Spectroscopy*. 1985; **17**: 33–67.

[115] Barnes A.B., Paëpe G.D., Van Der Wel P.C.A. *et al.* 'High-field dynamic nuclear polarization for solid and solution biological NMR'. *Applied Magnetic Resonance*. 2008; **34**(3–4): 237–263.

[116] Zhang Z., Huang Y., Smith P.E.S., Wang K., Cai S., and Chen Z. 'High-resolution heteronuclear multi-dimensional NMR spectroscopy in magnetic fields with unknown spatial variations'. *Journal of Magnetic Resonance*. 2014; **242**: 49–56.

[117] Chinthalapalli S., Bornet A., Segawa T.F., Sarkar R., Jannin S., and Bodenhausen G. 'Ultrahigh-resolution magnetic resonance in inhomogeneous magnetic fields: Two-dimensional long-lived-coherence correlation spectroscopy'. *Physical Review Letters*. 2012; **109**: 047602.

[118] Aue W.P., Bartholdi E., and Ernst R.R. 'Two-dimensional spectroscopy. Application to nuclear magnetic resonance'. *Journal of Chemical Physics*. 1976; **64**: 2229–2246.

[119] Martin G.E and Zekter A.S. *Two-Dimensional NMR Methods for Establishing Molecular Connectivity*. New York, NY: VCH Publishers, Inc.; 1988. p. 59.

[120] Mateescu Gh. D. *2D NMR Density Matrix and Product Operator Treatment*. PTR Prentice Hall, Englewood Cliffs, NJ.

[121] Cournia Z., Allen T.W., Andricioaei I. *et al.* 'Membrane protein structure, function, and dynamics: A perspective from experiments and theory'. *The Journal of Membrane Biology*. 2015; **248**(4): 611–640.

[122] DeToma A.S., Salamekh S., Ramamoorthy A., and Lim M.H. 'Misfolded proteins in Alzheimer's disease and type II diabetes'. *Chemical Society Reviews*. 2012; **41**(2): 608–621.

[123] Moreno-Gonzalez I. and Soto C. 'Misfolded protein aggregates: Mechanisms, structures and potential for disease transmission'. *Seminars in Cell & Developmental Biology*. 2011; **22**(5): 482–487.

[124] Ellisdon A.M. and Bottomley S.P. 'The role of protein misfolding in the pathogenesis of human diseases'. *IUBMB Life*. 2004; **56**(3): 119–123.

[125] Stefani M. 'Protein misfolding and aggregation: New examples in medicine and biology of the dark side of the protein world'. *Biochimica et Biophysica Acta (BBA)-Molecular Basis of Disease*. 2004; **1739**(1): 5–25.

[126] Emwas A.-H., Roy R., McKay R.T. *et al.* 'NMR spectroscopy for metabolomics research'. *Metabolites*. 2019; **9**(7): 123.

[127] Larive C.K., Barding G.A., and Dinges M.M. 'NMR spectroscopy for metabolomics and metabolic profiling'. *Analytical Chemistry*. 2014; **87**(1): 133–146.

[128] Savorani F., Rasmussen M.A., Mikkelsen M.S., and Engelsen S.B. 'A primer to nutritional metabolomics by NMR spectroscopy and chemometrics'. *Food Research International*. 2013; **54**(1): 1131–1145.

[129] Kruk J., Doskocz M., Jodłowska E. *et al.* 'NMR techniques in metabolomic studies: A quick overview on examples of utilization'. *Applied Magnetic Resonance*. 2016; **48**(1): 1–21.

[130] Roessner U. and Bowne J. 'What is metabolomics all about?'. *BioTechniques*. 2009; **46**(5): 363–365.

[131] Duarte L.F. and Gil A.M. 'Metabolic signatures of cancer unveiled by NMR spectroscopy of human biofluids'. *Progress in Nuclear Magnetic Resonance Spectroscopy*. 2012; **62**: 51–74.

[132] Capati A., Ijare O., and Bezabeh T. 'Diagnostic applications of nuclear magnetic resonance–based urinary metabolomics'. *Magnetic Resonance Insights*. 2017; **10**: 1178623X17694346.

[133] Neild G.H., Foxall P.J., Lindon J.C., Holmes E.C., and Nicholson J.K. 'Uroscopy in the 21st century: High-field NMR spectroscopy'. *Nephrology Dialysis Transplantation*. 1997; **12**: 404–417.

[134] Beckonert O., Keun H., Ebbels T. *et al.* 'Metabolic profiling, metabolomic and metabonomic procedures for NMR spectroscopy of urine, plasma, serum and tissue extracts'. *Nature Protocols*. 2007; **2**: 2692–2703.

[135] Kim E., Kwon H., Nam H., Kim J., Park S., and Kim Y. 'Urine-NMR metabolomics for screening of advanced colorectal adenoma and early stage colorectal cancer'. *Scientific Reports*. 2019; **9**: 4786.

[136] Gupta A., Dwivedi M., Mahdi A.A., Gowda G.A.N., Khetrapal C.L., and Bhandari M. '1H-nuclear magnetic resonance spectroscopy for identifying and quantifying common uropathogens: A metabolic approach to the urinary tract infection'. *BJU International*. 2009; **104**(2): 236–244.

[137] Zhang Z., Smith P.E.S., and Frydman L. 'Reducing acquisition times in multidimensional NMR with a time-optimized Fourier encoding algorithm'. *The Journal of Chemical Physics*. 2014; **141**(19): 194201.

[138] Nanni E.A., Barnes A.B., Griffin R.G., and Temkin R.J. 'THz dynamic nuclear polarization NMR'. *IEEE Transactions on Terahertz Science and Technology*. 2011; **1**(1): 145–163.

[139] Becerra L.R., Gerfen G.J., Temkin R.J., Singel D.J., and Griffin R.G. 'Dynamic nuclear polarization with a cyclotron resonance maser at 5T'. *Physical Review Letters*. 1993; **71**(21): 3561–3564.

[140] Bajaj V., Farrar C., Hornstein M. *et al.* 'Dynamic nuclear polarization at 9T using a novel 250 GHz gyrotron microwave source'. *Journal of Magnetic Resonance*. 2003; **160**(2): 85–90.

[141] Kreischer K., Farrar C., Griffin R., Temkin R., and Vieregg J. 'A 250 GHz gyrotron for NMR spectroscopy'. *Proceedings of the 27th Int. IEEE Plasma Sci. Conf. Rec.*; 2000. p. 198.

[142] Khutoryan E.M., Idehara T., Kuleshov A.N. *et al.* 'Gyrotron output power stabilization by PID feedback control of heater current and anode voltage'. *Journal of Infrared, Millimeter, and Terahertz Waves*. 2014; **35**(12): 1018–1029.

[143] Glyavin M.Y., Denisov G.G., Kulygin M.L. *et al.* 'Stabilization of gyrotron frequency by reflection from nonresonant and resonant loads'. *Technical Physics Letters* 2015; **41**(7): 628–631.

[144] Melnikova M.M., Rozhnev A.G., Ryskin N.M. *et al.* 'Frequency stabilization of a 0.67-THz gyrotron by self-injection locking'. *IEEE Transactions on Electron Devices*. 2016; **63**: 1288–1293.

[145] Golubiatnikov G.Yu., Krupnov A.F., Lubyako L.V., *et al.* 'Gyrotron frequency control by a phase lock system'. *Technical Physics Letters*. 2006; **32**: 650–652.

[146] Khutoryan E.M., Idehara T., Kuleshov A.N. *et al.* 'Stabilization of gyrotron frequency by PID feedback control on the acceleration voltage'. *Journal of Infrared, Millimeter, and Terahertz Waves*. 2015; **36**(12): 1157–1163.

[147] Zotova I.V., Ginzburg N.S., Denisov G.G. *et al.* 'Frequency locking and stabilization regimes in high-power gyrotrons with low-Q resonators'. *Radiophysics and Quantum Electronics*. 2016; **58**(9): 684–693.

[148] Glyavin M.Y., Denisov G.G., Kulygin M.L. *et al.* 'Gyrotron frequency stabilization by a weak reflected wave'. *Radiophysics and Quantum Electronics*. 2016; **58**(9): 673–683.

[149] Hovav Y., Feintuch A., Vega S., and Goldfarb D. 'Dynamic nuclear polarization using frequency modulation at 3.34 T'. *Journal of Magnetic Resonance*. 2014; **238**: 94–105.

[150] Abdelmohsen M.A., Omar W.M., and Shaaban A. 'Rectal operative bed: ? tumor? post-management changes … positron emission tomography/computed tomography (PET/CT) can answer'. *Egyptian Journal of Radiology and Nuclear Medicine*. 2020; **51**(20): 10.1186/s43055-020-0139-z.

[151] Sun Y., Brauckmann O., Nixdorf D. *et al.* 'Imaging human teeth by phosphorus magnetic resonance with nuclear Overhauser enhancement'. *Scientific Reports*. 2016; **6**: 30756.

[152] Giacomelli G., Yoshitake T., Cahill L.C. *et al.* 'Multiscale nonlinear microscopy and wide field white light imaging enables rapid histological imaging of surgical specimen margins'. *Biomedical Optics Express*. 2018; **9**: 2457–2475.

[153] Idehara T., Sabchevski S.P., Glyavin M., and Mitsudo S. 'The gyrotrons as promising radiation sources for THz sensing and imaging'. *Applied Sciences*. 2020; **10**: 980.

[154] Karagoz B., Altan H., and Kamburoglu K. 'Terahertz pulsed imaging study of dental caries'. *Proceedings of Medical Laser Applications and Laser-Tissue Interactions VII*; Munich, Germany, Jul 2015. SPIEl; 2015. 95420N.

[155] Sleiman J. 'Terahertz imaging and spectroscopy: Application to defense and security in front of the examination panel'. *Eng.D. dissertation*, Université de Bordeaux, Bordeaux, France, 2016.

[156] Baek I.-K. 'Terahertz spectroscopic study on hydration dynamics of the human skin'. *Ph.D. dissertation*, Seoul National University, Seoul, South Korea, 2017.

[157] Bajwa N., Nowroozi B., Sung S. *et al.* 'Reflective THz and MR imaging of burn wounds: A potential clinical validation of THz contrast mechanisms'. *Proceedings of Terahertz Emitters, Receivers, and Applications III*; San Diego, CA, 2012. SPIE; 2013. 84960X.

[158] Smirnov S.V., Grachev Ya.V., Tsypkin A.N., and Bespalov V.G. 'Experimental studies of the possibilities of diagnosing caries in the solid tissues of a tooth by means of terahertz radiation'. *Journal of Optical Technology*. 2014; **81**: 464–467.

[159] Alabaster C.M. The microwave properties of tissue and other lossy dielectrics, PhD thesis, Cranfield University, 2004.

[160] Clothier R. and Bourne N. 'Effects of THz exposure on human primary keratinocyte differentiation and viability'. *Journal of Biological Physics*. 2003; **29**: 179–185.

[161] Zeni O., Gallerano G.P., Perrotta A., Romanò M., Lai A., and Messina G. 'Cytogenetic observations in human peripheral blood leukocytes following in vitro exposure to THz radiation: A pilot study'. *Health Physics*. 2007; **92**(4): 349–357.

[162] Zaytsev K.I., Dolganova I.N., Chernomyrdin N.V. *et al.* 'The progress and perspectives of terahertz technology for diagnosis of neoplasms: A review'. *Journal of Optics*. 2019; **22**(1): 013001.

[163] Sitnikov D.S., Ilina I.V., Revkova V.A. *et al.* 'System for long-term irradiation of living cell culture with high-intensity THz pulses'. *High Temperature*. 2020; **58**: 36–43.

[164] Borovkova M., Serebriakova M., Fedorov V. *et al.* 'Investigation of terahertz radiation influence on rat glial cells'. *Biomedical Optics Express*. 2017; **8**: 273–280.

[165] Mazor R., Korenstein-Ilan A., Barbul A. *et al.* 'Increased levels of numerical chromosome aberrations after *in vitro* exposure of human peripheral blood lymphocytes to radiofrequency electromagnetic fields for 72 hours'. *Radiation Research*. 2008; **169**(1): 28–37.

[166] Toptica. *Terahertz Technologies: Systems and Accessories* [online]. 2020. Available from https://www.toptica.com [Accessed 15 Jun 2020].

[167] TeraView. *Terahertz Applications: Pharmaceutical* [online]. 2020. Available from https://teraview.com/pharmaceutical [Accessed 15 Jun 2020].

[168] Pickwell E., Cole B.E., Fitzgerald A.J., Pepper M, and Wallace V.P. 'In vivo study of human skin using pulsed terahertz radiation'. *Physics in Medicine & Biology*. 2004; **49**(9): 1595–1607.

[169] Vilagosh Z., Lajevardipour A., and Wood A.W. 'Computational absorption and reflection studies of normal human skin at 0.45 THz'. *Biomedical Optics Express*. 2020; **11**: 417–431.

[170] Titova L.V., Ayesheshim A.K., Golubov A. *et al.* 'Intense picosecond THz pulses alter gene expression in human skin tissue in vivo'. *Proceedings of Terahertz and Ultrashort Electromagnetic Pulses for Biomedical Applications*; San Francisco, CA, Feb 2013. SPIE; 2013. 85850Q.

[171] Klier J., Torosyan G., Schreiner N.S. *et al.* 'Influence of substrate material on radiation characteristics of THz photoconductive emitters'. *International Journal of Antennas and Propagation*. 2015; **2015**: 540175.

[172] Taylor Z.D., Singh R.S., Culjat M.O. *et al.* 'Reflective terahertz imaging of porcine skin burns'. *Optics Letters*. 2008; **33**: 1258–1260.

[173] Mejía A.F.E., Bava J.A., and Tocho J.O. 'Image detection with pyroelectric sensors'. *Proceedings of the XVII Workshop on Information Processing and Control*; Mar del Plata, 2017. pp. 1–4.

[174] Bauer M., Rämer A., Chevtchenko S.A., *et al.* 'A high-sensitivity AlGaN/GaN HEMT terahertz detector with integrated broadband bow-tie antenna'. *IEEE Transactions on Terahertz Science and Technology*. 2019; **9**(4): 430–444.

[175] Saqueb S. and Sertel K. 'Multisensor compressive sensing for high frame-rate imaging system in the THz band'. *IEEE Transactions on Terahertz Science and Technology*. 2019; **9**(5): 520–523.

[176] Gao Y., Charles J.R., Yu G. *et al.* 'Design and measurement of a digital phase locked BWO for accurately extracting the quality factors in a biconcave resonator system'. *Journal of Infrared, Millimeter, and Terahertz Waves*. 2012; **33**: 357–365.

[177] Khutoryan E.M., Idehara T., Kuleshov A.N., *et al.* 'Gyrotron output frequency and power stabilization by PID feedback control on the acceleration and anode voltages'. *Proceedings of the 41st International Conference on Infrared, Millimeter, and Terahertz Waves*; Copenhagen, 2016. pp. 1–2.

[178] Safian R., Ghazi G., and Mohammadian N. 'Review of photomixing continuous-wave terahertz systems and current application trends in terahertz domain'. *Optical Engineering*. 2019; **58**(11): 110901.

[179] Karpowicz N., Zhong H., Xu J., Lin K.-I., Hwang J.-S., and Zhang X.-C. 'Comparison between pulsed terahertz time-domain imaging and continuous wave terahertz imaging'. *Semiconductor Science and Technology*. 2005; **20**(7): S293–S299.

[180] Vilagosh Z, Lajevardipour A, and Wood A.W. 'Computational phantom study of frozen melanoma imaging at 0.45 terahertz'. *Bioelectromagnetics*. 2019; **40**(2): 118–127.

[181] Danciu M, Alexa-Stratulat T., Stefanescu C. *et al.* 'Terahertz spectroscopy and imaging: A cutting-edge method for diagnosing digestive cancers'. *Materials (Basel)*. 2019; **12**(9): 1519.

[182] Dobroiu A., Yamashita M., Ohshima Y.N., Morita Y., Otani C., and Kawase K. 'The backward wave oscillator as a radiation source in terahertz imaging'. *Infrared and Millimeter Waves, Conference Digest of the 2004 Joint 29th International Conference on 2004 and 12th International Conference on Terahertz Electronics*; Karlsruhe, Germany, 2004. pp. 825–826.

[183] Boutaayamou M., Cerica D., and Verly J. 'Terahertz reflection imaging of paraffin-embedded human breast cancer samples: Some first results'. *Proceedings of the 13th International Joint Conference on Biomedical Engineering Systems and Technologies*; Valletta, Malta, Feb 2020. pp. 200–203.

[184] Chen G., Pei J., Yang F., Zhou X.Y., Sun Z.L., and Cui T.J. 'Terahertz-wave imaging system based on backward wave oscillator'. *IEEE Transactions on Terahertz Science and Technology*. 2012; **2**(5): 504–512.

[185] Dobroiu A., Yamashita M., Ohshima Y.N., Morita Y., Otani C., and Kawase K. 'Terahertz imaging system based on a backward-wave oscillator'. *Applied Optics*. 2004; **43**: 5637–5646.

[186] Wong T.M., Kahl M., Haring Bolívar P. *et al.* 'Computational image enhancement for frequency modulated continuous wave (FMCW) THz image'. *Journal of Infrared, Millimeter, and Terahertz Waves*. 2019; **40**: 775–800.

[187] Tripathi S.R., Sugiyama Y., Murate K., Imayama K., and Kawase K. 'Terahertz wave three-dimensional computed tomography based on injection-seeded terahertz wave parametric emitter and detector'. *Optics Express*. 2016; **24**: 6433–6440.

[188] Balbekin N.S., Kulya M.S., Belashov A.V. *et al.* 'Increasing the resolution of the reconstructed image in terahertz pulse time-domain holography'. *Scientific Reports*. 2019; **9**: 180.

[189] Woodward R.M., Cole B.E., Wallace V.P. *et al.* 'Terahertz pulse imaging in reflection geometry of human skin cancer and skin tissue'. *Physics in Medicine & Biology*. 2002; **47**(21): 3853–3863.

[190] Guillet J.P., Recur B., Frederique L. *et al.* 'Review of terahertz tomography techniques'. *Journal of Infrared, Millimeter, and Terahertz Waves*. 2014; **35**: 382–411.

[191] Sun Y., Sy M., Wang Y., Ahuja A., Zhang Y., and Pickwell-Macpherson E. 'A promising diagnostic method: Terahertz pulsed imaging and spectroscopy'. *World Journal of Radiology*. 2011; **3**(3): 55–65.

[192] Theofanopoulos P.C., Sakr M., and Trichopoulos G.C. 'Multistatic terahertz imaging using the radon transform'. *IEEE Transactions on Antennas and Propagation*. 2019; **67**(4): 2700–2709.

[193] Theofanopoulos P.C. and Trichopoulos G.C. 'A novel THz radar imaging system using the radon transform'. *Proceedings of 2017 IEEE International Symposium on Antennas and Propagation & USNC/URSI National Radio Science Meeting*; San Diego, CA, 2017. pp. 1513–1514.

[194] Valzania L., Zhao Y., Rong L. *et al.* 'THz coherent lensless imaging'. *Applied Optics*. 2019; **58**: G256–G275.

Chapter 4
UWB antennas for medical imaging applications

Khalil H. Sayidmarie[1] *and Yasser A. Alsaidosh*[2]

4.1 Introduction

The introduction of the ultra-wideband (UWB) technology opened new horizons into wireless communications as it offered high data rates that were achieved by the transmission over a wide spectrum at a very low-power spectral density. One of the most important parts of the UWB systems is the antenna which is at the forefront of the system. Thus, the UWB antenna is required to have an acceptable gain and radiation pattern across the whole UWB frequency range. This, in turn, means that the input impedance of the UWB antenna must be almost constant within the UWB frequency range to minimize reflections from the antenna that reduces the delivered power. Although the UWB antenna can be realized in either planar or nonplanar structures, the planar design is preferable due to its small size, mechanical rigidity, and easier integration. Therefore, this chapter considers planar UWB antennas that were proposed to serve many applications, including UWB imaging.

4.2 Medical imaging systems

The microwave imaging systems utilize the differences in the electrical properties of the region to be imaged and the surrounding. For example, tumor detection relies on the fact that malignant cells have different dielectric properties from those of healthy tissues. Therefore, the transmission and reflection of microwaves through the imaged region are used to reconstruct an image. This image has to display clearly the differences in the electrical properties across the intended region. The shown variations should have adequate spatial resolution such that a better localization is achieved. Of equal importance is that the image should present minimal changes, defined as image contrast to convey adequate diagnostic information.

In the microwave imaging systems, whether they are for general applications or for particular medical applications, the antennas are very important parts that are at the forefront of the imaging system. The transmit/receive antennas have to be

[1]College of Electronic Engineering, Nineveh University, Nineveh, Iraq
[2]College of Engineering, University of Duhok, Duhok, Iraq

mechanically scanned across a two-dimensional region to acquire enough data to reconstruct a meaningful image. Another more convenient alternative to mechanical scanning is to operate the system over a certain band of frequencies that is necessary to attain the required image resolution. Thus, mechanical scanning can be replaced by frequency scanning. Very narrow pulses can also be sent through the suspected area of human tissue. Frequency- and time-domain operations are considered dual concepts in electrical systems in general and in imaging systems, and thus data acquisition can be performed in either of the two domains. Other modalities of microwave imaging use a number of antennas arranged on a ring around the region to be imaged, and the transmit/receive response is acquired over a wide band of frequencies [1–4].

In order to obtain a high spatial resolution, the antennas must be able to radiate signals over a broad range of frequencies while maintaining the fidelity of the waveform over the operation band. Therefore, there is a need for UWB antennas that are compact, efficient, and properly matched across the operation band.

4.3 Fractal UWB antennas

Since the adoption of UWB systems by the federal communications commission in 2002, extensive work has been performed on the development of the UWB antennas. Among the important features of the UWB antennas are their very wide bandwidth (3.1–10.6 GHz), small size, moderate gain, and even planar structure. These features are very desirable in the microwave imaging systems. The microstrip printed antenna can offer such features if the problem of the narrow bandwidth is solved. Many solutions were presented, such as using various shapes for the patch to attain enough aspect or area to furnish multimode surface current on the conducting surface. This will result in multiband resonances that extend the bandwidth to cover the entire UWB range. In the following sections, two solutions are presented.

A large impedance bandwidth (BW) can be achieved by exploiting the concept of multi-resonance elements, such as deploying a few printed monopole antennas [5]. Another technique utilized the fractal concept to produce a multiband performance covering a wider band [6]. This technique and others were mixed with few methods such as corner trimming, tapered ground plane, and gradual change of the width of the feed line that achieve matching across a wider band. Obviously, when more than one idea is used in the same design, it will not be easy to differentiate between their effects, and hence their benefits may not be fully utilized. A tree-shaped monopole, formed by staggering a number of squares and thus can be considered a fractal geometry, was presented in [7] for the enhancement of the antenna bandwidth.

In this section, the fractal concept is applied using patches of rectangular and triangular shapes to generate fractal with two iterations into the design of a new UWB monopole named fractal monopole antenna. The repetition of the shape results in a multi-resonance operation that leads to a wider bandwidth compared to the single (conventional) monopole antennas [8,9].

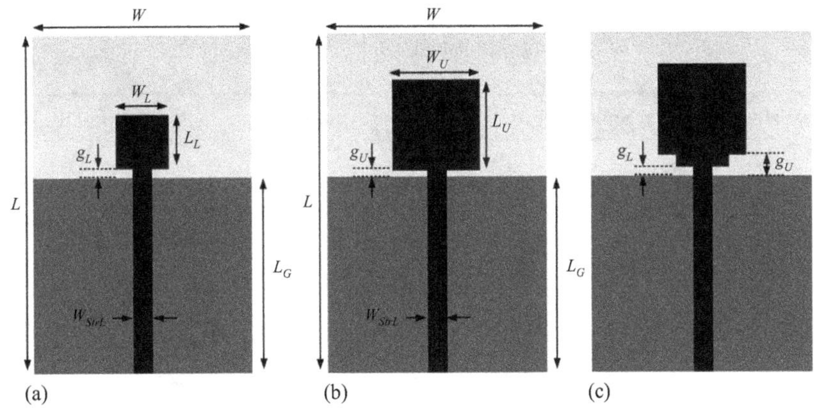

Figure 4.1 Geometry of the rectangular monopoles, showing small (a), large (b), and fractal monopole (c) [9]

4.3.1 The fractal rectangular monopole antenna

The fractal concept is applied here to the rectangular monopole [8,9]. The geometries, shown in Figure 4.1(a)–(c), illustrate the small patch, large patch, and the combined patches (double rectangle) or fractal monopole. These antennas were designed using the FR4 substrate whose parameters and design dimensions are as listed in Table 4.1. The parameters g_L, g_U, W_{StrL}, and the ratio between the dimensions of the large and small rectangles have been optimized manually to achieve better matching for the fractal monopole. The ratio of sizes $L_U/L_L = W_U/W_L = 1.666$, which is the used scaling factor.

The variations of the reflection coefficients with frequencies for the three antennas are illustrated in Figure 4.2. It is obvious that the larger rectangle has better performance at the lower side of the band, while the smaller rectangle has better performance across the higher frequencies of the band.

Combining the large and small rectangles that have two different resonance frequencies, corresponding to their sizes, has produced a multi-resonance performance. This explains the achieved bandwidth enhancement for the fractal rectangular monopole across the UWB frequency range and beyond. The response has a first band extending from 2.58 to 12.26 GHz, which exceeds the UWB requirement. The second band extends from 12.53 GHz up to more than 18 GHz.

The two rectangles give two responses that are superpositioned to yield the composite response of the fractal monopole. The idea of superposition can be considered the first-degree approximation here since it ignores the mutual coupling between the two patches. The current distributions at the resonance frequencies are illustrated in Figure 4.3, where it can be seen that the current density at the large rectangle is higher over the lower frequencies, and it is higher on the small rectangle at the upper frequencies. These results confirm that the larger rectangle influences the lower part of the band of operation, while the smaller rectangle works on the upper part of the band.

Table 4.1 Comparison of design parameters and performance of the small, large, and fractal rectangular monopoles [9]

Parameter (mm)	Small patch	Large patch	Fractal patch
L	48	48	48
L_L	7.2	–	7.2
L_U	–	12	12
L_G	26	26	26
W	40	40	40
W_L	7.2	–	7.2
W_U	–	12	12
W_{StrL}	2.6	2.6	2.6
g_L	1.2	–	1.2
g_U	–	0.8	2.8
FR4 substrate (GHz)	Thickness = 1.6 mm, ε_r = 4.3, loss tangent = 0.025, copper thickness = 0.035 mm		
f_{min}	4.4	3.27	2.58
f_{max}	>18	12.11	12.26
BW	>13.6	8.84	9.68
f_{max}/f_{min}	>4.09:1	3.70:1	4.75:1

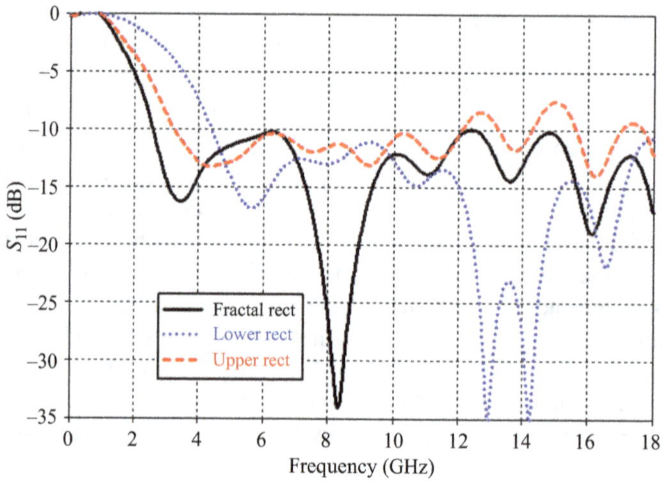

Figure 4.2 Variations of the reflection coefficients with frequencies for small, large, and fractal rectangular monopole antennas [9]

The phase responses of the reflection coefficients were found from the calculated reflection coefficients as arg(S_{11}). Figure 4.4 shows the phase responses for the two patches, where it can be seen that both phases have the same trend of variation. To have a better insight into the obtained results, the difference between the two responses, i.e.,

phase of the large patch – phase of the small patch

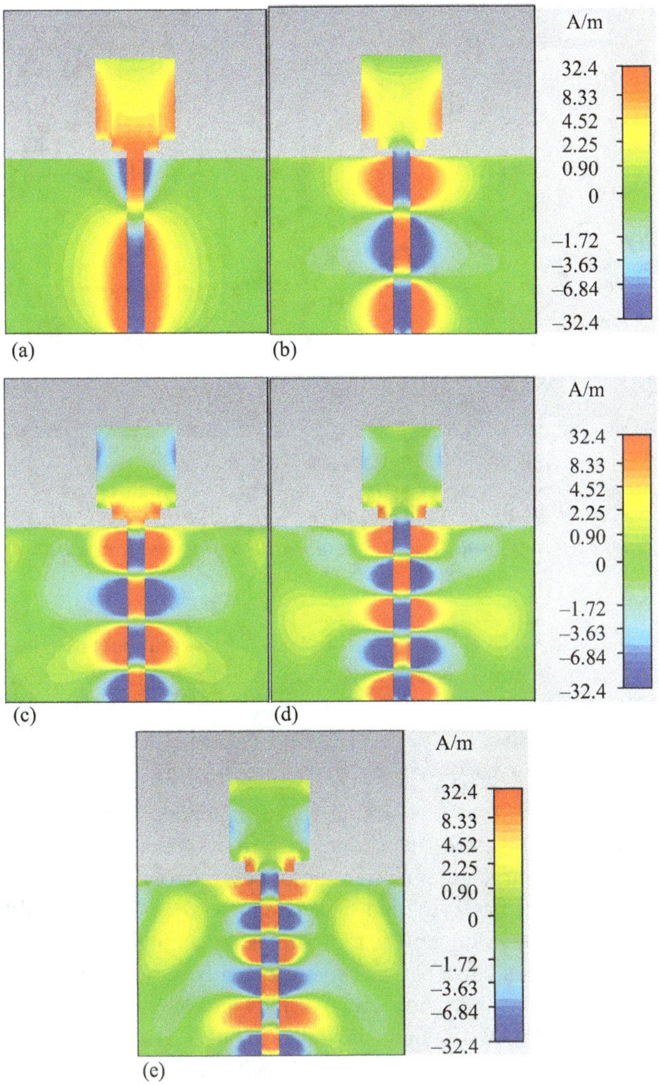

Figure 4.3 The surface current distribution of the fractal rectangular monopole antenna at the resonance frequencies of (a) 3.45, (b) 8.28, (c) 11.07, (d) 13.62, and (e) 16.14 GHz [8]

was calculated and displayed on the same figure (black continuous line). The results show that across the frequency range of 2–4 GHz, there is a general reduction in the magnitude ($|S_{11}|$) of the reflection coefficient, as well as smaller ripples in the phase response. Then the improvement in ($|S_{11}|$) diminishes at about 5 GHz, where there is no phase difference. In the range of 7–9 GHz, there is another negative peak in the phase difference. Therefore, there is a dip in $|S_{11}|$. Finally,

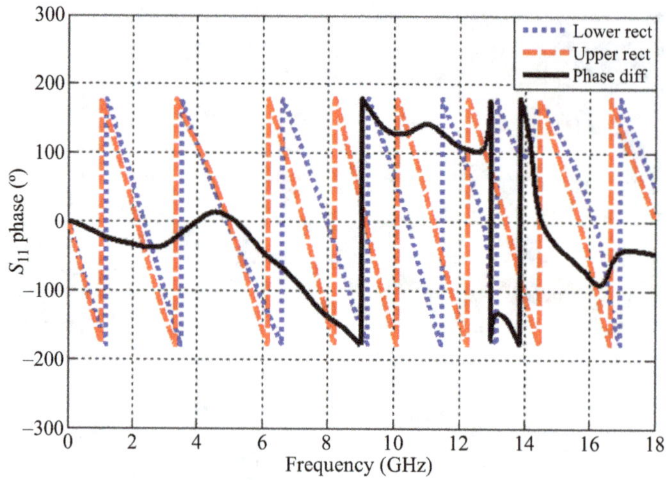

Figure 4.4 Variations of the reflection coefficient phases with frequencies for small, large, and fractal rectangular monopole antennas [9]

in the range of 12–15 GHz, the reduction in $|S_{11}|$ is marginal because the magnitude of the small patch response is too low to contribute to the reduction as shown in Figure 4.2.

4.3.2 The fractal triangular monopole antenna

The proposed idea in the previous section was also applied to the triangular monopole [8,9], where the suggested fractal antenna is a combination of two triangles of different sizes. The two triangular (lower and upper) monopoles have been designed as shown in Figure 4.5(a) and (b), and their parameters are listed in Table 4.2. The performance of the fractal monopole was optimized by tuning the design dimensions. When applying the fractal concept here, one has to choose whether the two triangles have a common vertex (as in Figure 4.5(c)) or they have equal slopes of the sides (as in Figure 4.5(d)), and the two designs were investigated. The design of the common vertex offers two different slopes of the triangle sides, and hence it is anticipated that the design will give a better performance. Figure 4.6 shows the magnitude of the reflection coefficients $|S_{11}|$ for the common vertex configuration for lower, upper, and fractal monopoles. The figure shows that the response of the fractal monopole shares almost the same performance with that of the lower triangle at higher frequencies, while it shares the same performance of the upper triangle at the lower part of the band. Thus, each of the two triangles covers a part of the frequency of the fractal monopole, as they behave as multi-resonance elements. The achieved result of using the fractal monopole is a wider bandwidth.

The phases of the reflection coefficients have been calculated using a similar procedure to that used in the previous section and then displayed in Figure 4.7. It is obvious that there are two negative peaks in the frequency range from 10 to

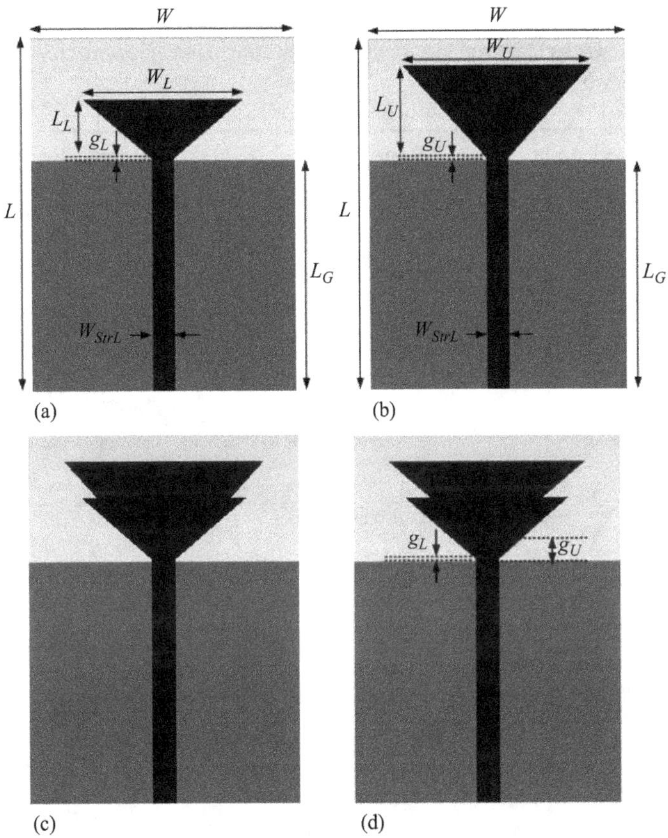

Figure 4.5 Geometry of the triangular monopole antennas, showing lower triangular monopole (a), upper triangular monopole (b), fractal triangular monopole with the same vertex (c) and same slope (d) [9]

16 GHz. Therefore, good reduction can be noticed in the magnitude of the reflection coefficient $|S_{11}|$ of the fractal triangle monopole.

In the other fractal design, the monopole sides have the same slope, and it was investigated, and the obtained results are compared with those of the common vertex monopole, as shown in Figure 4.8. It is obvious that the common vertex configuration shows enhanced performance for the frequencies above 9 GHz as compared to that designed with the same slope. These results are due to the fact that the common vertex shape offers two slopes, and hence one more degree of design freedom. However, the other design of the same slope has inherently one slope. The slope of the lower part of the monopole highly influences the electric field in the active region between monopole and the ground plane. Figures 4.9 shows the current distributions for the triangular monopole with the common vertex, while Figure 4.10 shows that for the monopole with the same slope at their corresponding

Table 4.2 Comparison of the design parameters and obtained frequency characteristics of the lower, upper, and fractal triangular monopole antennas [9]

Parameter (mm)	Lower	Upper	Fractal common vertex	Fractal same slope
L	40	40	40	40
L_L	6.6	–	6.6	6.6
L_U	–	10.6	10.6	10.6
L_G	26.2	26.2	26.2	26.2
W	30	30	30	30
W_L	18	–	18	18
W_U	–	22	22	22
W_{StrL}	3	3	3	3
g_L	0.2	–	0.2	0.2
g_U	–	0.2	0.2	2.7
FR4 substrate (GHz)	Thickness = 1.6 mm, ε_r = 4.3, loss tangent = 0.025, copper thickness = 0.035 mm			
$f_{\min}$	3.79	2.67	2.72	2.72
$f_{\max}$	9.03	5.64	>18	11.82
BW	5.24	2.97	15.28	9.1
$f_{\max}/f_{\min}$	2.38:1	2.11:1	6.62:1	4.35:1

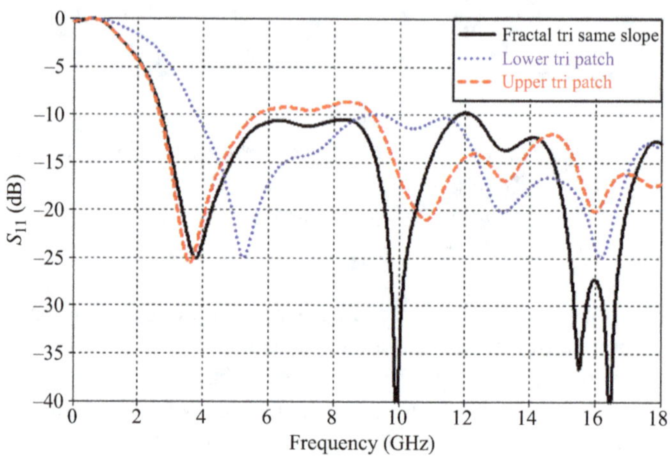

Figure 4.6 Variations of the reflection coefficients with frequencies for lower, upper, and fractal monopole with same slope monopole antennas [9]

resonant frequencies. The two figures show that at the lower frequencies the current has higher density on the large portions on the triangular patches, while at the higher frequencies larger current density is noticed at the smaller portion on the triangular patch. This fractal shape offers many possibilities for the current to be

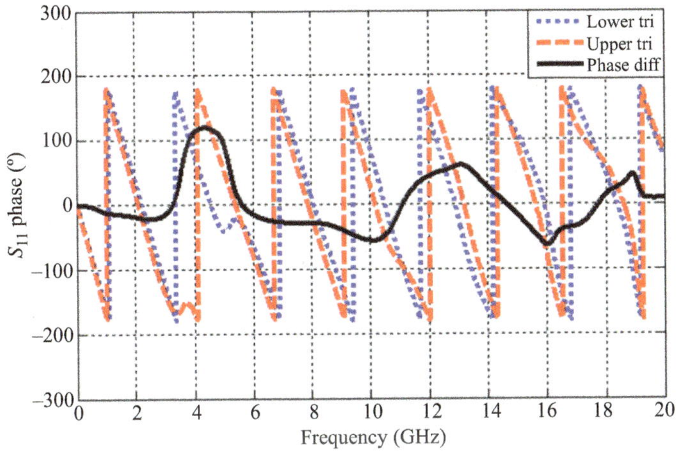

Figure 4.7 Variations of the reflection coefficient phases with frequencies for lower, upper, and fractal triangular monopole antennas [9]

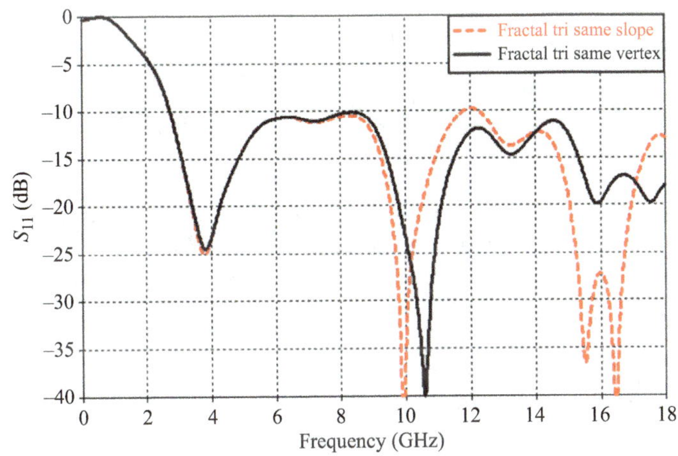

Figure 4.8 Comparison of reflection coefficient curves for the same slope and the common vertex fractal triangular monopole antennas [9]

distributed in half-wavelength forms, where the wavelength at the operating frequency corresponds to certain dimension of the monopole.

4.4 The self-complementary UWB antennas

The self-complementary ideas date back to the 1940s when Yasuto Mushiake suggested using the self-complementary principle to design constant impedance

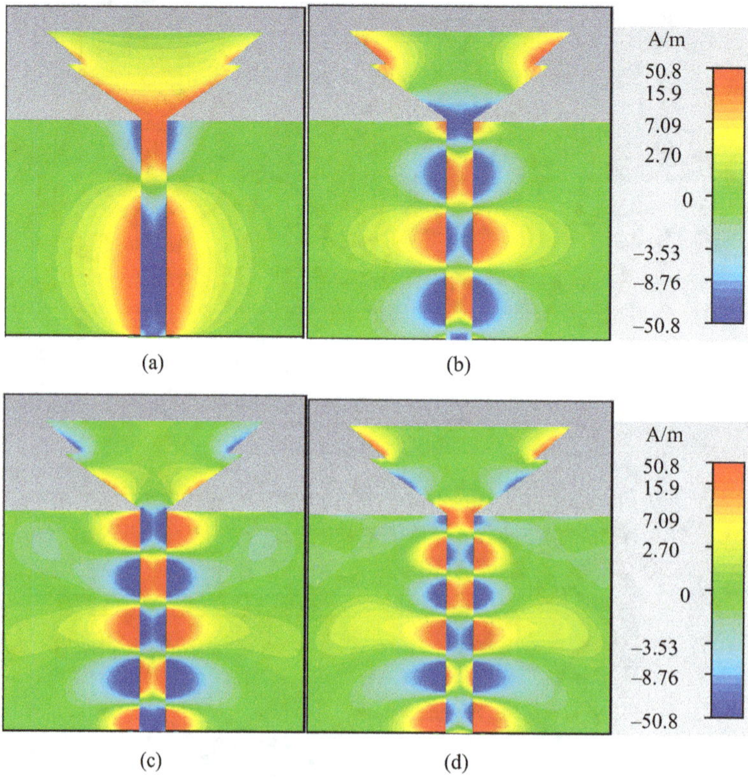

Figure 4.9 The surface current distribution of the common vertex fractal triangular monopole antennas at the resonance frequencies of (a) 3.8, (b) 10.58, (c) 13.22, and (d) 15.82 GHz [8]

antennas [10], and then Booker in 1946 extended and generalized the Babinet principle considering the vector nature of the electromagnetic (e.m.) fields [11]. In the 1950s, a major breakthrough was achieved by Rumsey in designing the frequency-independent antennas [12]. In 2009, Guo *et al.* applied the self-complementary concept into the design of UWB antennas with extended bandwidth [13], but the capabilities of the idea were not fully utilized. Although microstrip antennas inherently suffer from bandwidth limitation, which raises difficulties in using them in UWB designs, good classical broadbanding techniques can be used in the design of the planar UWB antennas.

The last decade has witnessed significant research activities in the field of UWB antennas. Among a large number of UWB antenna configurations are a planar volcano-smoke slot antenna [14,15], triangular monopole [16], circular, and elliptical disk monopoles [17,18]. The dipole geometry was also investigated to obtain the UWB characteristics, where square, triangular, circular, and other shapes for the two arms have been used [19,20]. Most of the presented designs have

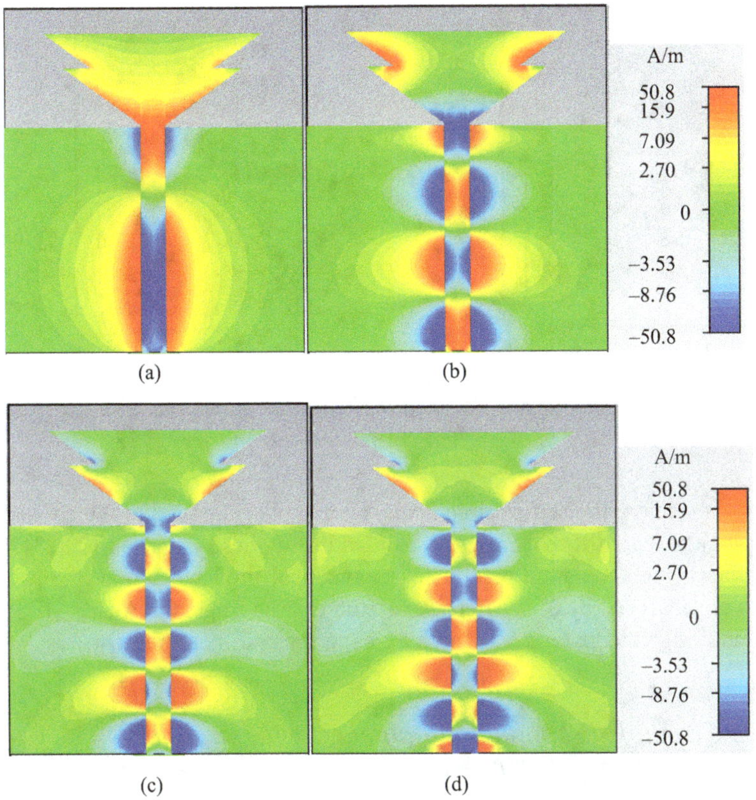

Figure 4.10 The surface current distributions of the same slope fractal triangular monopole antennas at the resonance frequencies of (a) 3.78, (b) 9.92, (c) 15.52, and (d) 16.46 GHz [8]

benefited from the recent powerful e.m. simulation software to get designs by sort of trial and error methods. The desired UWB characteristics were obtained by tailoring corners, tips, slots, or adding parasitic elements. Other designs have used optimization techniques such as particle swarm optimization procedure [21] to get the proper dimensions and shapes. Some of the published designs have very complicated geometries, and dimensions that are sensitive to the fabrication tolerances, and thus may not be realized practically. Nevertheless, some other methods that can be exploited were, unfortunately, rarely used. One of these methods uses the principle of self-complementary antennas. An antenna built in a complementary structure of magnetic and electric currents exhibits real impedance that is almost independent of frequency [10]. Some researchers had applied this principle into the design of UWB antennas with a good bandwidth, as that by Guo *et al.* [13]. However, the efforts seemed to obtain miniaturization rather than enhancing the impedance bandwidth.

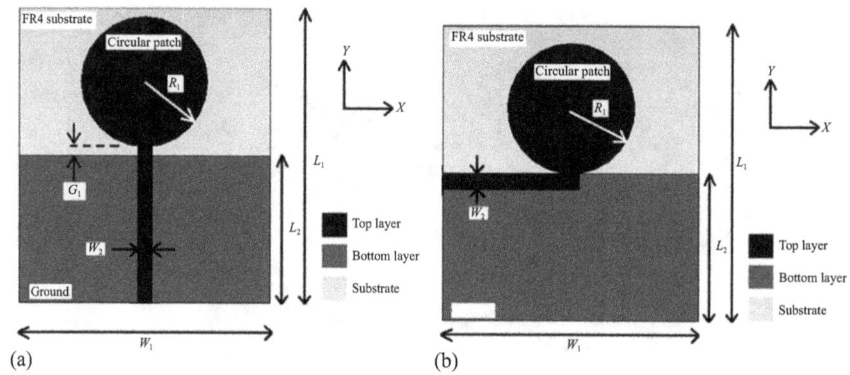

Figure 4.11 Geometry of the conventional circular monopole antenna-i (a) and the modified one with bent-feeder antenna-ii (b) [22]

In this section, the self-complementary principle is applied to the circular disk and triangular patch to enhance the bandwidth of these antennas [22,23]. For a validation of the simulation results before practical implementation, the proposed designs are analyzed by CST Microwave Studio^{TM} package, the Ansoft HFSS. The proposed designs have been validated by experimental measurements.

4.4.1 Circular disk monopole antenna with straight microstrip feed line—antenna-i

The first proposed design of the UWB antenna is a monopole having a circular shape, as shown in Figure 4.11(a). For the disk monopoles, it is difficult to identify the resonating modes of the antenna on the Smith chart in the traditional way and the criterion is that at resonance the reactance vanishes to zero, and the resistance approaches 50 Ω. However, dips in the reflection coefficient ($|S_{11}| \ll -10$ dB), which indicate the best impedance matching at certain frequencies, can indicate the resonances. The first resonance frequency can be determined by the diameter of the disk, which is about 1/4 the wavelength in air [16]. By considering the effects of feed-gap length and the relative dielectric constant of the substrate, a correction factor was given in [24].

The geometry of the printed monopole antenna that is illustrated in Figure 4.11 (a) has been simulated assuming a dielectric FR4 substrate of 1.6-mm thickness, a relative permittivity of 4.3, and a dielectric loss tangent of 0.025. As aforementioned, the first resonant frequency is determined by the diameter of the disk, which is about 0.25 of λ in the air [17]. Accordingly, if the lower frequency is chosen to be 3.1 GHz and taking the effect of the substrate into account by using $k = 1.15$ for an FR4 substrate [25], then $R_1 = 10.5$ mm, and to ensure a lower frequency starting before 3.1 GHz, the disk radius R_1 has been chosen to be 11.5 mm. The microstrip feed-line width was set at $W_2 = 2.6$ mm. Other design parameters and the resultant frequency characteristics are shown in the second column of Table 4.3.

Table 4.3 The design parameters and obtained frequency characteristics of the three designed antennas [22]

Parameter (mm)	Antenna-i	Antenna-ii	Antenna-iii
L_1	52	52	52
L_2	26	26	26
W_1	46	46	46
W_2	2.6	2.8	2.8
R_1	11.5	11.5	11.5
R_2	–	–	11.5
G_1	1.5	–	–
G_2	–	–	1.0
FR4 substrate (GHz)	Thickness = 1.6 mm, ε_r = 4.3, loss tangent = 0.025, copper thickness = 0.035 mm		
f_{min}	1.63	5.014	1.86
f_{max}	12.2	11.5	17.77
BW	10.57	6.486	15.91
f_{max}/f_{min}	7.48:1	2.29:1	9.55:1

Figure 4.12 shows the simulated reflection coefficient (red dotted line) of antenna-i. Figure 4.12 and Table 4.3 show that the obtained frequency range extends from 1.63 to 12.2 GHz, which means a bandwidth ratio of 7.48:1. The input impedance is shown on the Smith chart of Figure 4.13(a). On the chart, the points nearest to the center (best matched) have been marked on the zoomed VSWR = 2 circle. These points occur at the resonance frequencies of 2.43, 5.36, 8.06, 10.99, 13.66, 16.34 GHz, which correspond to the six dips in the reflection coefficient curve (red dotted line) shown in Figure 4.12. The radiation patterns in the three principal planes are plotted in Figure 4.14, for selected frequencies of 3, 5, 7.5, and 10 GHz.

4.4.2 Circular dipole antenna with bent microstrip feed line—antenna-ii

The feed line in the previous design, antenna-i, was then bent by 90 degrees on the same plane and ran parallel to the edge W_1 of the ground plane, as shown in Figure 4.11(b). Such bending is to prepare for the suggested design that will be discussed in the next section. The design parameters and obtained performance are also listed in the third column of Table 4.3. Figure 4.12 shows the obtained reflection coefficient compared to that of the straight feed-line monopole. The obtained frequency range extends from 5.014 to 11.5 GHz, leading to a bandwidth ratio of 2.29:1. The variation of input impedance is shown in Figure 4.13(b), where the points nearest to the center (having best matching) have also been marked on the zoomed VSWR = 2 circle. These points occur at resonance frequencies of 7.08, 10.1, 14.24, and 16.78 GHz, which correspond to the four dips in the reflection coefficient pattern shown in Figure 4.12.

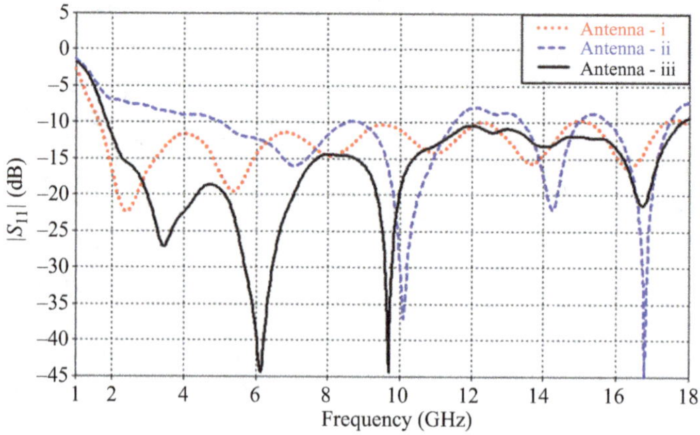

Figure 4.12 Variations of the reflection coefficients with frequencies for antenna-i, antenna-ii, and antenna-iii [22]

4.4.3 Self-complementary circular dipole antenna with bent microstrip feed line—antenna-iii

The proposed antenna has been developed according to the procedure illustrated in Figure 4.15 so as to deploy the self-complementary principle. In this design, the lower copper rectangle works as a ground plane for the disk arm, as a slot boundary for the other arm of the dipole, as well as for the microstrip feed line. The bending of the feed line provided the chance to feed the dipole at its center, and diverting the feed line away from the circular slot. Moreover, this design provides a direct connection to one arm and aperture coupling to the slot arm at the same time.

Figure 4.16 shows a detailed design and parameters of the proposed self-complementary dipole antenna. The design parameters are listed in the fourth column of Table 4.3. The reflection coefficient of the simulated antenna is shown in Figure 4.12, which shows that the performance of the self-complementary antenna is better than those of the previous monopoles. The bandwidth has been extended to cover the frequencies from 1.86 to 17.77 GHz, which means a better bandwidth ratio of 9.55:1. The input impedance performance is shown in Figure 4.13(c). The Smith chart shows the points nearest to the center (best matched points) as marked on the zoomed VSWR = 2 circle. These points occur at four resonance frequencies of 3.45, 6.12, 9.68, and 16.72 GHz, which correspond to the four dips in the reflection coefficient curve (continuous black line) that is shown in Figure 4.12. Figure 4.17 shows the radiation patterns in the three principal planes for selected frequencies of 3, 5, 7.5, and 10 GHz. In this antenna, a very wideband operation range, which covers more than the UWB range, has been achieved, while a good radiation pattern approaching omnidirectional shape is maintained across the extended frequency range.

The gain and radiation efficiency were calculated from the simulations of antenna-iii and displayed in Figure 4.18. The efficiency decreases with frequency

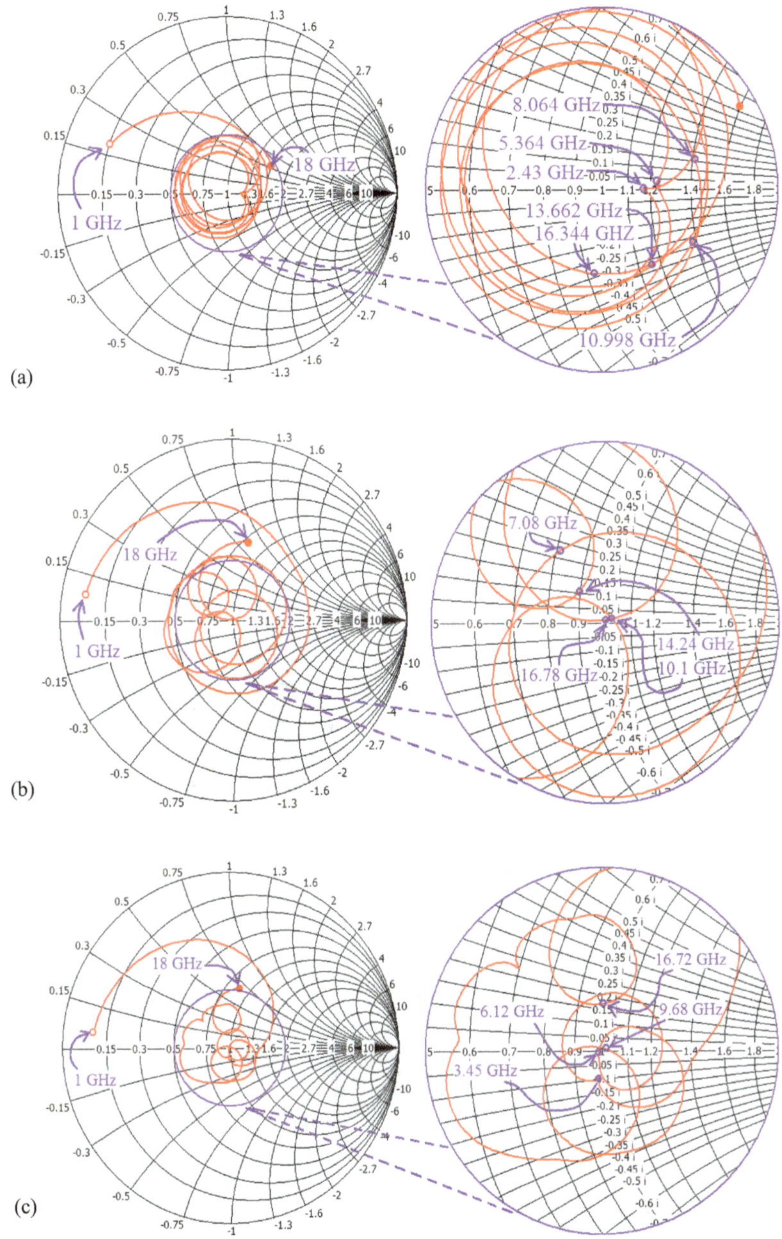

Figure 4.13 Input impedance variations for (a) antenna-i, (b) antenna-ii, (c) antenna-iii, showing the zoomed (VSWR = 2) circle on the right [22]

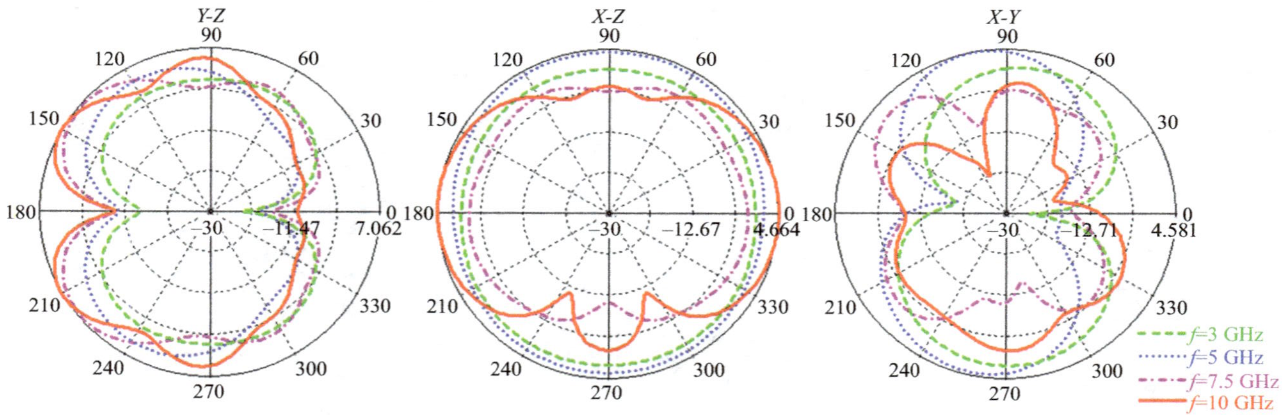

Figure 4.14 Radiation patterns of antenna-i in the three principal planes [22]

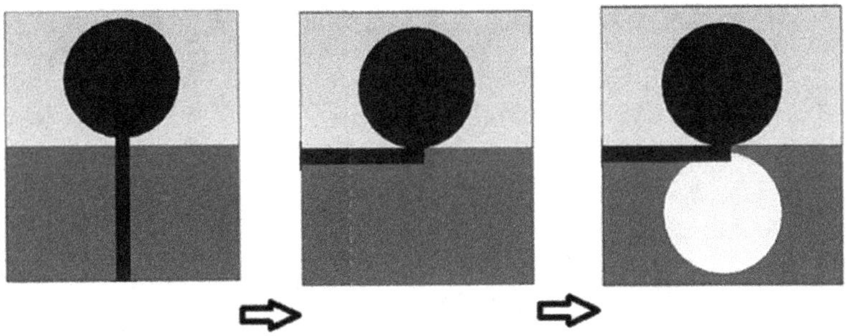

Figure 4.15 Development of the design for the microstrip-fed self-complementary disk/slot dipole antenna [22]

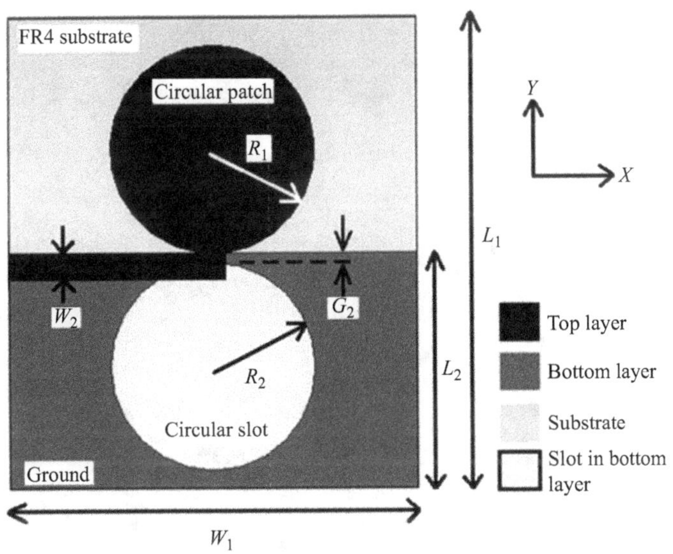

Figure 4.16 Geometry of the proposed self-complementary circular dipole antenna, antenna-iii [22]

due to increasing losses of the FR4 substrate. The gain increases for frequencies up to about 10 GHz due to the increased size/wavelength ratio but then starts to drop slightly as affected by the loss of the substrate and copper.

4.4.4 Experimental validations

To verify the simulated results for the antenna, the self-complementary dipole antenna-i and antenna-iii have been fabricated using the same substrate and design parameters listed in the second and fourth columns of Table 4.3, as shown in Figure 4.19(a) and (b), respectively. The manufacturing was done using a computer numerical control printed circuit board cutting machine. The Rohde and Schwarz

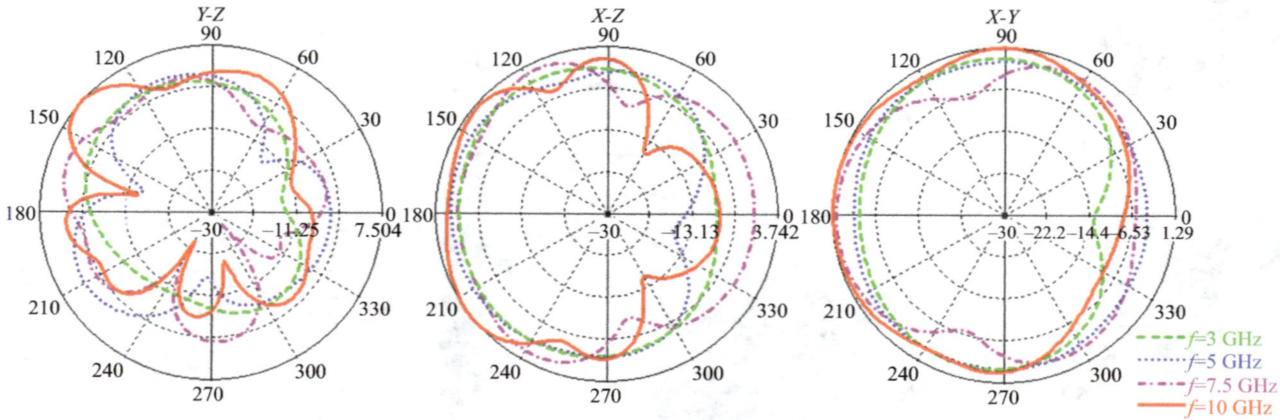

Figure 4.17 Radiation patterns in the three principal planes at the frequencies of 3, 5, 7.5, and 10 GHz for antenna-iii [22]

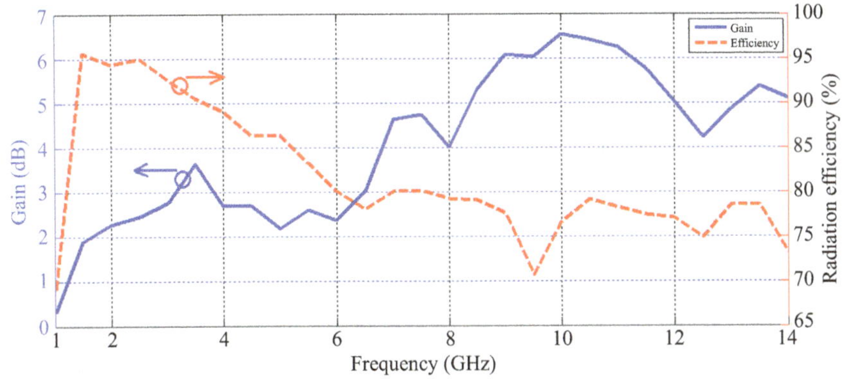

Figure 4.18 Variations of the simulated gains and efficiencies with frequencies for antenna-iii [22]

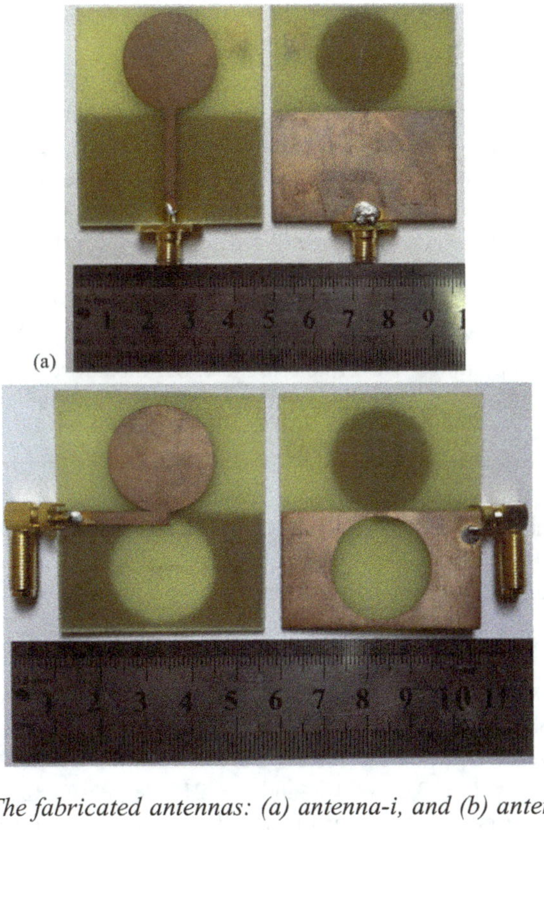

Figure 4.19 The fabricated antennas: (a) antenna-i, and (b) antenna-iii [22]

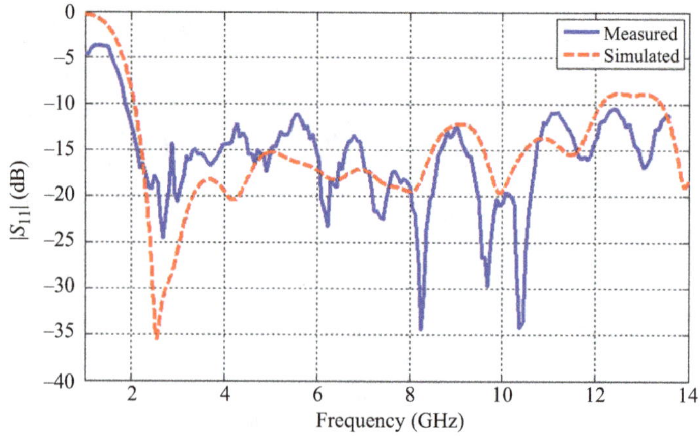

Figure 4.20 Measured and simulated variations of the reflection coefficients with frequencies for the fabricated self-complementary dipole antenna-iii [22]

ZVL13 vector network analyzer (VNA) has been used to measure the reflection coefficient over the frequency range of 1–13.6 GHz.

The simulated and measured variations of the reflection coefficient for antenna-iii are displayed in Figure 4.20. It can be seen that the antenna is matched across the frequency range, which extends from 1.882 GHz, as compared to 1.86 GHz for the simulation, to above 13.6 GHz. The latter value is the upper limit of the bandwidth of the used network analyzer; thus, it was not possible to examine the antenna beyond this value. The measured reflection coefficient shows six deep ($|S_{11}|<-20$ dB) dips, which are related to the six frequencies at which the antenna is in near resonance. However, the simulated reflection coefficient result, which is also plotted in Figure 4.20 for comparison, shows only three clear deeper dips for the same frequency range. Nevertheless, the experimental result complies with the criteria of less than -10-dB reflection coefficient over the range of 1.882 GHz to more than 13.6 GHz.

For further investigations, the phase of the measured reflection coefficient was obtained from the recorded VNA measurements. Figure 4.21 shows the phase response of antenna-iii. The variation of the unwrapped phase with frequency $\Phi(f)$ shows a mainly linear trend with relatively small imposed ripples. This variation can be represented by the following relation:

$$\Phi(f) = \Phi_0 + k(f - f_1) + \text{higher order terms for } f \geq f_1 \tag{4.1}$$

where Φ_0 is a constant term; k represents the phase slope in units of degrees/GHz; f and f_1 are frequencies in GHz, where f_1 is the frequency at which the phase equals the constant term Φ_0. For the results shown in Figure 4.21, it was found that $\Phi_0 = 212$ degrees, $f_1 = 3.016$ GHz, and $k = 215$ degrees/GHz give a good representation of the first two terms of (4.1). After subtracting the first two estimated

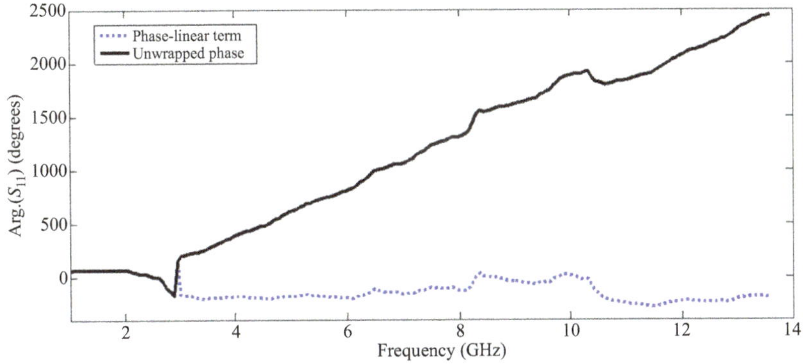

Figure 4.21 Variations of the reflection coefficient phases with frequencies for the self-complementary dipole antenna-iii: dotted curve shows the phase after subtracting the constant and linear terms of (4.1) [22]

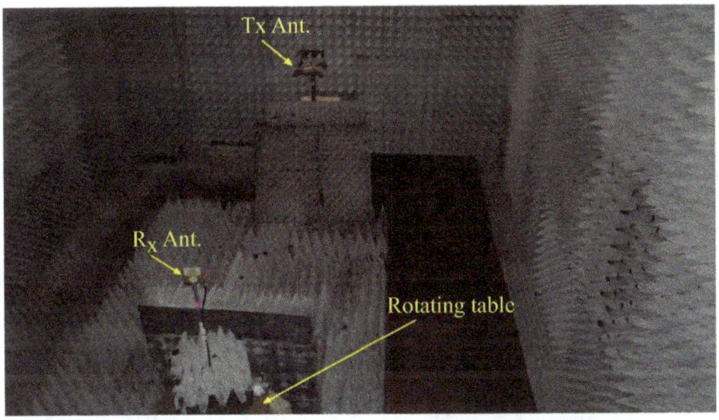

Figure 4.22 The radiation pattern measurement inside the anechoic chamber showing the rotating table, T_X and R_X antennas [8]

terms from (4.1), the resulting phase variation is also shown (dotted) in Figure 4.21. The phase ripples are now easily visible, and they clearly mark the regions of the abovementioned resonances. Therefore, the phase curve can give better insight into the study of matching and return loss variation of the investigated antenna.

Further experimental evaluations for each of antenna-i and antenna-iii were the far-field radiation patterns that were measured inside an anechoic chamber that is shown in Figure 4.22. The radiation patterns have been measured for E and H planes at different frequencies, using an Anritsu MS2665C spectrum analyzer of a frequency range of (9 kHz to 21.2 GHz). Figures 4.23 and 4.24 show the measured radiation patterns compared with the simulation results obtained from the CST simulations, for antenna-i and antenna-iii, respectively. The results show almost omnidirectional radiation patterns, especially in the H plane.

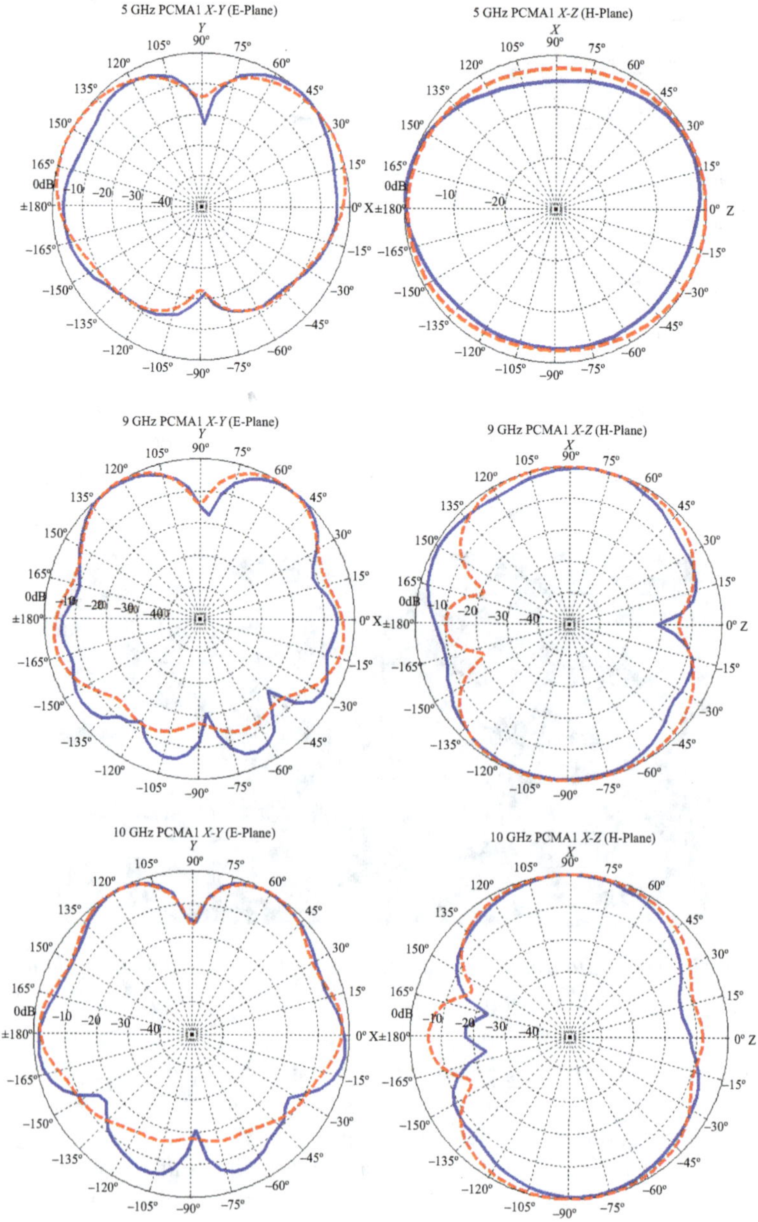

Figure 4.23 Measured (——) and simulated (– – –) radiation patterns in E *and* H *planes, for antenna-i, at the frequencies 5, 9, and 10 GHz [8]*

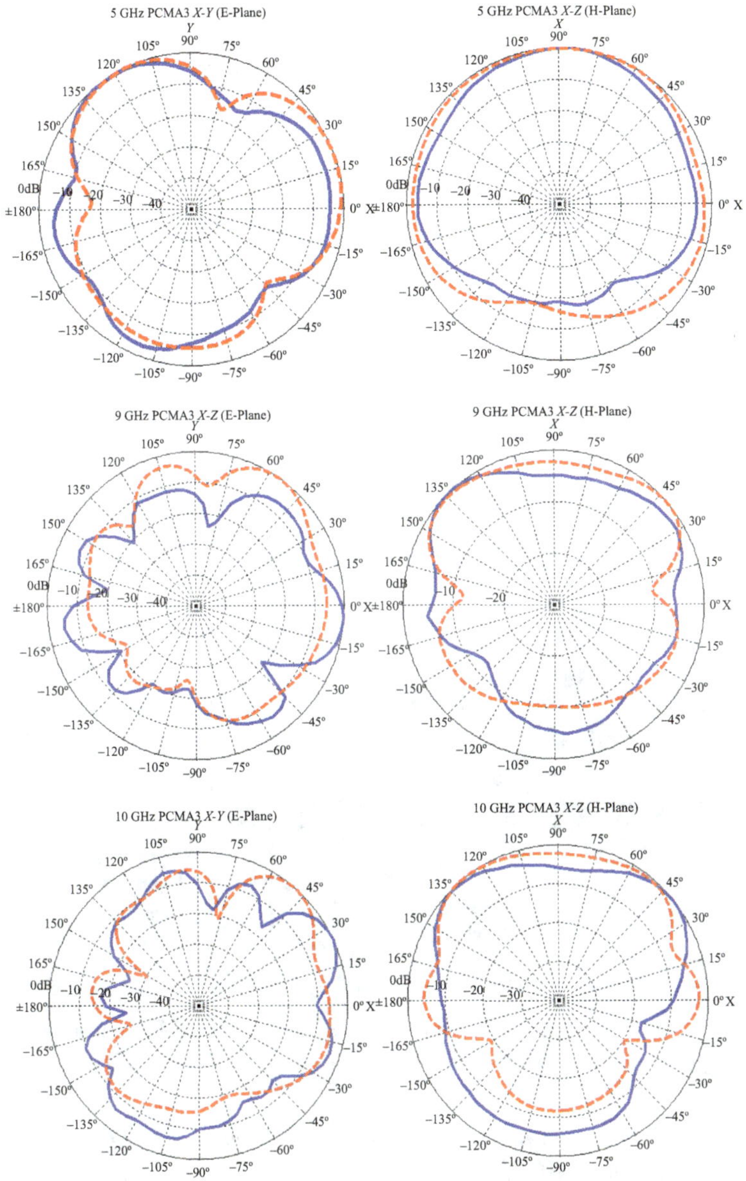

Figure 4.24 Measured (—) and simulated (– – –) radiation patterns in E *and* H *planes, for antenna-iii, at the frequencies 5, 9, 10, and 12 GHz [8]*

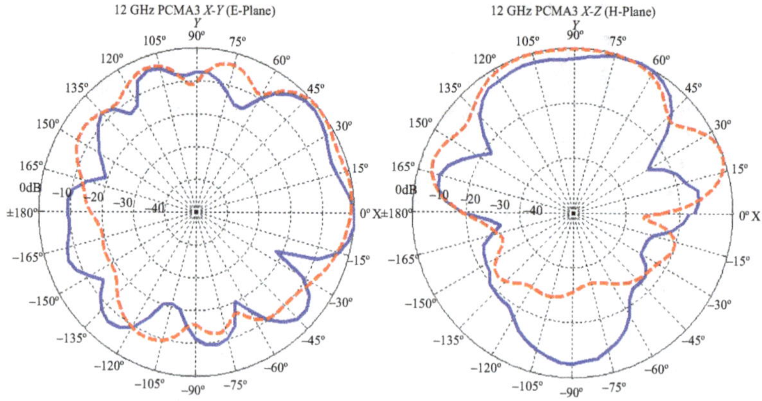

Figure 4.24 (Continued)

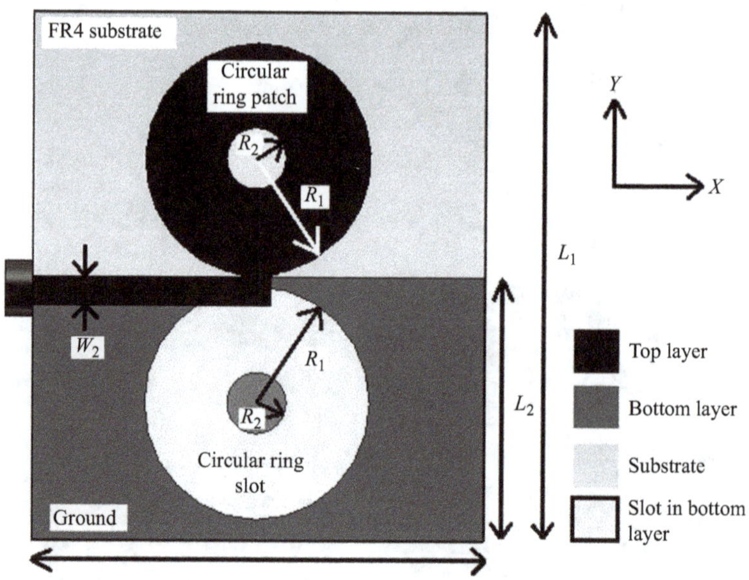

Figure 4.25 Geometry of the proposed self-complementary ring dipole antenna-iii [23]

4.4.5 Further developments

The self-complementary principle was also utilized for the design of ring-shaped antennas, as seen in Figure 4.25 [23]. This design, which has the form of a circular ring, followed that published in [23] and presented in Section 4.4.3. The ring shape offers another degree of design freedom represented by the value of the inner radius

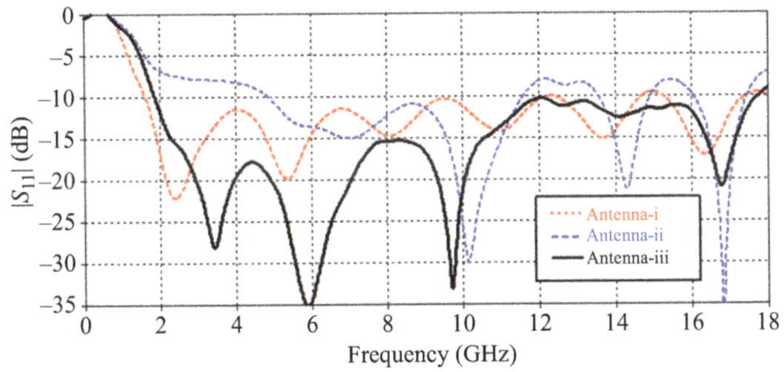

Figure 4.26 The variations of the reflection coefficients with frequencies for conventional ring monopole (antenna-i), bent-feed ring monopole (antenna-ii), and self-complementary antenna (antenna-iii) [23]

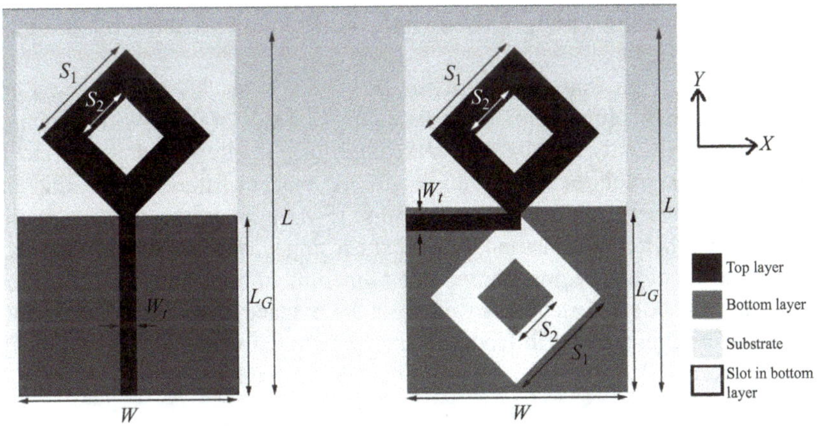

Figure 4.27 Geometry of the planner square ring monopole and the proposed self-complementary antenna SCPSMA2 [26]

of the ring. The obtained reflection coefficient response of the proposed antenna is compared with those for the conventional ring dipole, and bent-feed dipole, as shown in Figure 4.26. The radiation pattern shows similar performances.

A recent publication has applied the ring-shaped monopole into the design of self-complementary antenna [26]. The square-shaped ring monopole antenna was developed into a self-complementary configuration as shown in Figure 4.27, by following the design procedure in [22,23]. This antenna, which was designed for breast cancer detection, showed enhanced bandwidth that was smaller than that achieved by the circular ring and circular disk.

4.5 Self-complementary planar bow-tie antenna for UWB applications

One of the important types of antennas that are used in many broadband applications is the bow-tie antenna, which has undergone many design variations to enhance its performance. One of these attempts was to reduce its quality factor by resistively loading the bow-tie antenna. Small late-time ringing in the time-domain response and reduced antenna dimensions were achieved [27]. Another improvement was to apply the Sierpiński fractal on the bow-tie arms to initiate multi-resonant narrow bands of frequencies that lead to enhanced bandwidth [28].

Due to the complexity of the many design parameters, many bow-tie antennas designs were limited to bandwidths of about 2 GHz [29–32], while other designs have achieved a dual-band operation [33,34]. Another bow-tie antenna has been tuned for just a certain frequency [35]. Other researchers tried to increase the impedance bandwidth and have achieved about 4-GHz bandwidth in the X-band, but it is still less than the UWB requirements [36]. An array has been formed by using four bow-tie elements fed by e.m. coupling microstrip patch antenna, but the achieved bandwidth was limited to a small range of 2.7–3.3 GHz [37].

After a thorough examination of the bow-tie antenna literature, it was concluded that the main problem is that of matching each side of the bow-tie antenna to the feeding port (usually the 50-Ω (SMA) connector). The bow-tie antenna, like the biconical antenna, requires to be fed via a 300-Ω balanced transmission line [38]. Therefore, in order to feed the dipole by 50-Ω (SMA) connector, the designer has implemented either of two methods. The first is using a balun transformer, which is somewhat difficult to be implemented due to its limited bandwidth and sometimes it requires a complicated shape, as well as an extra space [39,40]. The second way uses a multi-section microstrip feed line having different widths or a feed line with gradually increased width, to work as an impedance transformer for matching the bow-tie antenna to the (SMA) connector [19,41].

In their attempts to improve the bow-tie antenna, some researchers have placed this antenna inside a slot in the ground plane, but this arrangement also needs the abovementioned matching techniques, or at least the balun transformer. Although some designs have succeeded in achieving antenna matching over the entire UWB range, but it was on account of a long list of design parameters, which in turn added complexity to the design procedure [42,43]. Other researchers have formed the bow-tie slot antenna in the ground plane of a certain monopole antenna and achieved a limited bandwidth of about 2 GHz [44].

In an attempt to overcome all the abovementioned difficulties, a novel self-complementary bow-tie planar antenna (SCBT antenna) has been designed [45]. The modification has been applied to both arms of the bow-tie (patch and its complementary slot), producing a fractal self-complementary bow-tie antenna (FSCBT antenna). Better return loss performance has been achieved, as will be shown in the next section.

4.5.1 Design methodology

The traditional bow-tie (TBT) antenna is usually designed by choosing suitable dimensions, keeping in mind the need to feed the antenna via a balanced 300-Ω line source. If it is desired to feed the antenna by a 50-Ω SMA connector, a microstrip feed line must be designed to work as an impedance transformer with variable width or a number of stepped sections. The main aim of the work presented in the following sections is to design new types of bow-tie antennas that do not need the impedance transformer at front end, while offering adequate bandwidth, and very convenient coupling to SMA connectors.

4.5.2 The traditional bow-tie antenna (TBT antenna)

A TBT antenna has been designed to cover the entire UWB range using a CST simulation tool, with dimensions optimized by trial and error, as shown in Figure 4.28. The design parameters are shown in Table 4.4. The antenna was fed by a discrete port having an impedance of 300 Ω, and the simulation results showed that its reflection coefficient response covers more than the UWB range (2.688 GHz, up to more than 12 GHz), as depicted in Figure 4.29. The antenna has achieved the required UWB range; however, it will need a matching section if it is desired to be fed via an SMA connector.

4.5.3 The self-complementary bow-tie antenna (SCBT antenna)

The proposed SCBT antenna was designed by implementing the self-complementary principle [10]. The design idea stems from developing the

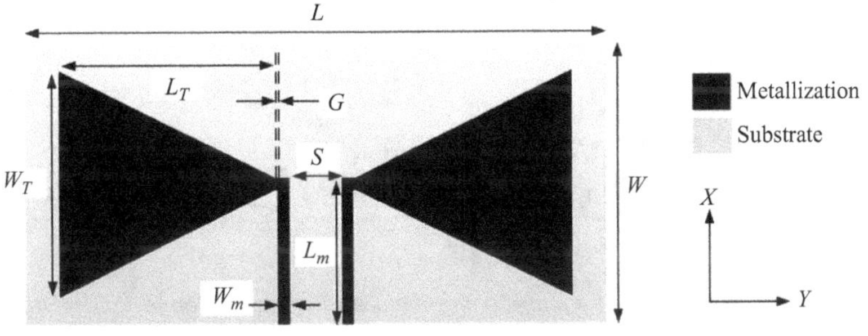

Figure 4.28 Geometry of the traditional bow-tie antenna (TBT antenna) with balanced feed

Table 4.4 Design parameters of the traditional bow-tie antenna (TBT antenna)

Parameter (mm)	L	L_T	L_m	W	W_T	W_m	S	G
	65	23.6	15.65	30	24	1.3	5.8	0.4
Substrate	Thickness = 1.6 mm, ε_r = 4.3, copper thickness = 0.035 mm, and loss tangent = 0.025							

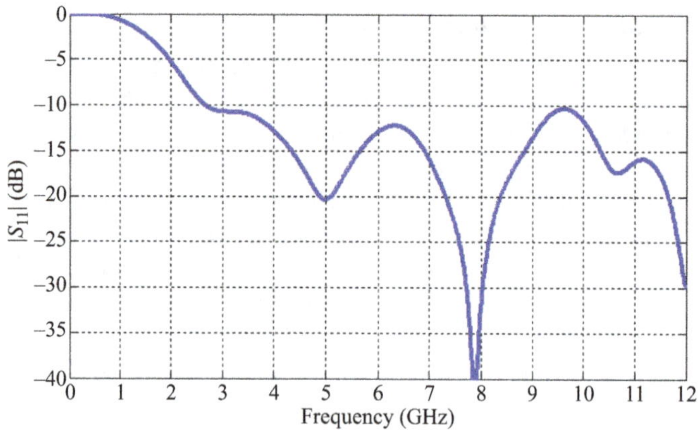

Figure 4.29 Variation of the simulated reflection coefficient versus frequency for the TBT antenna shown in Figure 4.28

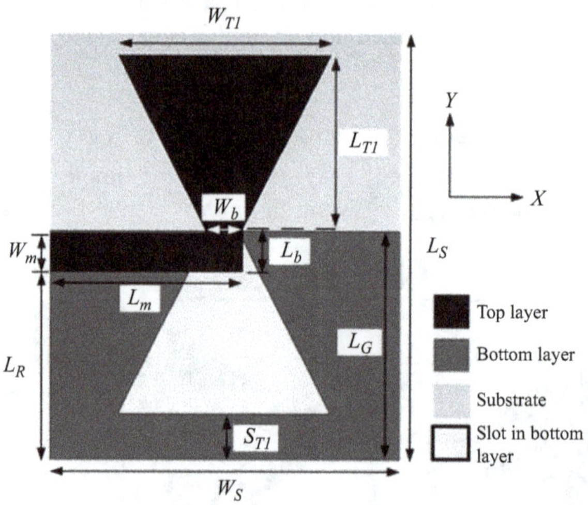

Figure 4.30 Geometry of the self-complementary bow-tie antenna (SCBT antenna)

triangular monopole antenna by adding an opposite triangular slot on its ground plane so as to form the other arm of the dipole, while at the same time the micro-strip feed line is bent by 90 degrees, as illustrated in Figure 4.30.

The relations proposed in [24] were applied to estimate the lower frequency of operation f_L. The closer shape to the proposed SCBT antenna is the triangular monopole antenna, and the corresponding relations given in [24] are as follows:

$$f_L = \frac{7.2}{(L + r + p) * k} \text{ (GHz)} \tag{4.2}$$

$$r = \frac{W}{4\pi} \tag{4.3}$$

$$L_T = \frac{\sqrt{3}W_T}{2} \tag{4.4}$$

$$k = \sqrt{\varepsilon_{eff}}. \tag{4.5}$$

where p is the feed-probe length (neck length) or the gap between the radiating patch and the ground plane (in cm). r is the radius of the equivalent cylindrical monopole (in cm). L_T is the height of the equivalent cylinder, which is taken equal to that of the triangular monopole (patch) (in cm). W_T is the base of the triangular patch (in cm). ε_{eff} is the effective dielectric constant, which can be calculated from the relative dielectric constant of the substrate (ε_r) and air as

$$\varepsilon_{eff} = \frac{\varepsilon r + 1}{2} \tag{4.6}$$

The SCBT antenna introduced here has been designed using triangular shape and dimensions, as shown in Figure 4.30. The values of various parameters computed from the previous equations, and using an FR4 substrate having $\varepsilon_r = 4.3$ with a loss tangent of 0.025, are listed in the following:

$$W_T = W_{T2} = 18\ \text{mm}, r = 1.43\ \text{mm}, L_T = L_{T1} = 15.56\ \text{mm}.$$

Substituting the previous values into (4.2)–(4.6), f_L is found to be equal to 2.539 GHz. However, L_T is chosen as 14.6 mm to increase the value of the lower frequency f_L slightly. The other dimensions for this antenna have been optimized by simulations using the CST software package, and the final design parameters are listed in Table 4.5.

The simulated results of the reflection coefficient are shown in Figure 4.31 (the red dashed curve), which indicates a lower edge frequency f_L of 2.75 GHz. The results of the simulation show that SCBT antenna has a wide range of operating frequency 2.75–11.58 GHz, which exceeds the UWB requirements, and has a bandwidth ratio of 4.21:1.

Table 4.5 Design parameters of the self-complementary bow-tie antenna (SCBT antenna) that is shown in Figure 4.27

Parameter (mm)	L_s	L_{T1}	L_m	L_b	L_G	L_R	W_S	W_{T1}
	36	14.6	16.6	3.6	19.2	15.8	30	18
Parameter (mm)	W_m	W_b	S_{T1}	$p = L_b - W_m$				
	3.2	3.2	3.9	0.4				
Substrate	Thickness = 1.6 mm, $\varepsilon_r = 4.3$, copper thickness = 0.035 mm, loss tangent = 0.025							

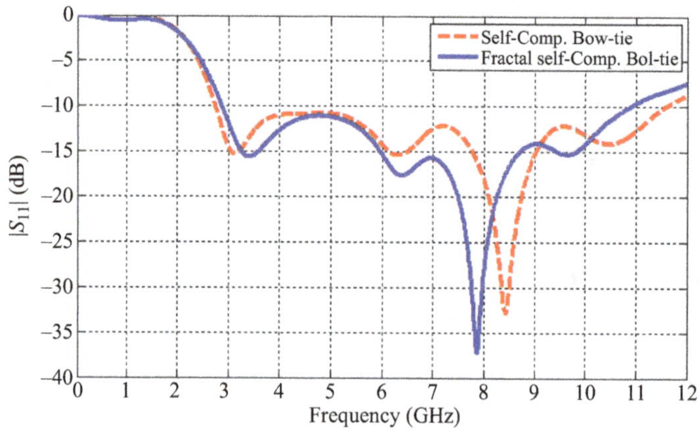

Figure 4.31 Variations of the reflection coefficients with frequencies for SCBT antenna and FSCBT antenna [44]

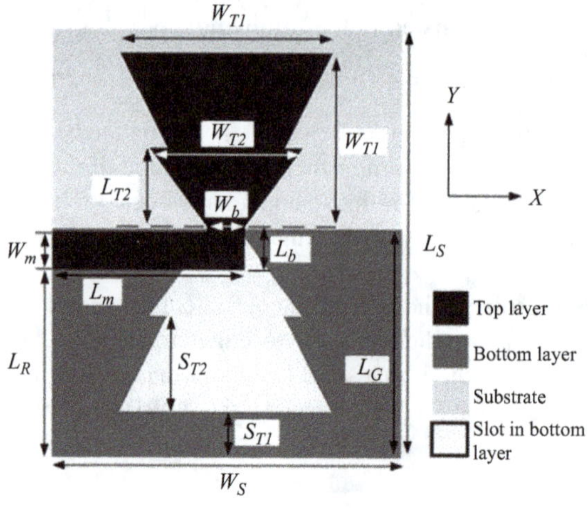

Figure 4.32 Geometry of the FSCBT antenna [44]

4.5.4 *The fractal self-complementary bow-tie antenna (FSCBT antenna)*

The obtained benefits from the fractal designs using the rectangular and triangular monopoles, which have been demonstrated in Section 4.3 [8] encouraged applying the same concept here to the SCBT antenna to achieve an enhanced design named FSCBT antenna. The triangular radiating patch and its complementary slot are fractally repeated using a proper scale factor. Figure 4.32 shows the proposed antenna and its design parameters, whose values are listed in Table 4.6 [44].

Table 4.6 Design parameters of the fractal self-complementary bow-tie antenna (FSCBT antenna) that is shown in Figure 4.32

Parameter (mm)	L_s	L_{T1}	L_m	L_{T2}	L_b	L_G	L_R	W_S	W_{T1}
	36	14.6	16.6	6.6	3.6	19.2	15.8	30	18
Parameter (mm)	W_{T2}	W_m	W_b	S_{T1}	S_{T2}	$p = L_b - W_m$			
	13	3.2	3.2	3.9	8	0.4			
Substrate	Thickness = 1.6 mm, $\varepsilon_r = 4.3$, copper thickness = 0.035, and loss tangent of 0.025								

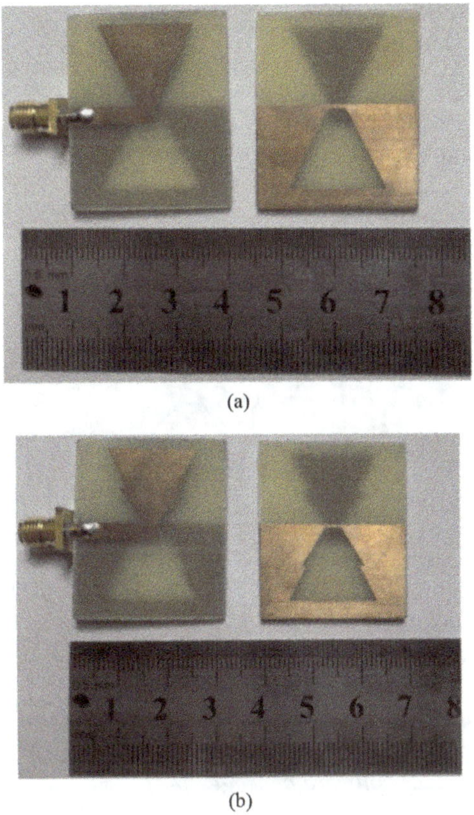

Figure 4.33 Fabricated (a) SCBT and (b) FSCBT antennas [44]

As depicted in Figure 4.31 (the solid blue curve), the simulation results show a reflection coefficient bandwidth of 2.88 GHz to about 10.89 GHz, which fully covers the UWB range. From this investigation, it has been noticed that the FSCBT antenna has lower reflection coefficient values over most of the band, because of utilizing the self-complementary feature as well as the fractal repetition of the

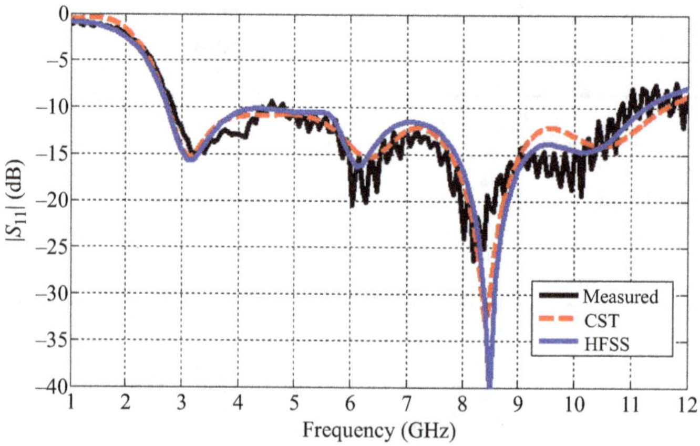

Figure 4.34 Measured (——) reflection coefficient versus frequency for SCBT antenna, compared to simulated one using: (a) CST (– – –) and (b) HFSS (——) software packages [44]

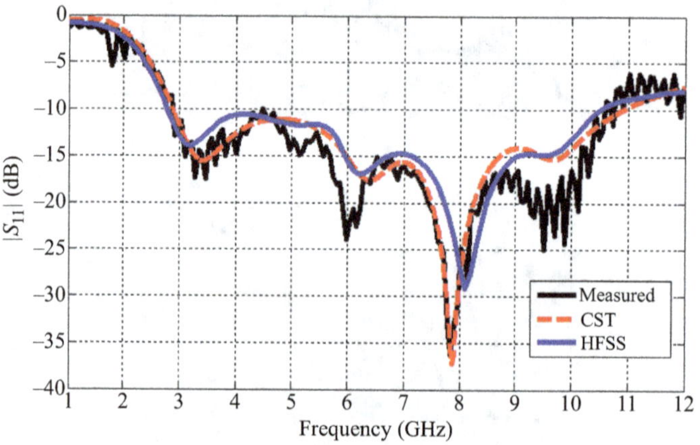

Figure 4.35 Measured (——) reflection coefficient versus frequency for FSCBT antenna, compared to simulated one using: (a) CST (– – –) and (b) HFSS (——) software packages [44]

triangular shape as has been introduced in [9,44]. In comparison with the results of the TBT antenna, both SCBT and FSCBT antennas are easier in design and implementation, smaller in size, and wider in bandwidth. They neither need baluns nor impedance matching sections because they are fed directly via a 50-Ω right-angle bent feed line.

Two prototypes for the SCBT and FSCBT antennas were fabricated on an FR4 substrate as shown in Figure 4.33 and were tested to verify the results of the simulations. Figures 4.34 and 4.35 show the measured reflection coefficient

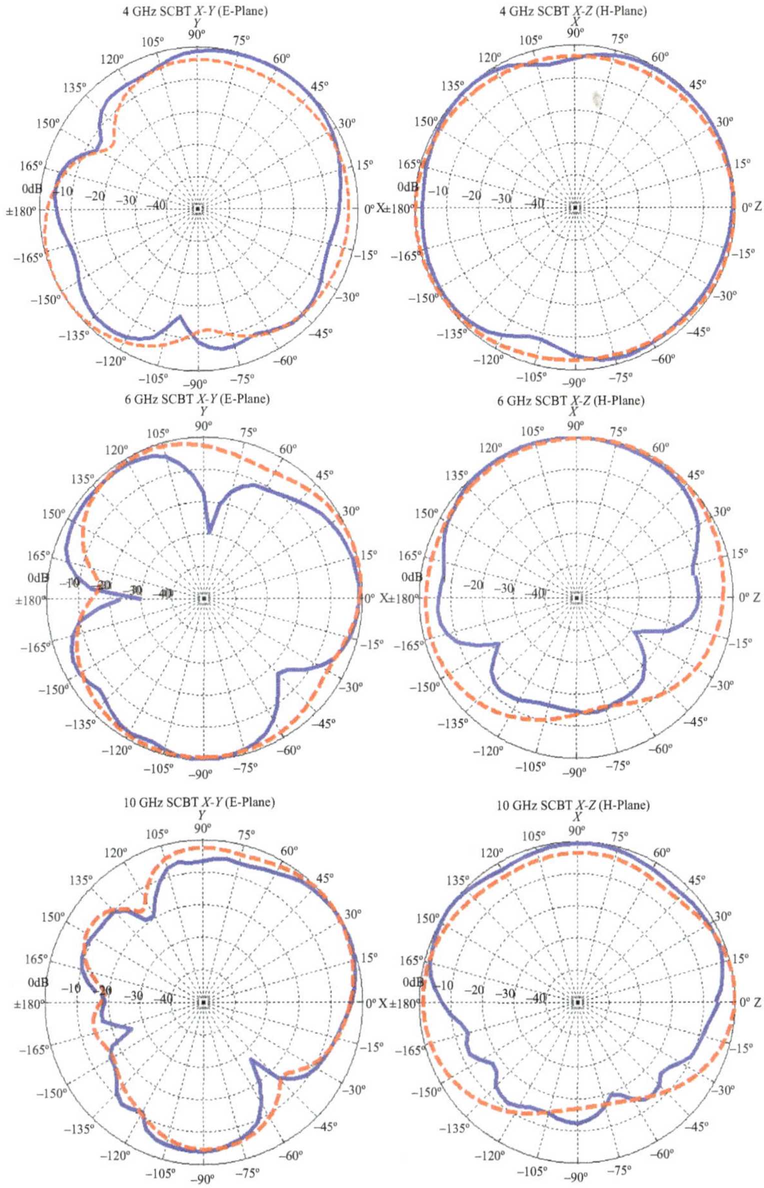

Figure 4.36 Measured (——) and simulated (– – –) radiation patterns of the SCBT antenna in E *and* H *planes, for the three frequencies 4, 6, and 10 GHz [44]*

responses of the SCBT and FSCBT antennas, respectively. Again, simulation results have been acquired from HFSS software package in addition to CST, as other verification, before fabrication. A very good agreement between the results

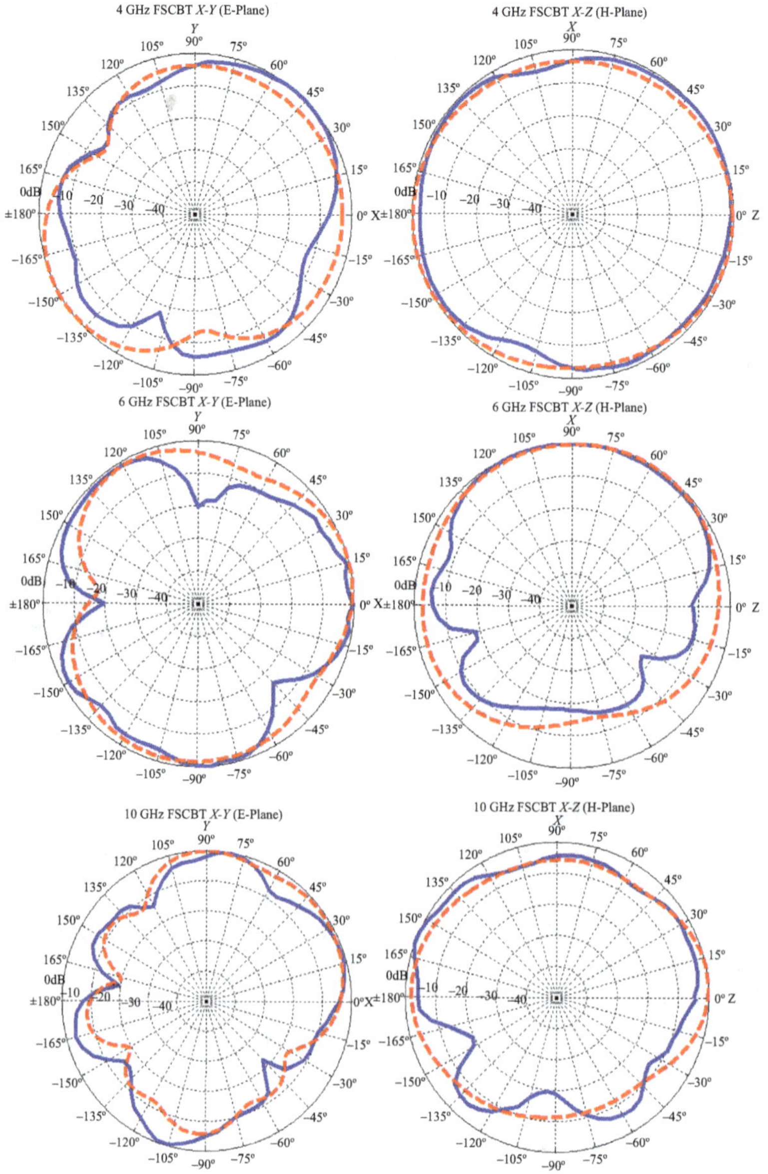

Figure 4.37 Measured (__) and simulated (_ _ _) radiation patterns of the FSCBT antenna in E *and* H *planes, for the three frequencies 4, 6, and 10 GHz [44]*

obtained from the two software packages is noticed, and the experimental responses show very good agreement with those obtained from the simulations.

The radiation patterns were measured inside an anechoic chamber, for both of *E* and *H* planes at frequencies of 4, 6, and 10 GHz. Figures 4.36 and 4.37 show the

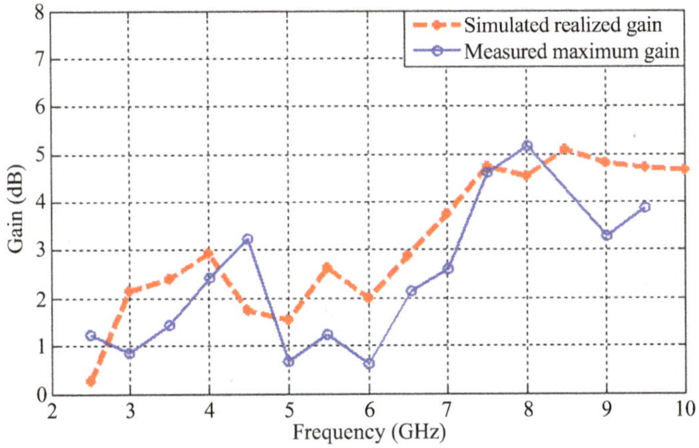

Figure 4.38 Simulated realized gain and measured maximum gain for the FSCBT antenna [44]

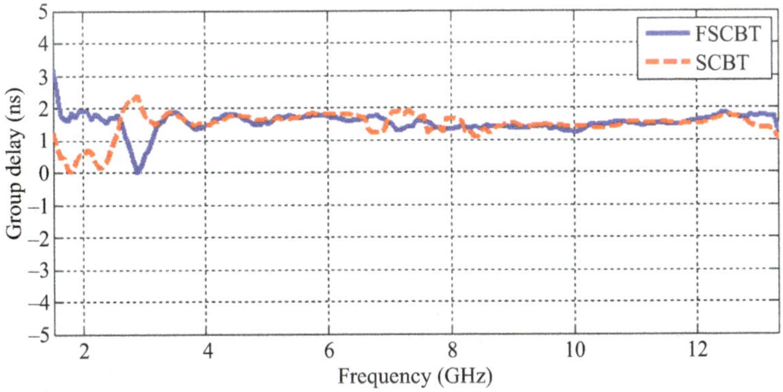

Figure 4.39 Measured group delay for SCBT and FSCBT antennas [8]

measured radiation patterns compared to the simulation results, for SCBT and FSCBT antennas, respectively. The results show almost omnidirectional radiation patterns, especially in the *H* plane.

Figure 4.38 shows the simulated realized gain results and measured maximum gain for the FSCBT antenna, which indicates the general trend of increased gain with frequency. Examining Figures 4.31 and 4.38 with more insight, it can be seen that in the range of 6–10 GHz, the gain of the FSCBT antenna shows an increase with frequency due to the good reduction in the reflection coefficient (down to about −15 dB). In Figure 4.38, the measured maximum gain curve for the FSCBT antenna can be noticed to be comparable to that of the simulated realized gain in the overall shape, with some deviations less than 1.5 dB. The difference can be attributed to the fact that the direction of the maximum radiated field has been noticed to change slightly when the frequency of operation was varied.

The group delay for each of the two fabricated antennas was measured in order to assess the time response of the proposed antennas. The time response is an important factor when the antenna is used in pulsed imaging systems. In each case, the two similar antennas were placed side-by-side, at a separation distance of 30 cm, and arranged to work in transmitting/receiving configuration. The group delay was calculated from the measured phase variation with frequency by differentiating the measured phase with respect to the frequency, and the results are shown in Figure 4.39. The two responses are almost constant over the UWB frequency range, indicating practically linear phase change with frequency. The FSCBT antenna shows a smoother response that indicates a nearly linear phase variation and hence better time response. The frequency range of the measurements was limited to 13.6 GHz, which was the upper working frequency of the used VNA (Rohde and Schwarz ZVL13).

References

[1] S. A. Rezaeieh, A. Zamani, K. S. Bialkowski, G. A. Macdonald and A. M. Abbosh, "Three-dimensional electromagnetic torso scanner", *Sensors*, vol. 19, p. 1015, 2019.

[2] M. T. Islam, M. Z. Mahmud, M. T. Arikul-Islam, S. Kibria, and M. Samsuzzaman, "A low cost and portable microwave imaging system for breast tumor detection using UWB directional antenna array", *Scientific Reports*, vol. 9, p. 15491, 2019 https://doi.org/10.1038/s41598-019-51620-z.

[3] A. S. M. Alqadami, N. Nguyen-Trong, B. Mohammed, A. E. Stancombe, M. T. Heitzmann, and A. Abbosh, "Compact unidirectional conformal antenna based on flexible high-permittivity custom-made substrate for wearable wideband electromagnetic head imaging system", *IEEE Transactions on Antennas and Propagation*, vol. 68, no. 1, pp. 183–194, 2020.

[4] B. A. J. Mohammed, A. M. Abbosh, and P. Sharpe, "Planar array of corrugated tapered slot antennas for ultrawideband biomedical microwave imaging system", *International Journal of RF and Microwave Computer-Aided Engineering*, vol. 23, pp. 59–66, 2013.

[5] K. Ray and G. Nikhare, "Analysis of harmonic and off-band response of a dipole antenna", 8th International Conference on Electromagnetic Interference and Compatibility, INCEMIC2003, pp. 367–370, 2003.

[6] M. Al-Husseini, A. Ramadan, A. El-Hajj Karim, and Y. Kabalan, "Design of a compact and low-cost fractal-based UWB PCB antenna", 26th National Radio Science Conference (NRSC2009), pp. 1–8, Mar. 17–19, 2009.

[7] H. Song, H. An, J. Lee, J. Park, and J. Kim, "Design of the tree-shaped UWB antenna using fractal concept", Korea-Japan Microwave Conference, pp. 73–76, Nov. 19 2007.

[8] Y. A. Fadhel, "Design and Implementation of Ultra Wide Band Antennas for Imaging Applications", Ph.D. Thesis, College of Engineering, University of Mosul, 2013.

[9] K. H. Sayidmarie and Y. A. Fadhel, "UWB fractal monopoles of rectangular and triangular shapes", *Proceeding of MAPE2011*, Beijing, China, pp. 709–712, 2011.

[10] Y. Mushiake, "Self-complementary antennas", *IEEE Antennas and Propagation Magazine*, vol. 34, no. 6, pp. 23–29, 1992.

[11] H. G. Booker, "Slot aerials and their relation to complementary wire aerials (Babinet's principle)", *Journal of the Institution of Electrical Engineers – Part IIIA*, vol. 93, pp. 620–626, 1946.

[12] V.H. Rumsey, "Frequency independent antennas", *IRE International Convention Record*, vol. 5, no. 1, pp. 114–118, 1957.

[13] L. Guo, X. Chen, and C. Parini, "Study of a miniaturized quasi-self-complementary UWB antenna in frequency and time domain", *Radio Engineering*, vol. 18, no. 4, pp. 381–387, 2009.

[14] J. Yeo, Y. Lee, and R. Mittra, "Wideband slot antennas for wireless communications", *IEE Proceedings – Microwaves, Antennas and Propagation*, vol. 151, pp. 351–355, 2004.

[15] C. Ying, G. Li, and Y. Zhang, "An LTCC planar ultra-wideband antenna", *Microwave and Optical Technology Letters*, vol. 42, pp. 220–222, 2004.

[16] C. Lin, Y. Kan, L. Kuo, and H. Chuang, "A planar triangular monopole antenna for UWB communication", *IEEE Microwave and Wireless Components Letters*, vol. 15, no. 10, pp. 624–626, 2005.

[17] J. Liang, C. Chiau, X. Chen, and C. Parini, "Study of a printed circular disc monopole antenna for UWB systems", *IEEE Transactions on Antennas and Propagation*, vol. 53, no. 11, pp. 3500–3504, 2005.

[18] L. Wang, W. Wu, X.-W. Shi, F. Wei, and Q.-L. Huang, "Design of a novel monopole UWB antenna with a notched ground", *Progress in Electromagnetics Research C*, vol. 5, pp. 13–20, 2008.

[19] T. Karakolak and E. Topsakal, "A double-sided rounded bow-tie antenna (DSRBA) for UWB communication", *IEEE Antennas and Wireless Propagation Letters*, vol. 5, no. 1, pp. 446–449, 2006.

[20] X. N. Low, Z. N. Chen, and T. S. P. See, "A UWB dipole antenna with enhanced impedance and gain performance", *IEEE Transactions on Antennas and Propagation*, vol. 57, no. 10, 2009.

[21] L. Lizzi, G. Oliveri, P. Rocca, and A. Massa, "Planer monopole UWB antenna with UNII1/UNII2 WLAN-Band Notched characteristics", *Progress in Electromagnetics Research B*, vol. 25, pp. 277–292, 2010.

[22] K. H. Sayidmarie and Y. A. Fadhel, "Self-complementary circular disk antenna for UWB applications", *Progress In Electromagnetics Research C*, vol. 24, pp. 111–122, 2011.

[23] Y. A. Fadhel and K. H. Sayidmarie, "Self-complementary ring planer antenna of very wideband operation", *Proc. of ISAP2011*, Jeju, Korea, Oct. 25–28 2011.

[24] K. P. Ray, "Design aspects of printed monopole antennas for UWB applications", *International Journal of Antennas and Propagation*, vol. 2008, 8 pages, 2008.

[25] M. A. Matin, "*Ultra wideband Communications: Novel Trends – Antennas and Propagation*", Published by InTech, Croatia, pp. 177–183, Jul. 2011.

[26] H. N. M. Salih, M. Fiebich, and Y. A. Fadhel Alsaidosh, "Design of a self-complementary planar rectangular monopole antenna for breast cancer detection", *Technology Reports of Kansai University*, vol. 62, no 05, pp. 2353–2364, 2020.

[27] A. A. Lestari, A. B. Suksmono, A. Kurniawan, E. Bharata, A. G. Yarovoy, and L. P. Ligthart, "Modified bow-tie antenna for efficient transmission of UWB pulses", *Proc. of ISAP'04*, Sendai, Japan, pp. 521–524, 2004.

[28] A. H. Yamini, and M. Soleimani, "Multiband behavior of wideband Sierpiński fractal bow-tie antenna", *The European Conference on Wireless Technology*, Paris, France, pp. 503–506, Oct. 2005.

[29] C. H. Ng, S. Uysal, and M. S. Leong, "Microstrip bowtie patch antenna for wireless indoor communications", *Radio and Wireless Conference, RAWCON'98*, Colorado Springs, pp. 205–207, Aug. 1998.

[30] E. Rufus, Z. C. Alex, and P. V. Chaitanya, "A Modified bow-tie antenna for microwave imaging applications", *Journal of Microwaves, Optoelectronics and Electromagnetic Applications*, vol. 7, no. 2, pp. 115–122, 2008.

[31] A. M. Gomaa, D. A.-E. Mohamed, and M. A. Mangoud, "Double-sided printed triangular bow-tie antenna for UWB communications", *Proceeding of the 17th International Conference on Computer Theory and Applications*, Alexandria, Egypt, Aug. 2007.

[32] G. Zheng, A. Z. Elsherbeni, and C. E. Smith, "A coplanar waveguide bow-tie aperture antenna", Antennas and Propagation Society International Symposium, San Antonio, Texas, pp. 564–567, Aug. 2002.

[33] A. Mehdipour, C. W. Trueman, A. R. Sebak, and S. V. Hoa, "Carbon-fiber composite t-match folded bow-tie antenna for RFID applications", Antennas and Propagation Society International Symposium, Charleston, SC, 2009.

[34] R. K. Joshi and A. R. Harish, "A Modified bow-tie antenna for dual band applications", *IEEE Antennas and Wireless Propagation Letters*, vol. 6, pp. 468–471, 2007.

[35] K. R. Mahmoud, "Design optimization of a bow-tie antenna for 2.45 GHz RFID readers using a hybrid BSO-NM algorithm", *Progress in Electromagnetics Research, PIER*, vol. 100, pp. 105–117, 2010.

[36] A. A. Eldek, A. Z. Elsherbeni, and C. E. Smith, "Wideband microstrip-fed printed bow-tie antenna for phased-array systems", *Microwave and Optical Technology Letters*, vol. 43, no. 2, pp. 123–126, 2004.

[37] F. Zhang, F.-S. Zhang, Y.-B. Yang, and Z. Zhang, "Wide band antenna array using bowtie-shaped microstrip patch antenna", ICMMT 2010 Proceedings, Chengdu, China, pp. 424–427, May 2010.

[38] J. D. Kraus, "*Antennas for all applications*", Tata McGraw-Hill, Inc., New Delhi, 2nd ed., pp. 634, 67, 1988.

[39] R. Persico, N. Romano, and F. Soldoviero, "Design of a balun for a bow tie antenna in reconfigurable ground penetrating radar systems", *Progress in Electromagnetics Research C*, vol. 18, pp. 123–135, 2011.

[40] S. Kubota, X. Xiao, N. Sasaki, K. Kimoto, and T. Kikkawa, "Characteristics of UWB bow-tie antenna integrated with balun for breast cancer detection", *Antennas and Propagation Society International Symposium*, Charleston, SC, 2009.

[41] A. A. Eldek, A. Z. Elsherbeni, and C. E. Smith, "Wide-band modified printed bow-tie antenna with single and dual polarization for C– and X-Band applications", *IEEE Transactions on Antennas and Propagation*, vol. 53, no. 9, pp. 3067–3072, 2009.

[42] J. Liu, D. Zhao, and B.-Z. Wang, "A Beveled and slot-loaded planar bow-tie antenna for UWB application", *Progress in Electromagnetics Research M*, vol. 2, pp. 37–46, 2008.

[43] S. Sadek and Z. Katabay, "Ultra wideband CPW bow-tie antenna", International Conference on Electromagnetics in Advanced Applications, Torino, pp. 261–263, 2009.

[44] S.-J. Wu, and T.-G. Ma, "A slotted bow-tie antenna with reconfigurable CPW-to-slotline transition for pattern diversity", Proc. of ISAP2007, Niigata, Japan, pp. 720–723, Aug. 2007.

[45] K. H. Sayidmarie and Y. A. Fadhel, "A planar self-complementary bow-tie antenna for UWB applications", *Progress in Electromagnetics Research, PIER C*, vol. 35, pp. 253–267, 2013.

Chapter 5

Antennas and wearable sensors for biomedical diagnostics and therapeutic applications

Sachin Kumar[1,2] *and Lulu Wang*[1]

5.1 Introduction

Microwaves are electromagnetic radiations with frequencies ranging from 300 MHz to 300 GHz. They can be used for diagnosis, treatment, and prevention of the diseases. Using an antenna, the signals can be transmitted wirelessly over a distance that facilitates the remote treatment of the patient at home, and thus reducing the cost. Remote monitoring and treatment are already implemented for endoscopy, glucose level, insulin pumps, and other body fluids [1,2].

Due to the increasing interest in the body communication systems with time, an IEEE 802.15 standardization group was set up to standardize the in-body, on-body, and off-body communications. The in-body equipment communicates between the biomedical device implanted inside the body (e.g., wireless capsule endoscopy) and the nodes present on the body. The off-body communication happens between the wearable sensors and the nearby receiver unit [3]. Body-centric communications form an integral part of personal area networks and body area networks.

Recent technological developments in wireless sensor networks and wireless communications facilitated the design of lightweight, tiny, intelligent, and low-cost medical sensor nodes that can be placed strategically on the human body to create a wireless body area network (WBAN). WBAN helps in monitoring various physiological parameters of the body and provides real-time feedback to the patient.

5.2 Diagnostic technologies/techniques

5.2.1 Wireless body area network

A wireless sensor network comprising of communication and medical technologies and present in and around the human body is known as WBAN [4–6]. It contains

[1]Biomedical Device Innovation Center, Shenzhen Technology University, Shenzhen, China
[2]Department of Electronics and Communication Engineering, SRM Institute of Science and Technology, Chennai, India

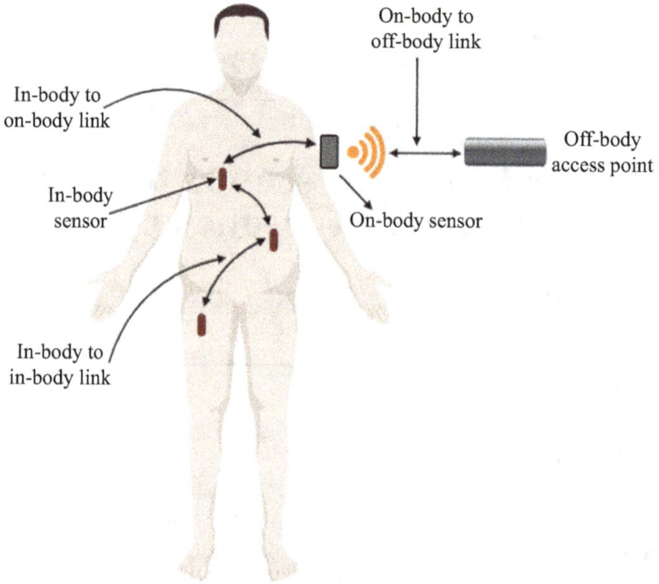

Figure 5.1 Schematic of a WBAN system

miniaturized sensors for monitoring physical activity, health, and emergency situations and acts as a connecting link between the electronic and physical domains. It is one of the emerging technologies that can be used for medical as well as nonmedical applications [7,8].

WBAN provides several advantages as compared to traditional healthcare monitoring systems. First, it uses portable compact sensors for monitoring and thus allowing mobility to the patients. Second, it continuously measures and monitors the different physiological parameters of the body. Data collected by the biosensors can be transmitted to the remote servers for the analysis of results and storage for future use.

WBAN consists of a gateway node or hub to connect with the external receiver system through communication networks such as WLAN, Bluetooth, Wi-Fi, dedicated network, mobile phone, and standard telephone networks. WBAN uses a high-speed data-transfer network to transfer the patient's data securely from one node to another [9]. Several communication standards were defined by the IEEE 802.15 Task Group 6 (TG6) to standardize communication between different devices in the networks [10].

Mainly three types of medical devices are present in the WBAN (see Figure 5.1)—implantable, ingestible, and wearable devices.

5.2.1.1 Implantable devices

Implantable devices are implanted or placed inside the human body using catheter-based procedures or surgical operations. They are made up of three functional units: sensors for collecting data of different parameters, communication unit for transferring data between the implanted device and the external receiver unit, and stimulators for performing required operations [11].

5.2.1.2 Ingestible devices

Some monitoring devices, known as ingestible, are swallowed by the patients and are generally used to monitor and diagnose diseases of the gastrointestinal tract [12]. An ingestible device consists of a camera, biosensors, and batteries that can last up to 24 h. After ingesting, it moves through the entire gastrointestinal tract and collects and transmits data of different physiological parameters, real-time images, videos, and can even deliver drugs. Capsule endoscopy is an example of the ingestible device [13].

5.2.1.3 Wearable devices

Wearable devices are externally worn by the patients to measure and monitor different physiological parameters of the human body. They can be used to monitor heart rate, temperature, glucose level, and other biochemical parameters of different body organs [14–16]. The recorded data can be transferred to the external hub using the data telemetry link. Compared to implantable and ingestible devices, the communication between devices is simple in the case of wearable as it is placed on the body. The wearable gadget/device battery can also be replaced easily, whenever required. Various applications of wearable devices include monitoring of heart rate in patients with cardiac irregularities, artificial limb movements, and monitoring of glucose levels in diabetic patients [17,18].

5.2.2 Implantable electronic medical devices

Implantable electronic devices provide improved diagnosis and treatment of various diseases and therefore are being used by a large number of people worldwide. These devices have even outperformed the nonimplantable devices in many aspects. For example, an insulin pump implanted near the pancreas showed better insulin infusion as compared to the traditional insulin injections given externally [19]. The implantation location of the device in the body depends on the functionality of the implanted gadget. Some devices are implanted superficially, which makes the implantation procedure easy and allows easy access to the implanted device, whereas some other devices are placed close to the target organ to be monitored. Some of the implants used are described in the following sections.

5.2.2.1 Biosensors and drug delivery systems

Biosensors are implanted under the skin to monitor biochemical properties and physiological conditions in the patients. A glucose monitoring sensor keeps track of the blood glucose level and an insulin injector is used to inject insulin, whenever required.

5.2.2.2 Cardiac implants

Cardiac implants include implantable cardioverter-defibrillator (ICD) and pacemakers and are the most widely used implantable devices [20]. They have different accelerometer and impedance sensors that can continuously monitor heart conditions. They monitor the cardiac rhythm and provide electrical pulses at the required positions and intensities.

5.2.2.3 Cochlear implants

Cochlear implants help people with poor hearing or deaf people to intercept and understand spoken languages [21]. These implants replace the damaged parts of the ear to redirect sound signals to the hearing nerves directly.

5.2.2.4 Neurostimulators

Neurostimulators are used to stimulate different parts of the brain and are generally placed on the skull. They help in treating different neurological diseases such as chronic depression, epilepsy, and Parkinson's disease by providing low amplitude electrical signals. Neurostimulators have better results than medicines [22–24].

5.2.2.5 Retinal implants

Retinal implants consist of microelectrodes and microelectronics that are implanted in the retina of the eye to give partial vision to blind people affected by photo-receptor cell degeneration [25]. These devices stimulate retinal nerve cells to produce visual perception through the brain. In addition to the implantable devices listed before, many other implantable devices are under research and development; for example, gastric pacemakers may be implanted in the abdomen to treat obese people and gastroparesis disease can be treated by using mild electric pulses [26].

5.3 Implant communication technologies

Implantable devices need to communicate with an external unit/base station for device monitoring and data transfer. The device monitoring provides updates on the battery condition and the time to repair the battery. Data transfer facilitates online control and review of information by physicians looking after patient's wellbeing. Once the data conversion process has been completed, the original data can be removed from the memory to provide room for new data tracking.

Implantable devices also communicate between themselves to facilitate synchronized and efficient operations. The data obtained from various implant sensors offer a deeper picture of the patient's condition and provides an appropriate and effective treatment to the patient. A comparison of different implant communication technologies is presented in Table 5.1. Some of the challenges faced in the implant communication systems are as follows:

- **Data rate:** Capsule video endoscopy needs a high data rate for seamless transmission of images and videos of the gastrointestinal tract to the external base station. For high data rate communication, the ultrawideband (UWB) may be used, but it results in high losses in propagation. Therefore, it is important to establish a trade-off between the data rate and the frequency.
- **Frequency spectrum regulations:** The demand for medical frequency spectrum is increasing with time. The frequency bands available currently include

Table 5.1 Performance comparison of different implant communication technologies

Communication technology	Method of propagation	Frequency	Data rate	Communication distance (cm)	Path loss	Power consumption	Standard
Inductive coupling	Magnetic field	<50 MHz	<1 Mbps	<5	High	Low	None
Intra body	Electric field	<20 MHz	<100 kbps	<10	Low	Moderate	IEEE 802.15.6
Molecular	Action potential	<1 kHz	<10 bps	<0.1	Ultra high	Ultra low	None
Optical	Infrared	300 GHz to 430 THz	<100 Mbps	<1	Very high	High	None
Radio frequency	Radio wave	402–405, 433.1–434.8, 868–868.6, 902.8–928, 2,400–2,500 MHz	<2 Mbps	<20	Moderate	High	MICS, ISM
Ultrasound	Ultrasonic	<3 MHz	<250 kbps	<10	High	High	None

industrial, scientific and medical (ISM), wireless medical telemetry service, medical implant communication system (MICS), and UWB [12]. The problem of interference is seen due to the increasing number of medical devices resulting in the interruption of vital services. In addition, the unlicensed ISM band can also be used for some nonmedical purposes that can lead to more communication interference.

- **Power consumption:** The life of the implantable device is determined by the battery used in it. The battery replacement process is a cumbersome task, and therefore the electronic circuitry of the implantable device should be designed in such a way as to consume less power. Wireless power transmission (WPT) is an alternative for recharging batteries, but its development is still in the infant stage and will not recharge the batteries of deep tissue implants [27]. Also, the use of WPT systems is restricted by the threshold values of the specific absorption rate (SAR) for the human body. If the power exceeds the SAR value, then it is not permitted to be used because it can create unnecessary heat, which can result in human tissue injury.
- **Security:** Privacy and security of the patient's information are important factors to take into consideration. Communication between the implantable devices and the external receiver units need to be highly secure to avoid any eavesdropping attempts.

5.3.1 Inductive coupling communication

In inductive coupling, the data and energy transmission takes place due to the mutual coupling between the primary and secondary coils [28]. The magnetic flux has better penetration at lower frequencies; therefore effective communication is achieved on them [29]. The magnetic field produced by the current flow in the primary/transmitter coil of the implant produces a current in the secondary coil of the implant.

Antennas are not required for signal propagation in inductive coupling communication, and thus the size of the implant can be decreased to a larger extent. Also, the use of inductive power transfer requires less battery power, which decreases the size of the battery. However, the inductive coupling only allows short-distance communication between the implants in the human body, as the magnetic field intensity decreases significantly with distance [30]. Moreover, even a small misalignment of the coils reduces coupling to a large extent. Therefore, this type of coupling communication is not suitable where the alignment of the implant is not fixed in the body and for implants located in deep corporal tissues. The inductive coupling offers limited bandwidth, and therefore it is not suitable for high data rate applications. Research has been done on the use of graphene nano-coils to increase the data rate, but further tests are needed on its impact on the body prior to practical use. Main parameters such as magnetic field strength and frequency of operation need to be tuned to ensure that this method is safe for patients, based on the approved SAR values.

Inductive coupling is used for neural implants, retinal implants, and cochlear implants. The inductive coupling should not be used for deep implants such as multi-node leadless pacemaker systems as implant displacement can occur due to the cardiac movements, resulting in the misalignment of the inductor coils, which will disturb the communication link.

5.3.2 Intra-body communication

Intra-body communication (IBC) uses a pair of electrodes on the transmitter side to generate a current and electric field, which propagates through the tissues. Similarly, the receiver consists of a pair of electrodes to receive transmitted information. The signal is propagated through the lossy and conductive human tissues for communication. IBC uses low power signals that work in a lower frequency region ranging from tens of kilohertz to tens of megahertz, where the skin serves as a nonconductive layer to prevent signal leakage outside the body. These properties make this communication robust to security breaches and enhance the security and privacy of the implantable device.

Based on the method used for signal coupling (for transmission within the human body), IBC can be divided into two categories—galvanic coupling and capacitive coupling. In galvanic coupling, the current flows via a direct path between a pair of electrodes at the transmitter and receiver [31]. The current density tends to decrease with the increasing distance between the transmitter and receiver electrodes. The galvanic coupling is suitable for communication between the in-body and the in-body implants and is least affected by the environmental noise. In capacitive coupling, the signal is coupled through the transmitter and receiver electrodes, but the signal return path is created by a common ground electrode outside the human body [32]. Capacitive coupling is used for on-body to on-body communication as a return path is established outside of the human body.

5.3.3 Molecular communication

Molecular communication uses molecules to encode, transmit, and receive in-body information. It encodes data in molecular characteristics such as release time, ratio, concentration, and type. It takes inspiration from nature and aims to emulate the way biological cells are communicated. It enables the design of smaller nanoscale implants, which are biocompatible by nature.

Molecular communication can be used for nanomachines that are used to detect the physiological properties of the human body and to deliver drugs. It also facilitates contact between different nanomachines of nanoscale implants present within the body. Molecular communication seems promising, but a lot of effort is still needed in this direction. The designing of these networks is difficult due to very small nanoscale dimensions and the stochastic nature of biochemical reactions [33]. Moreover, it involves molecules as the fundamental building blocks, which makes it different from conventional communication.

5.3.4 Optical communication

Optical communication involves the transmission of signals using infrared waves. It consists of a laser diode that converts the electrical signal at the transmitting end to the infrared signal. This communication consumes less power and thus increases the life of the implants. However, it suffers from the disadvantage of line-of-sight communication, which is not always available between the implants in the body, and due to high losses, communication is possible at a very short distance.

5.3.5 Radio frequency communication

Radio frequency (RF) communication consists of a transmitting antenna that radiates the signal in the form of electromagnetic waves, which are collected at the receiver antenna for further processing [34].

5.3.6 Ultrasound communication

Ultrasound communication involves the propagation of mechanical waves, from the transmitter to the receiver, within the human body. Piezoelectric transducers are used at the receiving end to convert mechanical waves to electrical signals. Ultrasound communication suffers from the disadvantage of high-energy absorption and high attenuation within the human body, resulting in biological tissue heating. However, the data obtained using this approach is controversial and inconsistent.

5.4 Cardiac pacemakers

Cardiovascular diseases are caused by the malfunctioning of the conduction mechanism of the heart and are one of the leading causes of death worldwide. These disorders can lead to disruption of blood pumping and adversely affect the efficiency of the heart, leading to cardiac arrest. Implantable electronic cardiovascular devices help to restore the natural rhythm of the heart and enhance the quality of life.

Cardiovascular implants can be grouped into the following categories:

- **Implantable cardioverter-defibrillators (ICD)**
  These implants are used to monitor and treat fast heart rhythm by giving anti-tachycardia shocks [35].
- **Tachycardia pacemakers**
  These implants are used to detect and treat a condition of bradycardia, where the heart rate slows down to less than 60 beats/min [36]. Tachycardia pacemaker continuously monitors the heart rate, and if it drops below a certain threshold, the pacemaker starts to pace the heart rate.
- **Cardiac resynchronization therapy devices**
  These devices are used to treat the condition when the right and left ventricles of the heart are out of synchronization [37]. A continuous wave of small and undetectable electrical pulses is sent to both the ventricles of the heart to synchronize their beating pattern, which improves ventricular contraction and pumping action.

5.4.1 Conventional pacemaker

The first cardiac pacemaker was implanted in the United States and Sweden in the 1960s, extending the life of patients by nearly 18 months [38]. Since then, pacemakers have experienced a great deal of progress in their design, implementation, and implantation processes.

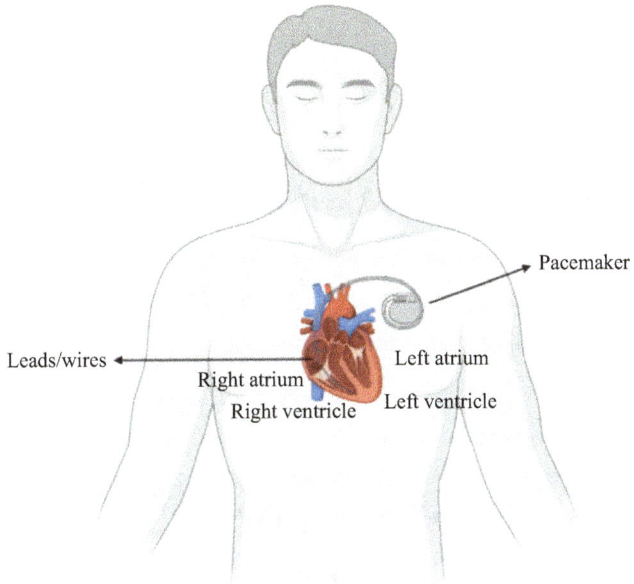

Figure 5.2 Pacemaker implanted in the human body

The first pacemakers featured only a timer and a battery-less sensor, data storage memory, and signal transmission communication equipment. A pacemaker consists of a biocompatible metallic can with an electrical pulse generator containing a lithium battery and its associated electrical circuits. The pacemaker is implanted in the subcutaneous pocket of the shoulder bone through surgery, as shown in Figure 5.2. The electrical circuitry uses one to three metallic wires or leads to connect the can to the heart chambers. The sensors present at the tip of the leads detect the irregularity in the heart and regulates the heartbeat by sending electrical pulses from the can to the heart. The pacemaker pulse generators need to be checked regularly at least twice or thrice a year. They must be replaced once every 5–10 years, depending on the life of the battery used in the can.

Conventional pacemakers are effective, but they suffer from some shortcomings primarily associated with the subcutaneous can or transvenous lead. These include hematoma, pocket infection, pneumothorax, cardiac perforation, and lead dislodgement [39]. Some other long-term complications include tricuspid regurgitation, venous obstruction, insulation failure, and lead breakage. The formation of endocarditis is another major concern with a high mortality rate [40,41]. Leads are seen to be the weakest link in traditional pacemakers, and thus, the advent of leadless pacemakers is seen to solve these complications.

5.4.2 Leadless pacemaker

The emergence of the concept of a leadless pacemaker was first seen in 1970 [42]. The schematic diagram of a leadless pacemaker is shown in Figure 5.3. Devices are

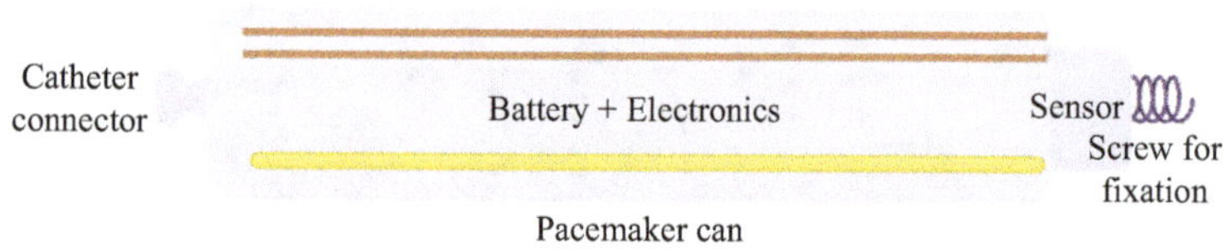

Figure 5.3 Schematic of a leadless pacemaker capsule

placed in the right ventricular wall using a catheter delivery system and offer ventricular simulation only.

The available leadless pacemakers stimulate only one chamber and are unable to perform synchronous atrioventricular pacing. Technology to stimulate multiple chambers of the heart and provide cardiac resynchronization is sought and will be the optimum solution [43].

5.5 Microwaves for medical applications

The standard imaging technologies such as computed tomography (CT), magnetic resonance imaging (MRI), ultrasound, and X-ray are being used for tumor detection, bone imaging, cancer diagnosis, appendicitis, musculoskeletal disorders, trauma, and infectious diseases. Some of these methods use ionizing radiation and provide significant clinical information and high-resolution images with good contrast.

The MRI provides high-resolution, but it is a costly and time-taking procedure. X-ray and CT scans use ionizing radiations for examination and therefore have the risk of cancer. The diagnostic ultrasound technique is preferred as it does not use ionizing radiation. However, it is unable to penetrate bones and air as it involves strong reflections resulting in acoustic shadows [44]. Also, this procedure requires a skilled operator to perform the examination and is less sensitive to certain regions such as the detection of retroperitoneal hematoma. The use of microwaves for medical applications helps to reduce the risks and problems associated with these technologies. Microwave methods are less harmful than CT scans and mammography due to the use of nonionizing electromagnetic waves. In addition, microwave techniques offer a noninvasive diagnosis, thus minimizing discomfort, patient recovery time, and improving the effectiveness of the procedure. Microwave techniques allow a disease to be detected early and increase accuracy and diagnostic performance. The primary applications of microwaves in the medical area include medical diagnosis, telemetry, and treatment, as shown in Figure 5.4. The main applications of the microwave method are explained in the following subsections.

5.5.1 Microwave medical diagnosis

The use of nonionizing electromagnetic waves for imaging and sensing medical applications in the microwave frequency range is increasing as it is more affordable and poses a low risk to human health compared to the imaging methods mentioned before. Microwave methods are based on the different signal-scattering behavior that

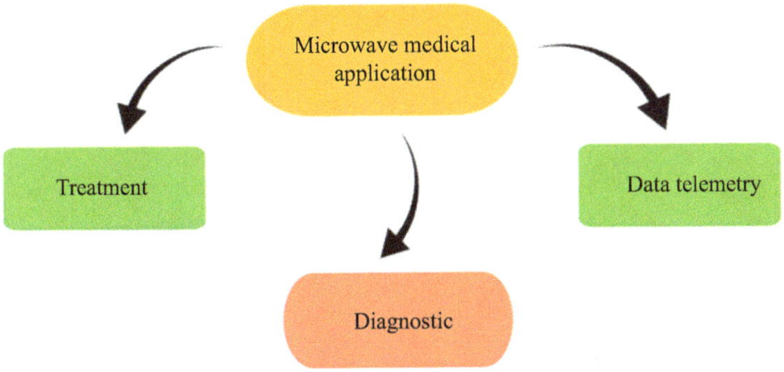

Figure 5.4 Applications of microwaves in medicine

is caused by the difference in dielectric properties (conductivity and relative permittivity) of the healthy and diseased tissue [45–47]. The image can also be formed by the differences in the permittivity and the high scattering positions that are generally seen in the case of a tumor formed inside the body. The microwave sensing and imaging spectrum used in medical diagnostics covers various applications such as stroke, fluid accumulation, blood flow, blood pressure, heartbeat detection, and traumatic brain injury [48–50]. Mainly two approaches are used for medical diagnosis using microwave methods of radio detection and ranging (radar) and microwave tomography (MWT) imaging. Both radar-based and MWT-based imaging employs wideband antennas, matching homogenous medium, and imaging algorithms to produce body image [51,52]. MWT requires the reconstruction of the dynamic distribution of permittivity using the reverse electromagnetic scattering solution.

5.5.2 Data telemetry

The data transmission mechanism between the implanted device and the external receiver/base station wirelessly using electromagnetic waves is known as data telemetry. In recent times, the use of healthcare products such as implanted devices for remote healthcare monitoring has been increased. Data telemetry helps in continuous monitoring and data transmission in different applications such as cochlear implants, diabetic glucose level monitoring, and deep brain stimulation [53,54]. In cochlear implant applications, an antenna is connected externally to the ear, which transmits audio signals directly to the cochlear implant receiver. Similarly, readings measured by an implanted glucose biosensor are passed to an external receptor system using an antenna during blood glucose monitoring. Data telemetry is also used for applications such as body temperature, intracranial pressure, heart rate, and blood pressure.

Microwave is the best technology available for data telemetry between the implanted and the external devices. Microwave allows wireless transmission through the tissues of the human body and the external receiver device and thus considerably increases the quality of life compared to conventional wire-based systems. Capacitive and galvanic couplings are two approaches used for data transmission.

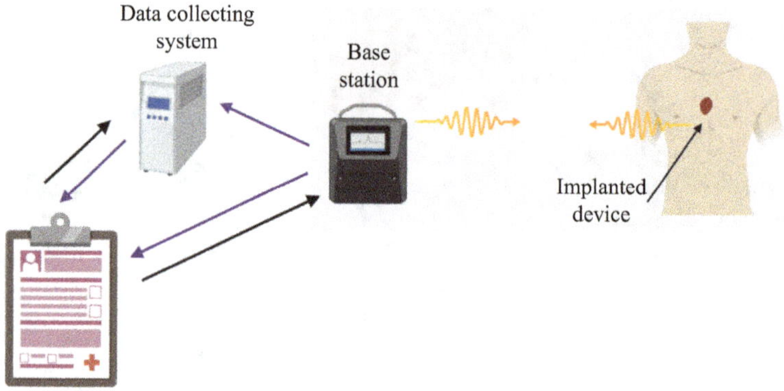

Figure 5.5 Schematic of the healthcare monitoring system

The use of wearable sensors and implantable devices, such as antennas, pacemakers, and swallowable pills, to monitor different parameters of the body is increasing. In general, such devices consist of a power supply unit and a transceiver system that facilitates the transmission of recorded signals wirelessly to the external receiver unit present outside the human body.

Figure 5.5 illustrates the model of the human healthcare monitoring system. This system is used to collect and transmit information (of different body parameters) to an external base station and consists of the following components.

5.5.2.1 Base station

The base station is generally composed of the following:

1. A controller module that collects and stores readings of different parameters of the body. It also controls the operation of the entire monitoring system.
2. A networking device for connecting the transmitter and the receiver terminals.
3. A receiver terminal to receive the transmitted signals and store the parameter readings.

5.5.2.2 Propagation medium

For the transmission of signals from the implant to the receiver base station, a medium/channel is needed.

5.5.2.3 Human body

The dispersive, complex, and highly lossy nature of the human body affects the manner in which the implantable devices are designed, realized, characterized, and analyzed in order to accurately transmit signals to the external receiver unit.

5.5.2.4 Implantable antennas

An antenna is one of the main components of RF-linked medical devices that allow communication between the implantable medical device and the external control unit. Patch antennas are preferred as they are flexible in conformability, shape, and design, which allow a small design and easy integration of a communicative antenna into a medical implant device [55–57].

5.5.2.5 Electronic circuitry

The electronic components of the implant determine the overall functionality of the device, define the specifications for operating power, and provide signal processing and data transmission. The battery is often used as a power source and the battery life defines the working duration of the implant. Several solutions, such as wireless power transfer, internal power supplies, or energy harvesting, may be used to increase the life of the implant [58,59].

5.5.2.6 Biosensors and bioactuators

The biosensors and bioactuators are the key components of the medical implant device that determines the operation and location of the implant in the human body. They can be used for various applications, including the monitoring of different parameters such as glucose measurement, pH, temperature, or they can serve as active systems for drug delivery applications.

5.5.2.7 Insulations

The components of the medical implant system should be properly insulated with a biocompatible material before being implanted in the human body to prevent any kind of adverse reaction inside the human body. The insulating layers are located either on the surface of the human skin or around the antenna, and the presence of an insulating layer often increases the transmission of electromagnetic waves between the implantable device and the base station.

5.6 Microwave medical treatment

Microwave medical treatment uses a thermal effect to destroy malignant cells. Microwave radiation is used to produce heat, thus increasing the local temperature of the malignant tissues to kill them. This method is more effective and reliable compared to other treatments such as surgical, ionizing radiation (X-ray), and toxins (chemotherapy) [60,61]. Microwave can also be used to treat hepatocellular carcinoma by heating and killing the hepatocells in blood clots (microwave coagulation therapy). Other microwave methods, such as microwave ablation, hyperthermia, and microwave thermotherapy, are also used for treatment [62–64].

5.7 Telemedicine: challenges and opportunities

The use of telecommunications to transmit patient information remotely to healthcare clinics is known as telemedicine. It allows monitoring of the health and diseases of the patients while continuing their treatment at home. Because of rapid technological advancements, telemedicine can be extended to video, audio, pictures, live streaming, and interactive teleconference systems. These technologies

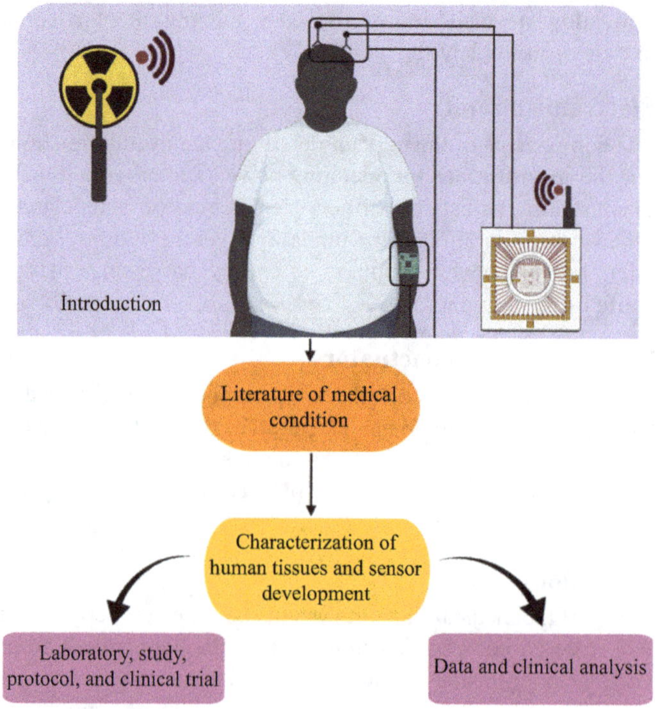

Figure 5.6 Illustration of telemedicine using microwaves

will contribute to the delivery of health services to rural and suburban communities. It also facilitates the collaboration of urban and rural healthcare professionals and keeps them up-to-date with all the latest developments in the field of healthcare.

The vision of telemedicine using microwaves is shown in Figure 5.6. Telemedicine can be used to monitor diseases such as stroke, asthma, burns, and cardiovascular. It is also used to relay vital signs such as respiration rate, blood glucose, blood pressure, and heart rate to a remote healthcare clinic that can help prompt timely medical action, if needed. From this perspective, a combination of microwave medical diagnostics and data telemetry effectively leads to an integrated and robust healthcare system.

5.8 Future perspectives

A lot of effort has been made in the study of in-body sensor networks. The body sensor network appears to be a promising technology to deliver an effective and personalized healthcare system to the patients. But there are still many issues that need to be tackled in order to successfully incorporate and take full advantage of the WBAN system. Several factors, such as power requirements, size, operating frequency, and biocompatibility issues, need to be addressed in the design of in-body devices. Addressing the limitations of in-body sensors will lead to new therapeutic applications, which will reduce medical costs for both patients and the community.

Another challenge is to optimize the power requirements of the implant in order to have long-lasting battery life. Energy harvesting and wireless power transfer need to be used to recharge the batteries used in the implant in order to run these devices for a lifetime. However, there is still no robust solution for WPT for deep tissue implants in an efficient manner. Moreover, implantation of implant devices and charging of batteries without damaging the surrounding biological tissues are problems yet to be addressed. Catheter technology helps to place implants in the cardiac chamber, but expertise is needed for the proper implantation process. Since the implanted device remains within the body for a long period of time, body tissues grow around them with time, making the implantation process more difficult and tricky.

The ongoing research in the development of a wireless system for the transfer of data between implants and external peripheral devices is important for effective communication between different devices. Patient data collected from various implant sensors could be fed to systems equipped with artificial intelligence algorithms. In the future, the devices will be connected to the Internet to form a network known as the "Internet of Implants." Though in-body sensor networks have been developed to monitor physiological conditions and provide medical treatment, their applications can be expanded in the future to military and interactive gaming.

References

[1] Wessels D. 'Implantable pacemakers and defibrillators: Device overview and EMI considerations'. *Proceedings of the IEEE International Symposium on Electromagnetic Compatibility*; Minneapolis, USA, August 2002. pp. 911–915.

[2] Chow E.Y., Morris M.M., and Irazoqui P.P. 'Implantable RF medical devices: The benefits of high-speed communication and much greater communication distances in biomedical applications'. *IEEE Microwave Magazine*. 2013;14(4):64–73.

[3] Kim J. and Rahmat-Samii Y. 'Implanted antennas inside a human body: Simulations designs, and characterizations'. *IEEE Transactions on Microwave Theory and Techniques*. 2004;52(8):1934–1943.

[4] Khan J.Y., Yuce M.R., Bulger G., and Harding B. 'Wireless body area network (WBAN) design techniques and performance evaluation'. *Journal of Medical Systems*. 2012;36:1441–1457.

[5] Rathee D., Rangi S., Chakarvarti S.K., and Singh V.R. 'Recent trends in wireless body area network (WBAN) research and cognition based adaptive WBAN architecture for healthcare'. *Health and Technology*. 2014;4:239–244.

[6] Latré B., Braem B., Moerman I., Blondia C., and Demeester P. 'A survey on wireless body area networks'. *Wireless Networks*. 2011;17:1–18.

[7] Jovanov E., Milenkovic A., Otto C., and de Groen P.C. 'A wireless body area network of intelligent motion sensors for computer assisted physical rehabilitation'. *Journal of NeuroEngineering and Rehabilitation*. 2005;2:6.

[8] Cao H., Leung V., Chow C., and Chan H. 'Enabling technologies for wireless body area networks: A survey and outlook'. *IEEE Communications Magazine*. 2009;47(12):84–93.

[9] Kos A., Milutinović V., and Umek A. 'Challenges in wireless communication for connected sensors and wearable devices used in sport biofeedback applications'. *Future Generation Computer Systems*. 2019;92:582–592.

[10] Chavez-Santiago R., Sayrafian-Pour K., Khaleghi A. *et al.* 'Propagation models for IEEE 802.15. 6 standardization of implant communication in body area networks'. *IEEE Communications Magazine*. 2013;51(8): 80–87.

[11] Schulman J.H., Dell R.D., and Gord J.C. 'System of implantable devices for monitoring and/or affecting body parameters'. US6164284. 2000.

[12] Kiourti A., Psathas K.A., and Nikita K.S. 'Implantable and ingestible medical devices with wireless telemetry functionalities: A review of current status and challenges'. *Bioelectromagnetics*. 2014;35(1):1–15.

[13] Iddan G., Meron G., Glukhovsky A., and Swain P. 'Wireless capsule endoscopy'. *Nature*. 2000;405:417.

[14] Lee H., Song C., Hong Y.S. *et al.* 'Wearable/disposable sweat-based glucose monitoring device with multistage transdermal drug delivery module'. *Science Advances*. 2017;3(3):e1601314.

[15] Trung T.Q., Ramasundaram S., Hwang B., and Lee N. 'An all-elastomeric transparent and stretchable temperature sensor for body-attachable wearable electronics'. *Advanced Materials*. 2016;28(3):502–509.

[16] El-Amrawy F. and Nounou M.I. 'Are currently available wearable devices for activity tracking and heart rate monitoring accurate, precise, and medically beneficial?'. *Healthcare Informatics Research*. 2015;21(4):315–320.

[17] Mohammed S., Amirat Y., and Rifai H. 'Lower-limb movement assistance through wearable robots: State of the art and challenges'. *Advanced Robotics*. 2012;26(1–2):1–22.

[18] Cheng C.H., Chong P.F., and Wong K.S. 'Wearable device to assist with the movement of limbs'. US8409117 B2. 2013.

[19] Malasri K and Wang L. 'Securing wireless implantable devices for healthcare: Ideas and challenges'. *IEEE Communications Magazine*. 2009;47(7): 74–80.

[20] Bardy G.H., Smith W.M., Hood M.A. *et al.* 'An entirely subcutaneous implantable cardioverter–defibrillator'. *New England Journal of Medicine*. 2010;363:36–44.

[21] Ouellet C. and Cohen H. 'Speech and language development following cochlear implantation'. *Journal of Neurolinguistics*. 1999;12(3–4):271–288.

[22] Sette A.L., Seigneuret E., Reymond F. *et al.* 'Battery longevity of neurostimulators in Parkinson disease: A historic cohort study'. *Brain Stimulation*. 2019;12:851–857.

[23] Kassiri H., Tonekaboni S., Salam M.T. *et al.* 'Closed-loop neurostimulators: A survey and a seizure-predicting design example for intractable epilepsy treatment'. *IEEE Transactions on Biomedical Circuits and Systems*. 2017;11 (5):1026–1040.

[24] Paemeleire K. and Goodman A.M. 'Results of a patient survey for an implantable neurostimulator to treat migraine headaches'. *The Journal of Headache and Pain*. 2012;13:239–214.

[25] Chuang A.T., Margo C.E., and Greenberg P.B. 'Retinal implants: A systematic review'. *British Journal of Ophthalmology*. 2014;98:852–856.

[26] Alighaleh S., Cheng L.K., Angeli T.R. *et al.* 'A novel gastric pacing device to modulate slow waves and assessment by high-resolution mapping'. *IEEE Transactions on Biomedical Engineering*. 2019;66(10):2823–2830.

[27] Abdulfattah A.N., Tsimenidis C.C., Al-Jewad B.Z., and Yakovlev A. 'Performance analysis of MICS-based RF wireless power transfer system for implantable medical devices'. *IEEE Access*. 2019;7:11775–11784.

[28] Teshome A.K., Kibret B., and Lai D.T.H. 'A review of implant communication technology in WBAN: Progress and challenges'. *IEEE Reviews in Biomedical Engineering*. 2018;12:88–99.

[29] Bashirullah R. 'Wireless implants'. *IEEE Microwave Magazine*. 2010;11(7): S14–S23.

[30] Lee B. and Ghovanloo M. 'An overview of data telemetry in inductively powered implantable biomedical devices'. *IEEE Communications Magazine*. 2019;57(2):74–80.

[31] Song Y., Hao Q., Zhang K., Wang M., Chu Y., and Kang B. 'The simulation method of the galvanic coupling intrabody communication with different signal transmission paths'. *IEEE Transactions on Instrumentation and Measurement*. 2010;60(4):1257–1266.

[32] Lucev Ž., Krois I., and Cifrek M. 'A capacitive intrabody communication channel from 100 kHz to 100 MHz'. *IEEE Transactions on Instrumentation and Measurement*. 2012;61(12):3280–3289.

[33] Huang Y., Wen M., Yang L.-L., Chae C.-B., and Ji F. 'Spatial modulation for molecular communication'. *IEEE Transactions on Nanobioscience*. 2019;18(3):381–395.

[34] Kiourti A. and Nikita K.S. 'A review of implantable patch antennas for biomedical telemetry: Challenges and solutions [wireless corner]'. *IEEE Antennas and Propagation Magazine*. 2012;54(3):210–228.

[35] Young J.B., Abraham W.T., Smith A.L. *et al.* 'Combined cardiac resynchronization and implantable cardioversion defibrillation in advanced chronic heart failure: The miracle ICD trial'. *JAMA*. 2003;289(20):2685–2694.

[36] Brockway B.P., Dreher R.D., Huntwork D.E., Lindstedt B.S., Morrison D.C., and Mills P.A. 'Programmable multi-mode cardiac pacemaker'. US4562841A. 1986.

[37] Moss A.J., Hall W.J., Cannom D.S. *et al.* 'Cardiac-resynchronization therapy for the prevention of heart-failure events'. *New England Journal of Medicine*. 2009;361:1329–1338.

[38] Beck H., Boden W.E., Patibandla S. *et al.* '50th anniversary of the first successful permanent pacemaker implantation in the United States: Historical review and future directions'. *The American Journal of Cardiology*. 2010;106(6):810–818.

[39] Pakarinen S., Oikarinen L., and Toivonen L. 'Short-term implantation-related complications of cardiac rhythm management device therapy: A retrospective single-centre 1-year survey'. *Europace*. 2010;12(1):103–108.

[40] Maldari M., Albatat M., Bergsland J., Haddab Y., Jabbour C., and Desgreys P. 'Wide frequency characterization of intra-body communication for leadless pacemakers'. *IEEE Transactions on Biomedical Engineering*. 2020;67 (11):3223–3233.

[41] Miralles A., Moncada V., Chevez H., Rodriguez R., Granados J., and Castells E. 'Pacemaker endocarditis: Approach for lead extraction in endocarditis with large vegetations'. *The Annals of Thoracic Surgery*. 2001;72 (6):2130–2132.

[42] Bhatia N. and El-Chami M. 'Leadless pacemakers: A contemporary review'. *Journal of Geriatric Cardiology*. 2018;15:249–253.

[43] Bereuter L., Kuenzle T., Niederhauser T. *et al.* 'Fundamental characterization of conductive intracardiac communication for leadless multisite pacemaker systems'. *IEEE Transactions on Biomedical Circuits and Systems*. 2019;13(1):237–247.

[44] Metev S.M. and Veiko V.P. *Laser Assisted Microtechnology*. Berlin: Springer; 1998.

[45] Li X., Bond E.J., Van Veen B.D., and Hagness S.D. 'An overview of ultra-wideband microwave imaging via space-time beamforming for early-stage breast-cancer detection'. *IEEE Antennas and Propagation Magazine*. 2005;47(1):19–34.

[46] Fear E.C., Li X., Hagness S.C., and Stuchly M.A. 'Confocal microwave imaging for breast cancer detection: Localization of tumors in three dimensions'. *IEEE Transactions on Biomedical Engineering*. 2002;49(8):812–822.

[47] Semenov S.Y. and Corfield D.R. 'Microwave tomography for brain imaging: Feasibility assessment for stroke detection'. *International Journal of Antennas and Propagation*. 2008:254830.

[48] Obeid D., Sadek S., Zaharia G., and El Zein G. 'Multitunable microwave system for touchless heartbeat detection and heart rate variability extraction'. *Microwave and Optical Technology Letters*. 2010;52(1):192–198.

[49] Persson M., Fhager A., Trefná H.D. *et al.* 'Microwave-based stroke diagnosis making global prehospital thrombolytic treatment possible'. *IEEE Transactions on Biomedical Engineering*. 2014;61(11):2806–2817.

[50] Scapaticci R., Bucci O.M., Catapano I., and Crocco L. 'Differential microwave imaging for brain stroke followup'. *International Journal of Antennas and Propagation*. 2014:312528.

[51] Islam M.T., Mahmud M.Z., Islam M.T., Kibria S., and Samsuzzaman M. 'A low cost and portable microwave imaging system for breast tumor detection using UWB directional antenna array'. *Scientific Reports*. 2019;9:15491.

[52] Nikolova N.K. 'Microwave imaging for breast cancer'. *IEEE Microwave Magazine*. 2011;12(7):78–94.

[53] Qian H., Loizou P.C., and Dorman M.F. 'Phone-assistive devices based on Bluetooth technology for cochlear implant users'. *IEEE Transactions on Neural Systems Rehabilitation Engineering*. 2003;11(3):282–287.

[54] Karacolak T., Hood A.Z., and Topsakal E. 'Design of a dual-band implantable antenna and development of skin mimicking gels for continuous glucose monitoring'. *IEEE Transactions on Microwave Theory and Techniques*. 2008;56(4):1001–1008.

[55] Soontornpipit P., Furse C.M., and Chung Y.C. 'Design of implantable microstrip antenna for communication with medical implants'. *IEEE Transactions on Microwave Theory and Techniques*. 2004;52(8):1944–1951.

[56] Kiziltas G., Psychoudakis D., Volakis J.L., and Kikuchi N. 'Topology design optimization of dielectric substrates for bandwidth improvement of a patch antenna'. *IEEE Transactions on Antennas and Propagation*. 2003;51(10): 2732–2743.

[57] Zhou Y., Chen C.C., and Volakis J.L. 'Dual band proximity-fed stacked patch antenna for tri-band GPS applications'. *IEEE Transactions on Antennas and Propagation*. 2007;55(1):220–223.

[58] Tang Z., Smith B., Schild J.H., and Peckham P.H. 'Data transmission from an implantable biotelemeter by load-shift keying using circuit configuration modulator'. *IEEE Transactions on Biomedical Engineering*. 1995;42 (5):524–528.

[59] Valdastri P., Menciassi A., Arena A., Caccamo C., and Dario P. 'An implantable telemetry platform system for in vivo monitoring of physiological parameters'. *IEEE Transactions on Information Technology in Biomedicine*. 2004;8(3):271–278.

[60] Vrba J. and Oppl L. 'Prospective applications of microwaves in medicine'. *Proceedings of the 14th Conference on Microwave Techniques*; Prague, Czech Republic, April 2008. pp. 1–4.

[61] Roemer R.B. 'Engineering aspects of hyperthermia therapy'. *Annual Review of Biomedical Engineering*. 1999;1:347–376.

[62] Bansal R. 'Battling cancer: The latest on microwave hyperthermia'. *IEEE Microwave Magazine*. 2005;6(3):32–34.

[63] Diederich C.J. 'Thermal ablation and high-temperature thermal therapy: Overview of technology and clinical implementation'. *International Journal of Hyperthermia*. 2005;21(8):745–753.

[64] Simon C.J., Dupuy D.E., and Mayo-Smith W.W. 'Microwave ablation: Principles and applications'. *Radiographics*. 2005;25:69–83.

Chapter 6

Review of practical antennas for microwave and millimetre-wave medical imaging

Wasan H. Althubitat Al Amro[1] *and Boon-Chong Seet*[1]

With the proliferation of different cancerous diseases in the world and the limitations of the conventional methods for their early detection, radio-frequency medical imaging (RFMI) has emerged as a promising technique with attractive properties to overcome the detection challenges. Antennas play an essential role in RFMI as they directly impact the system detection efficiency. The parameters that need to be considered while designing the antenna for RFMI include operating bandwidth, directionality, gain, design complexity, and the cost of fabrication. This chapter reviews different practical antennas proposed in the literature for RFMI in microwave and millimetre-wave (mm-wave) regimes for the detection of breast cancer, lung cancer, lung fluid accumulation, skin cancer, brain tumour, and brain stroke.

6.1 Introduction

According to the World Health Organisation, breast cancer and lung cancer are the most common cancer in women and men, respectively [1]. Skin cancer is another prominent type of cancer that affects both genders, with New Zealand having one of the highest incidence rates in the world [2]. Breast cancer occurs when an abnormal and overgrowth of breast cells led to the formation of malignant (cancerous) tumour. The symptoms include a lump or swelling in the breast, abnormal nipple discharge, and changes to the nipple or breast shape and texture. Lung fluid accumulation is an acute respiratory system complication, which can occur inside the lung (pulmonary oedema) or around the lung (pleural effusion). The latter is commonly caused by lung cancer [3,4]. Skin cancer can be melanoma or non-melanoma. The former is more deadly as it can spread rapidly but is less common than the latter [5]. Brain tumour, even if benign (non-cancerous), can be life-threatening when located in deep and delicate part of the brain [6]. Brain stroke is generally caused by the lack of blood flow in the brain due to blood bleed or blood clot [7]. Both brain tumour and brain stroke can cause severe brain injuries [8].

[1]Department of Electrical and Electronic Engineering, Auckland University of Technology, Auckland, New Zealand

Early-stage detection of the aforementioned disease types plays an important role in controlling their prevalence. A reliable diagnosis at an early stage could greatly enhance the prognosis and the treatment outcomes. The first step of breast, brain, lung, and skin cancer detection is the physical examination or the conventional imaging techniques such as X-ray mammography, computed tomography (CT), ultrasound, and magnetic resonance imaging (MRI) [9]. X-ray mammography is the most popular detection method for early-stage breast cancer [10], while CT is most appropriate for lung cancer and fluid accumulation detection [11]. Using these methods, however, can be painful and difficult to pin-point the precise location of the tumour. X-ray mammogram is usually followed by ultrasound scanning to detect tumour sizes down to a few millimetres (mm), but it is still difficult to differentiate between benign and malignant tumours. MRI and CT are the common methods to identify pathological changes and structural variations of biological tissues such as brain, lung, and skin tissues [12], but they are not suitable for continuous monitoring of tumours due to high cost and high time consumption.

Medical imaging techniques using radio-frequency (RF) waves in the microwave and mm-wave regimes, which we referred to as RFMI, have been developed in the past two decades as a promising complementary technology for an early-stage detection of cancer and other serious diseases. The reconstructed image quality of the tumours and other abnormalities in the body by the RFMI system depend heavily on the characteristics of the used antennas such as the radiation pattern, gain, and operational bandwidth. For instance, using an antenna with high gain or directionality minimises the environmental noise effects and increases the signal penetration into the human target area, resulting in improved signal-to-noise ratio and consequently higher quality images. It is also desirable for the antenna to have an operational bandwidth of several GHz in order to achieve an image resolution down to millimetre scale. There are several advantages of RFMI over conventional imaging tools. First, it is less intrusive than X-ray mammography with no need for breast compression. Second, the produced radiation is non-ionised and thus is safer for pregnant women unlike CT and X-ray mammography [4,13]. Third, the amount of energy absorption by the human body from its radiation field is less and usually within a safe level of specific absorption rate [14]. Lastly, it is comparatively less expensive. These advantages of RFMI make it a prospective mechanism to overcome the limitations of traditional imaging methods.

In RFMI, the radio waves are scattered differently by the cancerous tissues because of their higher dielectric properties than the adjacent healthy tissues. Such dielectric discrepancy between different tissue types is the basic principle utilised by RFMI for cancer detection [15]. The scattered signals from human target area are acquired, pre-processed to reduce clutter produced by skin reflection and environmental background noise, and then used for reconstructing images of the target area through the application of signal processing.

The rest of the chapter is organised as follows. Section 6.2 discusses the different RFMI techniques and signal-processing algorithms. Sections 6.3–6.6 review current state-of-the-art antenna designs for detection of (i) breast cancer, (ii) brain cancer and stroke, (iii) lung cancer and fluid accumulation, and (iv) skin cancer, respectively. The antennas are discussed in terms of their performance, compactness, and the quality of reconstructed images. Section 6.7 concludes the chapter with some directions for future research.

6.2 RFMI techniques and signal-processing algorithms

RFMI techniques can be classified as active, passive, or hybrid [16]. Active RFMI is the most common technique, where human tissues are illuminated using low-power RF signals to reconstruct the images of the area under test, based on a contrast of the dielectric properties between cancerous and healthy tissues due to differences in their water, sodium, and protein content. Cancerous tissues can be malignant with higher sodium content than normal tissues that lead to high water retention and thus high permittivity and conductivity values; or benign with mainly fatty or adipose tissues that have lower dielectric properties than normal tissues [5]. On the other hand, the passive RFMI relies on the temperature contrast between cancerous and healthy tissues to reconstruct images. Distinctively, the lower thermo-regulatory potential of the cancerous tissues causes them to dissipate more heat than typical host tissues. This technique is referred to as *radiometry* performed with a radiometer. The hybrid RFMI techniques also use thermo-heating RF signals to illuminate the human issue. However, the detection is based on using an ultrasound transducer to detect the pressure waves generated due to heated tissue expansion, which are more significant for cancerous tissues. This difference in the level of generated pressure waves between cancerous and healthy tissues is used for reconstructing an image of the area. Examples of hybrid RFMI techniques include RF-induced ultrasound imaging, RF elastography, and thermo-acoustic tomography.

Active RFMI can be further classified into *tomography* (transmission–reflection imaging) and *ultra-wideband (UWB) radar*. Tomography is a non-linear scattering approach for reconstructing the dielectric profile of the target area using the incident and received fields, shape of the target area, and spatial distribution of electrical permittivity. Tomography imaging is based on the scattered RF field of a single frequency or multiple frequencies by transmitting a narrowband signal by a single antenna at a distinct location from the object, and the reflected signals are received by receiver antennas placed at the opposite location. If the target area tissue is cancerous and malignant, it would reduce the strength of the scattered signals, resulting in high permittivity and conductivity values. However, image reconstruction by tomography is an ill-posed inverse problem that is very prone to noise in the signal data [17].

On the other hand, UWB radar-based imaging is a linear scattering approach that transmits a short pulse towards a target area and measures the scattered pulse to create an image [18]. It is also referred to as *confocal medical imaging* (CMI) [19]. A cancerous malignant tissue will produce a spot with high intensity of energy due to high reflection. The antennas are used to transmit short pulses or modulated RF signal, and the scattered signals are received by either the same transmitting antennas or different receiver antennas located at different positions. Despite the

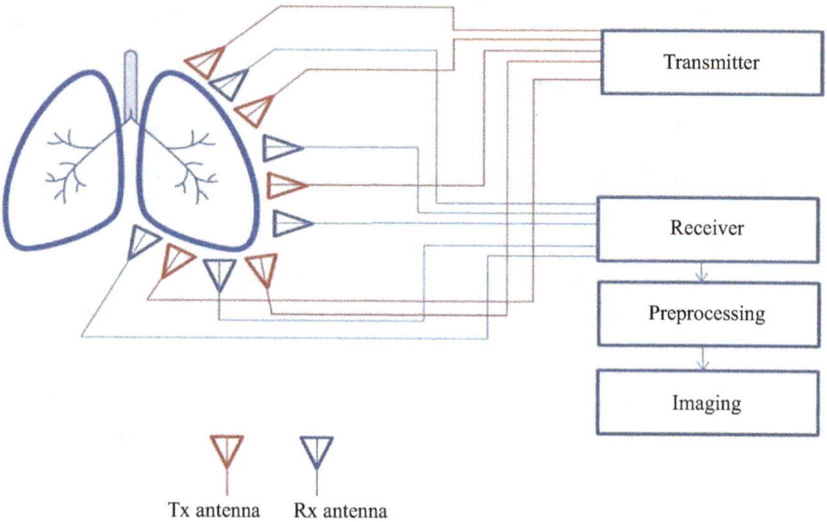

Figure 6.1 RFMI system architecture in example application for lung imaging

differences between these two active approaches, they share the same general architecture for imaging systems as shown in Figure 6.1.

In CMI, the target images can be reconstructed using radar-based beamforming algorithms. An effective reconstruction algorithm provides a precise localisation of tumours, while suppressing clutter and any residual artefacts from pre-processing stage. The algorithms implement coherent addition of the backscattered signals received after illuminating the target area with short UWB pulses. The algorithms can be classified as *data independent* (DI) or *data adaptive* (DA). To compensate path attenuation and dispersion, DI algorithms perform coherent addition using an assumed propagation model while DA algorithms estimate the propagation model from received signals and then utilise this model (applied with certain compensation factors) to perform coherent addition [20].

Different radar-based image reconstruction algorithms such as delay-and-sum (DAS), improved delay-and-sum (IDAS), delay-multiply-and-sum (DMAS), coherence factor based DAS (CF-DAS), channel ranked DAS (CR-DAS), and robust Capon beamformer (RCB) have been proposed in the literature, which can be used with both monostatic and multistatic UWB radar systems [20]. DAS, IDAS, DMAS, CF-DAS, and CR-DAS are DI algorithms, whereas RCB is a DA algorithm. Among these algorithms, DMAS exhibits the best overall performance in clutter reduction and tumour localisation. All the previously shown algorithms can be used to reconstruct two- (2D) or three-dimensional (3D) images. In most cases, 2D images can provide sufficient information, such as the existence of tumours, number of tumours, location, shape and size of detected tumours. However, if tumour depth is an important parameter, or there exist multiple tumours at the same location, then a 3D image is required. In dense fibro-glandular

Table 6.1 Hemispherical breast model parameters for a 2–4 GHz band

Layer	Thickness (mm)	Relative dielectric constant ε_r	Conductivity σ (S/m)
Skin	2	34.95	3.89
Fat	8	4.94	0.31
Glandular tissue	40	11–15	0.4–0.5

tissues, a 3D image can also provide more accurate detection and localisation of cancerous tissues than 2D images.

6.3 Antennas for breast cancer detection

Due to the increasing prevalence of breast cancer in women, antenna design for RFMI-based detection of breast tumours has attracted much attention. Typically, a breast phantom is used as a hemispherical model of breast tissue to evaluate the effectiveness of a proposed imaging system. Table 6.1 shows the parameters of the model, including thickness, relative dielectric permittivity, and conductivity for different layers of skin, fat, and glandular tissues that constitute the breast tissue [21]. The key types of antennas proposed in the literature for breast cancer detection include Vivaldi, fractal, and planar monopole antennas of semicircular, circular, rectangular, spiral, and triangular configurations. Their performance in terms of bandwidth, gain, radiation pattern, and compactness are discussed.

6.3.1 Vivaldi antennas

Vivaldi antennas are end-fire-type antennas that have been widely used in RFMI because of their wide operating bandwidth, high directional capability, and ease of fabrication. In general, a Vivaldi antenna is made up of a uniform slot with $\lambda/4$ length attached directly to an exponentially tapered slot. Hence, the Vivaldi antenna is also known as a tapered slot antenna. Recently, different methods have been used to enhance their directivity through better impedance matching and extend their operating frequency into lower bands by embedding slots in radiators to lengthen the path of the surface electric currents. In [21], the authors designed a Vivaldi antenna with three metal patches applied on the end-fire, which served as directors to increase the antenna gain by approximately 4 dBi. The proposed antenna is fabricated on 1-mm thick F4B substrate ($\varepsilon_r = 2.55$) with overall dimensions of $70\times79\times1$ mm^3, an operating frequency range of 2.4–13 GHz, peak gain of ~9.5 dBi at 12 GHz, and a consistent directional radiation pattern over the operating frequency range.

6.3.2 Fractal antennas

A fern-shaped fractal leaf configuration of antipodal Vivaldi antenna was presented in [22]. A good enhancement in the lower impedance bandwidth is offered, in which the lower frequency band is decreased in the second iteration of the leaf structure by 19% as compared with the first leaf structure. This reduction is accomplished by the reorientation of modes induced by current distribution. The antenna was fabricated on an FR4 substrate (ε_r = 4.4) with a total size of 50.8×62×0.8 mm^3 and operates at the frequency range of 1.3–20 GHz. There is a high directive gain of ~10 dBi and a stable radiation pattern. A good agreement between simulated and measured results of the proposed antenna is reported.

6.3.3 Planar monopole antennas

Several monopole antennas with different patch shapes have been widely used for RFMI because of their distinctive properties. The antenna classifications adopted in the literature for RFMI are described in the following subsections.

6.3.3.1 Circular and semicircular patch antennas

A multi-input–multi-output (MIMO) antenna with four circular radiating elements is proposed in [1]. The design approach to increase operational bandwidth is that of inserting slots into the ground plane, etching an elliptical slot into the patch, and laying out the ground plane in a staircase style. The designed antenna is printed on a 40×30×1.5 mm^3 FR4 substrate (ε_r = 4.4) and covers a bandwidth that spans the frequency range of 2.8–20 GHz. The results show a stable omnidirectional radiation pattern over the operational bandwidth.

In [9], the authors presented a semicircular patch antenna element and 16-element antenna array. The proposed structure improves impedance matching and operating bandwidth by the use of trapezoidal ground plane and the inclusion of semicircular slot in the patch. Fabricated on a Rogers RT5880 substrate (ε_r = 2.2) with dimensions of 41×42×1.575 mm^3, the proposed antenna exhibits a total bandwidth of 8.7 GHz over the frequency range of 2.3–11 GHz, peak gain of 5.8 dBi, and stable directional radiation pattern.

6.3.3.2 Rectangular, spiral, and triangular patch antennas

Two flexible 4×4 arrays are as follows: one with rectangular patch elements and the other with planar spiral elements are designed and fabricated on flexible 50 mm thick Kapton polyimide with an overall size of 20×20 mm^2 in [15] as shown in Figure 6.2. The rectangular patch antenna improves the impedance matching and bandwidth by cutting multiple steps at the lower patch corners and using a coplanar waveguide (CPW) network feeder. The single-arm spiral antenna is used to induce currents in both x and y directions equally, with the antenna being made of several rectangular components of equal length, positioned horizontally and vertically. The proposed rectangular and spiral antenna arrays can provide a wideband impedance bandwidth over the frequency range of 2–4 GHz. Figure 6.3(a) and (b) shows the S-parameters measurement set-up using a spiral antenna array on a breast mimicking phantom, and top view of the antenna array, respectively.

Several other rectangular patch antennas for breast imaging have been proposed in [10,13,23]. A rectangular patch antenna with cut slots at lower edges is

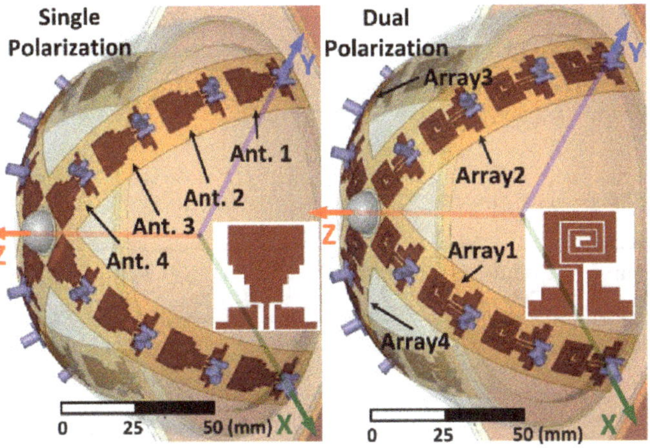

Figure 6.2 Overview of single-arm spiral and monopole antenna arrays for breast cancer detection [15]

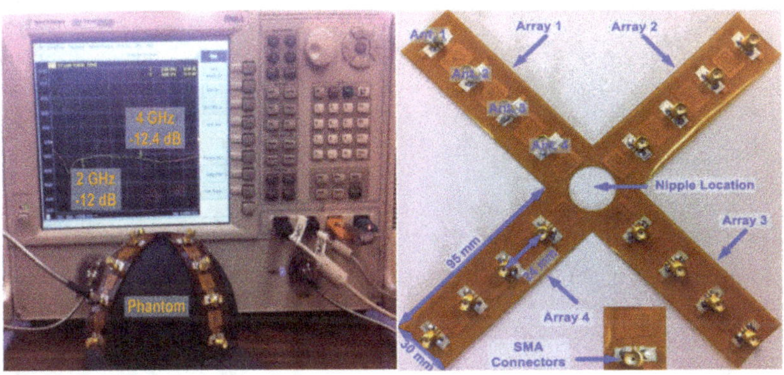

(a) (b)

Figure 6.3 (a) Antenna array on breast mimicking phantom and (b) top view of spiral antenna array [15]

reported in [23]. Fabricated on an FR4 substrate with a size of $36\times34\times1.6$ mm^3, the proposed structure achieves a wideband bandwidth over the frequency range of 2.4–4.7 GHz and is shown to be a good candidate for breast cancer detection at different depths. In [13], a structure consisting of a rectangular patch with stair-case configuration at the lower ends and extended distance between the patch and ground plane that significantly improve the performance is proposed. In [10], the authors introduced a planar rectangular monopole antenna backed by a reflector to reduce the unwanted backward radiation towards the human body. Both proposed antenna and reflector have the same dimensions of $50\times33\times1.635$ mm^3 implemented over an FR4 substrate. A unidirectional gain of 3.6 dBi is achieved over the operating frequency range of 2.5–6 GHz. Similarly, a triangular patch monopole antenna on an FR4 substrate operating in the frequency range of 0.5–3 GHz is proposed in [17]. A summary of the aforementioned antenna designs for breast cancer detection is given in Table 6.2.

Table 6.2 Summary of antenna designs for breast cancer detection

Ref.	Antenna type	Frequency (GHz)	Size (mm^3)	Gain (dBi)	Key features/Remarks
[1]	Circular patch	2.8–20	40×30×1.5	n/a	• MIMO antenna fabricated and tested on realistic phantom • Ultra-wide bandwidth for enhancing image resolution, but no reconstructed image produced • PCA method used in tumour detection
[9]	Semicircular patch	2.3–11	41×42×1.575	5.6	• A 16-element array to scan 240 locations and detect a tumour of diameter ≥5 mm • Ultra-wide bandwidth and directional radiation to enhance image resolution and signal penetration, respectively • Not tested on realistic phantom
[10]	Rectangular patch	2.5–6	50×33×1.635	3.8	• Proposed antenna backed by a reflector • Can detect a tumour size of 15×15×10 mm^3 in dense fibro glandular tissues • Tested on simulated not fabricated realistic phantom
[13]	Rectangular patch	2–4	n/a	n/a	• A 16-element array on wearable device to construct 2D tumour images • Proposed antenna size, gain, and radiation pattern not specified
[15]	Rectangular/ spiral patch	2–4	20×20×0.05	n/a	• A 4×4 array tested on a realistic phantom • Reported proposed antenna's reflection coefficient and efficiency but not its gain and radiation pattern

(Continues)

Table 6.2 (Continued)

Ref.	Antenna type	Frequency (GHz)	Size (mm^3)	Gain (dBi)	Key features/Remarks
					• No evaluation on image reconstruction
[17]	Triangular patch	0.5–3	n/a	n/a	• Tested on a realistic phantom to detect a tumour size of $\geq$16 mm • Proposed antenna size, gain, and radiation pattern not specified
[21]	Vivaldi	2.4–13	70×79×1	9.5	• Use metallic directors to increase gain at lower frequency range • Offers ultra-wideband bandwidth and high directive gain • Not tested on realistic phantom
[22]	Fractal	1.3–20	50.8×62×0.8	10	• Offers super-wideband bandwidth and high directive gain • Not tested on simulated or fabricated realistic phantom
[23]	Rectangular patch	2.4–4.7	36×34×1.6	n/a	• Tested on a realistic phantom to detect a tumour size of $\geq$16 mm at depths $\leq$30 mm in breast tissues • Proposed antenna gain and radiation pattern not specified

6.4 Antennas for brain cancer and stroke detection

Brain injury can be caused by traumatic and non-traumatic disorders such as brain cancer and brain stroke, respectively. Generally, strokes occurred due to blood flow deficiency as a result of either bleeding (haemorrhagic stroke) or clotting (ischemic stroke). The incidence of brain cancer and stroke is growing rapidly and posing a severe threat to human life. This motivates many researchers to develop different antennas for RFMI to detect brain tumour and stroke by contrasting the brain tissue dielectric properties. Table 6.3 shows the model parameters of a healthy human head phantom that consists of six layers: skin, fat, skull, dura, cerebrospinal fluid (CSF), and brain (mixture of grey and white matter). The relative dielectric constant and conductivity values are given for 1.6 GHz [24,25], which is the optimal imaging frequency for brain injury. In contrast, the dielectric properties of brain tumour and stroke are $\varepsilon_r = 59.7$, $\sigma = 1.91$ S/m, and $\varepsilon_r = 55$, $\sigma = 7$ S/m, respectively. The main types of antennas discussed here are planar monopole antennas of

Table 6.3 Human head model parameters

Layer	Thickness (mm)	Relative dielectric constant ε_r	Conductivity σ (S/m)
Skin	1	39.2	1.11
Fat	1.4	5.37	0.07
Skull	4.1	12	0.24
Dura	0.5	43.2	1.23
CSF	2	67.5	2.79
Brain	81	44	1.01

various configurations, including rectangular, modified circular, circular, triangular, trapezoidal, and bowtie. Their performances, such as in terms of antenna bandwidth, gain, radiation pattern, and compactness, are also discussed.

6.4.1 Antennas for brain cancer detection

6.4.1.1 Rectangular patch antennas

A rectangular microstrip patch antenna with symmetrical defected ground structure (DGS) is presented in [26]. This antenna is fabricated on a 0.812-mm thick Rogers's 4004 lossy substrate ($\varepsilon_r = 3.55$). A 30×22 mm DGS is incorporated to reduce the antenna loss at a resonant frequency of 5.8 GHz and extend its operating bandwidth to 1.9 GHz from 89 MHz obtained with a simple rectangular antenna. However, the antenna gain is reduced from 6.97 dB (simple rectangular antenna) to 3.496 dB (with DGS). Another rectangular patch antenna with dimensions $25.92 \times 31.017 \times 1.03$ mm^3 is proposed in [6] to detect brain tumour. A circular electromagnetic band gap (EBG) structure is incorporated on antenna's ground plane in order to enhance the reflection coefficient and imaging quality. Rogers R03003 with $\varepsilon_r = 3$ is chosen as the substrate. The antenna operates in the frequency range of 7.5–7.79 GHz with a flat gain of 6.7 dBi. A tumour of 5-mm radius can be detected in a simulated head phantom.

6.4.1.2 Circular and modified-circular patch antennas

A modified circular patch antenna fabricated on a 1.575-mm-thick Rogers Duroid RT5880 substrate ($\varepsilon_r = 2.2$) is presented in [27]. A 34.5×20-mm antenna structure is analysed, which operates in the frequency range of 3.1–10.6 GHz, providing an ultra-wide bandwidth with 7.573-dBi peak gain. A unidirectional radiation pattern is obtained by the utilisation of an aluminium plate reflector ($\varepsilon_r = 3.4$) with total dimensions of $50 \times 40 \times 2$ mm^3. The reflector is placed at the back side of the antenna to suppress undesired radiation lobes. Another UWB antenna array is made up of four identical circular patches of a 15-mm diameter is proposed in [28]. It is fabricated on a $45 \times 80 \times 1.5748$-mm^3 Taconic (TLY-5) substrate with $\varepsilon_r = 2.2$. The antenna has a frequency range of 2.6–13.1 GHz and a relative peak gain of 12.12 dB when measured on a phantom at different positions.

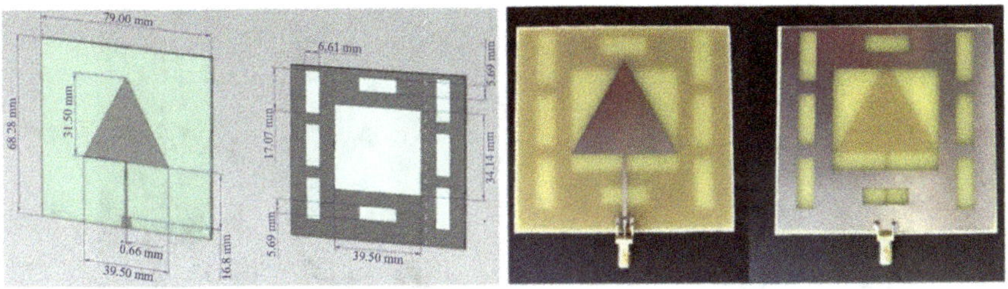

Figure 6.4 The front and back view of the designed (left) and fabricated (right) isosceles triangular patch antenna [7]

6.4.2 Antennas for brain stroke detection

6.4.2.1 Trapezoidal and triangular patch antennas

A trapezoidal patch antenna with CPW feeding network is reported in [29]. The antenna element is fabricated on a 70×30×0.2-mm^3 FR4 substrate. The operating frequency range of the antenna is between 1 and 4 GHz to ensure good penetration inside human head tissues. Since the radiation of monopole antennas is bidirectional, the back lobe radiation is suppressed by incorporating a lossy dielectric absorber EN-74 with a thickness of 19 mm where the antenna gain is doubled (5 dBi). Eight antenna elements are arranged in a hat-shaped structure that can be worn for head imaging. The simulated power distribution on a modelled head phantom is presented for two resonant frequencies of 1.5 and 3.5 GHz, which provides better penetration and better reconstructed image resolution, respectively. In [7], the authors presented an isosceles triangular patch antenna with a fractal ground plane as shown in Figure 6.4. It is fabricated on a 68.28×79×1.5-mm^3 FR4 substrate (ε_r = 4.7) and operates in the frequency range of 1.55–1.65 GHz. It is designed to detect haemorrhagic stroke which is modelled using a small tube containing blood-mimicking materials with circular cross-sectional radius of 5 mm and length of 35 mm. It is shown to be a good candidate for stroke detection through reconstructed images in both simulation and measurements. Figure 6.5 shows the measurement set-up for brain stroke detection using triangular patch antennas and brain-mimicking phantom. Another triangular antenna similarly fabricated on FR4 has dimensions of 70×50×1.55 mm^3 and an operating frequency range of 0.8–1.2 GHz is proposed in [30]. A triangular radiator, defected ground plane, and feedline with two stubs are the components of this antenna, which exhibits an omnidirectional radiation pattern. Both simulated and measured results indicate that it can identify the presence of a spherical stroke with radius of 12.5 mm.

6.4.2.2 Bowtie patch antennas

An inset fed meandered bowtie antenna with dimensions 18×18×0.5 mm^3 is proposed in [24]. It is fabricated on an FR4 substrate (ε_r = 4.3) and has an operating frequency range of 0.75–4 GHz. It is fed by a discrete port placed between two central vertices. To reduce the antenna size, a meandering technique is

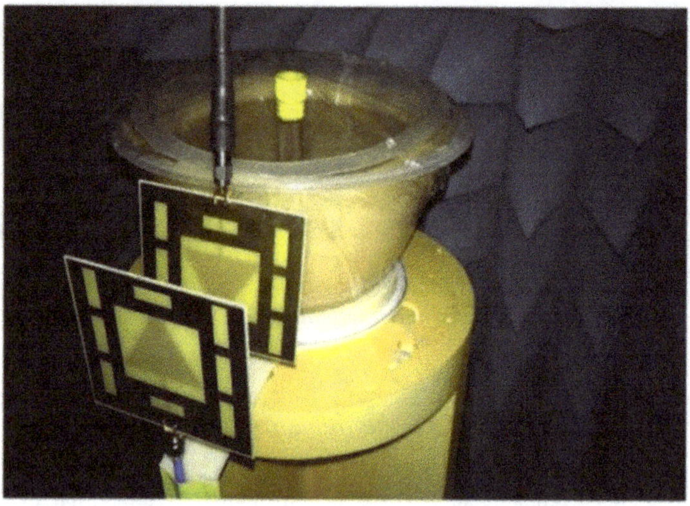

Figure 6.5 Measurement set-up for brain stroke detection [7]

implemented on the exterior region of the bowtie antenna. The bowtie elements are connected to each other using the meandered lines to create a long loop. The antenna element is tested on the head of a real human subject and the results indicate that the proposed antenna provides a good radiation efficiency and target penetration. A summary of the aforementioned antenna designs for a brain tumour and stroke detection is presented in Table 6.4.

6.5 Antennas for lung cancer and fluid accumulation detection

Lung cancer is another leading cause of cancer death. The accumulation of lung fluid is one end stage of lung cancer complication typically from stage III to IV, as well as the result of some other diseases. It is further classified into two types: pulmonary oedema where fluid accumulates inside the lung; and pleural effusion where the fluid accumulation occurs around the lung. Different antenna designs for lung cancer and fluid accumulation detection have been studied in literature through simulation and realistic phantoms of thoracic tissues that consist of multiple layers: skin, fat, muscle, rib bone, pleura, and lung. Their average dielectric properties are given in Table 6.5 for 2–14-GHz frequency range [31]. Materials mimicking a lung tumour ($\varepsilon_r = 54$, $\sigma = 2.5$ S/m) and fluid ($\varepsilon_r = 73$, $\sigma = 0.005$ S/m) are inserted within the thoracic phantom.

Various antenna designs for lung cancer and fluid accumulation detection have been proposed for RFMI systems. The main types are planar monopole antennas of different configurations such as circular, elliptical, cupcake-shaped, slot rotated, loop-dipole, folded, and metasurface antenna, which are discussed in the following subsections.

Table 6.4 Summary of antenna designs for brain tumour and stroke detection

Ref.	Antenna type	Frequency (GHz)	Size (mm^3)	Gain (dBi)	Key features/Remarks
[7]	Triangular patch	1.55–1.65	68.28×79×1.5	n/a	• For brain stroke detection • Narrow bandwidth of 0.1 GHz • No detailed characterisation of antenna features, e.g. gain
[6]	Rectangular patch	7.5–7.79	25.92×31.017×1.03	6.7	• For brain tumour detection • Circular EBG enhances reflection coefficient and image quality • Narrow bandwidth of 0.29 GHz • Not fabricated or tested on realistic phantom
[26]	Rectangular patch	4.85–6.75	n/a	3.497	• For brain tumour detection • DGS enhances antenna bandwidth and impedance matching but reduces antenna gain • Not fabricated or tested on a realistic phantom
[27]	Modified circular patch	3.1–10.6	34.5×20×1.575	7.573	• For brain tumour detection • Uses reflector to suppress backlobes and enhances antenna gain • Not tested on a realistic phantom
[28]	Circular patch	2.6–13.1	45×80×1.5748	12.12	• For brain tumour detection • Relatively low backlobe radiation • Tested only on simulated, not realistic phantom
[29]	Trapezoidal patch	1–4	70×30×0.2	5	• For brain stroke detection • An 8-element array in a hat-shaped wearable structure

(Continues)

Table 6.4 (Continued)

Ref.	Antenna type	Frequency (GHz)	Size (mm^3)	Gain (dBi)	Key features/Remarks
[30]	Triangular patch	0.8–1.2	70×50×1.55	n/a	• Antenna gain doubled by the use of dielectric absorber • Not tested on realistic phantom • For brain stroke detection • Radiation pattern is omnidirectional
[24]	Bowtie patch	0.75–4	18×18×0.5	n/a	• No detailed characterisation of antenna features, e.g. gain • For brain stroke detection • Tested on real human subject • No medical images generated

Table 6.5 Thoracic model parameters

Layer	Thickness (mm)	Relative dielectric constant ε_r	Conductivity σ (S/m)
Skin	3	33.036	6.273
Fat	2	9.35	1.317
Muscle	20	45.46	8.235
Rib bone	6	18.85	0.754
Lung	70	17.32	3.28

6.5.1 Antennas for lung cancer detection

A slot-rotated antenna designed for the frequency range of 1.5–3 GHz is utilised to circularly scan the artificial human torso phantom to detect lung tumour [32]. It has dimensions of 22×46×10 mm^3 and 2.6-dBi peak gain. The antenna scans the phantom at 12 different positions, and the produced images indicate its ability to accurately detect and localise the inserted tumour in the torso. In [16], a circular microstrip antenna is proposed and constructed on a 60×40×1.513-mm^3 FR4 substrate ($\varepsilon_r = 4.4$). The detection of lung tumour is studied for the frequency range of 3–4 GHz. The antenna performance is evaluated in terms of optimum distance between the antenna and phantom, the size of spherical tumour model, and tumour location. Results show that the antenna can detect tumour sizes of 4-mm radius or larger at a 10-mm optimum distance from the phantom where the lowest reflection coefficient is achieved. It is also shown to detect similarly sized tumours at different positions at a depth of 60 mm in the phantom where the upper and middle regions are more detectable than those at the lower region particularly at the model's lower edge corners.

An elliptical patch antenna with dimensions of $44 \times 44 \times 1.6$ mm^3 fabricated on an FR4 substrate to operate in a frequency range of 3–10.7 GHz is presented in [18]. The antenna is loaded with a box-shaped cavity to make it a directional antenna which is then tested using a thoracic model with an inserted tumour. Results show that the antenna can detect tumour particularly when placed in close proximity to the model. The authors in [31] proposed a cupcake-shaped antenna operating in the frequency range of 2.9–12 GHz. The antenna is fabricated on a $40 \times 30 \times 1.524$-mm^3 Roger RO4350 substrate ($\varepsilon_r = 3.66$) and evaluated on a thoracic model. It is found to exhibit an omnidirectional radiation pattern and can detect lung cancer from stage II onwards.

6.5.2 Antennas for lung fluid accumulation detection

In [3], a 7×5-unit-cell metasurface antenna with three rectangular microstrip-fed slot radiator is proposed as shown in Figure 6.6. The unit cell has dimensions of 46.875×46.875 mm^2, while that of the entire antenna are $337.5 \times 262.5 \times 22.5$ mm^3. It operates in the frequency range of 0.8–1.05 GHz and provides a gain of 8 dBi. Six PIN diodes are utilised to create three distinct beams by switching three radiating slots. The microstrip lines and slots are located on the opposite sides of a 1.6-mm-thick FR4 substrate ($\varepsilon_r = 4.3$), while the metasurface unit cells are configured into square shapes. The metasurface is printed on another 0.8-mm-thick FR4 substrate and is designed to increase the directivity and bandwidth of the antenna. This directional antenna is successfully tested to detect 20 mL of fluid (water) inside a realistic torso using generated images that differentiate between healthy and unhealthy cases. Figure 6.7 shows the measurement set-up for lung fluid accumulation detection using a mimicking torso phantom.

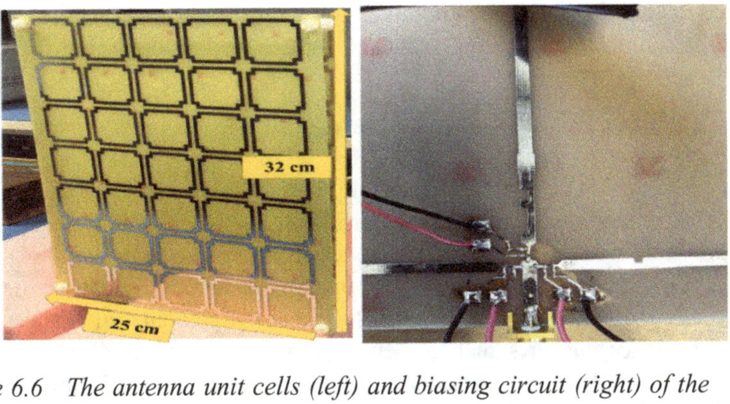

Figure 6.6 The antenna unit cells (left) and biasing circuit (right) of the fabricated metasurface antenna for lung fluid accumulation [3]

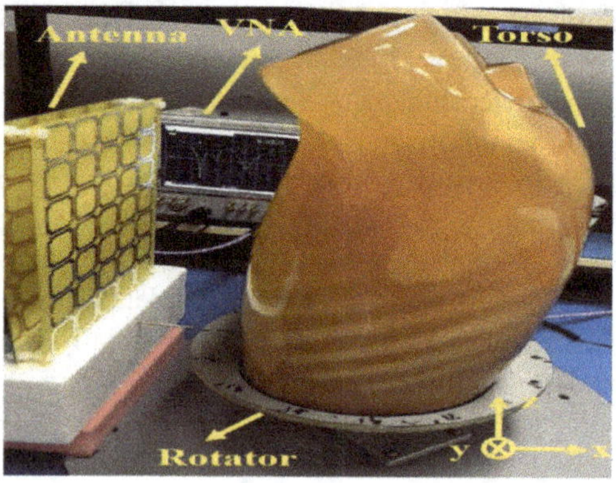

Figure 6.7 Measurement set-up for lung fluid accumulation detection [3]

A pattern reconfigurable loop dipole antenna for pleural effusion detection is proposed in [4]. It consists of one wavelength loop, a modified half wavelength bowtie-shaped dipole, and two parasitic directors to achieve an operating frequency range of 0.8–1.4 GHz and a high front-to-back ratio. The antenna has dimensions of $78\times130\times1.6$ mm^3 and shows a high directional radiation pattern with a peak gain of 5 dBi. It is fabricated on an FR4 substrate ($\varepsilon_r = 4.3$). Two PIN diodes are embedded across the parasitic directors to electronically control the current distribution, hence steering the radiation pattern.

Two linear arrays consisting of wideband antennas inserted into a foam-based bed and operating in the frequency range of 0.7–1 GHz for pulmonary oedema detection are presented in [11]. The array element comprises a meandered loop, an L-shaped monopole antenna, and a parasitic patch. They are printed and bonded to form a 3D structure using soldering and copper taping. The structure is fabricated on a 1.6-mm-thick FR4 substrate ($\varepsilon_r = 4.4$) and offers a directional radiation pattern, a moderate gain of 1.9 dBi, and a compact size of $20\times80\times48$ mm^3. Each 8×2 antenna array is tested with different water volumes inserted into the torso phantom. The generated images show the capability of the system to detect water contents as small as 1 mL. A summary of the aforementioned antenna designs is given in Table 6.6.

6.6 Antennas for skin cancer detection

Skin cancer detection using RFMI technique similarly relies on contrasting between the dielectric properties of cancerous skin tissues ($\varepsilon_r = 54$, $\sigma = 2.5$ S/m) and healthy ones ($\varepsilon_r = 39.2$, $\sigma = 1.11$ S/m). Unlike the detection of aforementioned diseases that require a deep penetration of the RF signal into human tissues, skin cancer detection requires only marginal signal penetration to detect the pathological changes in the skin layers. Hence, higher signal frequencies in mm-wave regime, i.e. between 30 and 300 GHz, which has a penetration depth of only 600 μm to 1.2 mm, have been explored recently for high-resolution imaging for skin cancer detection.

Table 6.6 Summary of antenna designs for lung tumour and fluid accumulation detection

Ref.	Antenna type	Frequency (GHz)	Size (mm^3)	Gain (dBi)	Key features/Remarks
[32]	Slot rotated	1.5–3	22×46×10	2.6	• For lung tumour detection • Tested on human torso phantom • Can detect and localise a tumour of dimensions 10×10×20 mm^3
[3]	Metasurface	0.8–1.05	337.5×262.5×22.5	8	• For fluid accumulation detection • Offer stable high gain and electronic beam scanning • Large antenna size and narrow operating bandwidth
[4]	Loop-dipole	0.8–1.4	78×130×1.6	5	• For pleural effusion detection • Electronically steerable tri-state radiation pattern • Not tested on realistic phantom • Detection efficacy not evaluated
[11]	3D loop, monopole and parasitic patch	0.7–1.0	20×80×48	1.9	• For pulmonary oedema detection • Tested on realistic torso phantom inserted with real lamb lung and injected with water • Can detect different levels of fluid accumulation • Antenna gain can be improved
[16]	Circular microstrip	3–4	60×40×1.513	n/a	• For lung tumour detection • Not fabricated or tested on realistic phantom • Can detect tumours of a 4-mm radius at a depth of 60 mm in, and a distance of 10 mm from a simulated phantom
[18]	Elliptical patch	3–10.7	44×44×1.6	n/a	• For lung tumour detection • Ultra-wide bandwidth, directional

(Continues)

Table 6.6 (Continued)

Ref.	Antenna type	Frequency (GHz)	Size (mm^3)	Gain (dBi)	Key features/Remarks
[31]	Cupcake shaped	2.9–12	40×30×1.524	n/a	• Not fabricated or tested on realistic phantom • Tested on simulated thoracic model • For lung tumour detection • Ultra-wide bandwidth • Can detect lung cancer from stage II • Not tested on realistic phantom

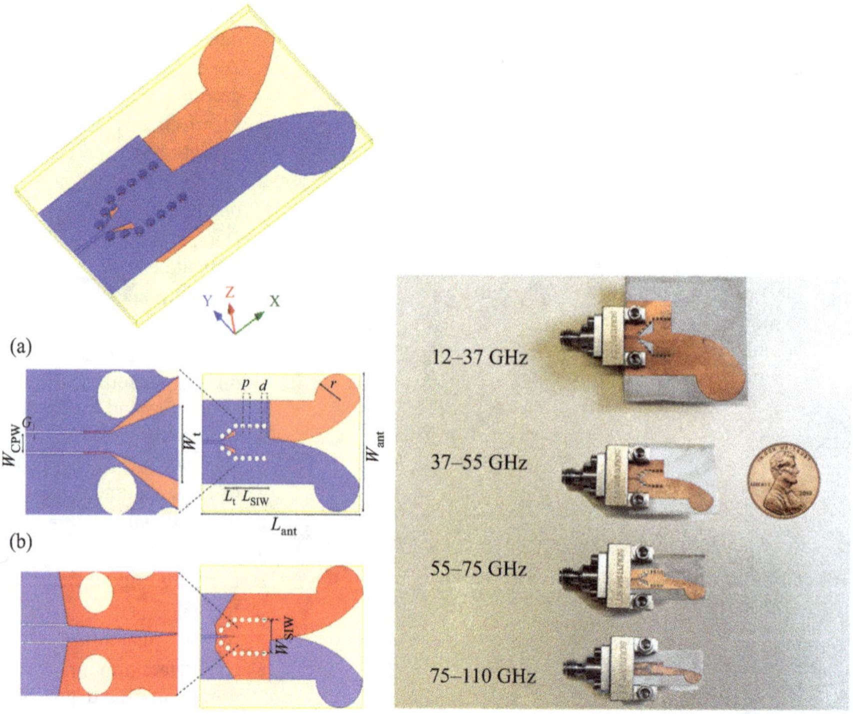

Figure 6.8 The designed (left) and fabricated (right) sub-band Vivaldi antennas [5]

In [5], four substrate-integrated waveguide-based antipodal Vivaldi antennas as shown in Figure 6.8, each operating in a different frequency range that extends into the mm-wave regime, are proposed. They are fabricated on an RT Duroid 6002 substrate of either 10 or 20 mm thicknesses, each having different dimensions as follows.

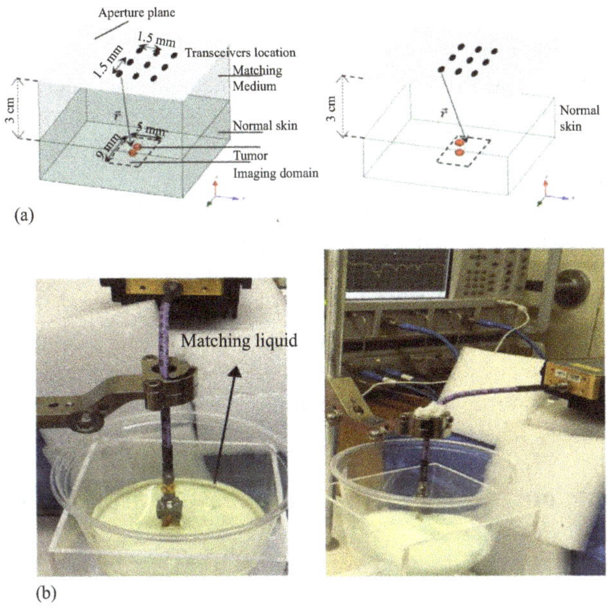

Figure 6.9 Measurement set-up for skin cancer detection: (a) schematic setup; (b) experimental set-up [5]

Table 6.7 Summary of antenna designs for skin cancer detection

Ref.	Antenna type	Frequency (GHz)	Size (mm^3)	Gain (dBi)	Key features/Remarks
[5]	Antipodal Vivaldi	12–110	Various	10–12	• Four antennas with distinct sub-bands to cover desired frequency range • Ultra-wide bandwidth, high stable gain, and 200 μm resolution
[33]	Hexagonal patch	6–12	44×48×6.2	6.5	• AMC improves antenna gain • Complex multi-layer structure • Not tested on realistic phantom • No medical images generated

Antenna 1 (12–37 GHz): 27.1×27.34×20 mm^3; Antenna 2 (37–55 GHz): 18.86×13.56×20 mm^3; Antenna 3 (55–75 GHz): 16.15×8.36×10 mm^3; and Antenna 4 (75–110 GHz): 14.44×4.46×20 mm^3. Collectively, the antennas provide an ultra-wide bandwidth of 98 GHz, a stable high gain of 10–12 dBi over the covered sub-bands and directional radiation pattern. Antennas 1 and 2 are fabricated on a 20-mm thick substrates, while Antennas 3 and 4 used 10-mm thick substrates. All antennas are evaluated on an artificial skin phantom embedded with spherical tumours of a 400-μm diameter. The resulting images show the antennas' promising potential for early-stage skin cancer detection. Figure 6.9 shows the measurement set-up for skin cancer detection using the sub-bands Vivaldi antennas.

The authors in [33] presented an artificial magnetic conductor (AMC)-based hexagonal patch antenna with CPW fabricated on a 2.2-mm thick felt fabric substrate ($\varepsilon_r = 1.22$). It consists of a hexagonal patch of dimensions 32×38 mm^2, which is separated from the AMC by a 2-mm thick foam layer. The AMC is fabricated on Zelt conductive fabric with dimensions of 44×48 mm^2 that consists of 4×4 unit cells with periodic hexagonal and rhombic shapes. Without AMC, the CPW-fed hexagonal patch antenna achieves a peak gain of 3.2 dB in the frequency range of 8–12 GHz. The addition of AMC increases the antenna's peak gain to 6.5 dBi due to the absorption of its back radiation. The antenna shows the ability to detect skin cancer in a simulated phantom based on contrasting reflection coefficients. Table 6.7 summarises the previous antenna designs for skin cancer detection.

6.7 Conclusion and recommendations for future work

The past decade has seen a rapid advancement of RFMI for biomedical applications such as for the detection of different cancer types and other critical diseases. It is one of the most promising biomedical imaging techniques owing to its non-invasiveness, non-ionising radiation with low illumination power level, relatively low-cost, and sustained reliability. This chapter focuses on the antenna element of the RFMI system, which is a key factor controlling the RFMI performance.

Different antennas have been proposed in the literature for different cancer and disease detection in different parts of the human body such as breast, brain, lung, and skin. Typically, imaging deep tissues require an antenna with a lower operating frequency than those for shallow ones. Furthermore, compact antennas are more desirable as more antennas can be employed to cover a given target area, thereby increasing the number of measurement points and consequently precision of detection. Moreover, increasing the bandwidth of the antenna will improve the resolution of reconstructed images. However, higher frequencies can result in lower penetration levels and are more susceptible to attenuation. Thus, to obtain good resolution and penetration with minimised attenuation, the designed antenna should have ultra-wide bandwidth and high gain. The latter can concentrate the radiated power on the area under test and increase the penetration depth. In addition, radiation sidelobes should be minimised to reduce interference with the main lobes of other antenna elements in the system and the possibility of clutter generation.

As a result, future improvements to enhance the RFMI performance can be made by designing antennas with the desired attributes of ultra-wide bandwidth, compact size, high gain, and directional radiation. Such antennas along with a suitable configuration to scan different parts of the body and an appropriate signal-processing algorithm will enable an RFMI system to detect different types of cancer and diseases at different depths with a good resolution and clutter reduction. For instance, employing a dual polarised antenna for RFMI could potentially enhance detection precision and allow a collection of more information from backscattered signals.

References

[1] Sharma M. K., Kumar M., Saini J. P., *et al.*, "Experimental Investigation of the Breast Phantom for Tumor Detection Using Ultra-Wide Band–MIMO Antenna Sensor (UMAS) Probe", *IEEE Sensors Journal*, Vol. 20, No. 12, 2020.

[2] Pondicherry A., Martin R., Meredith I., *et al.*, "The Burden of Non-Melanoma Skin Cancers in Auckland, New Zealand", *Australasian Journal of Dermatology*, 2018; doi:10.1111/ajd.12751.

[3] Darvazehban A, Rezaeieh S. A., Zamani A., *et al.*, "Pattern Reconfigurable Metasurface Antenna for Electromagnetic Torso Imaging", *IEEE Transactions on Antennas and Propagation*, 2019.

[4] Darvazehban A., Rezaeieh S. A. and Abbosh A., "Pattern-Reconfigurable Loop–Dipole Antenna for Electromagnetic Pleural Effusion Detection", *IEEE Transactions on Antennas and Propagation*, Vol. 68, No. 8, 2020.

[5] Mirbeik-Sabzevari A., Li S., Garay E., *et al.*, "Synthetic Ultra-High-Resolution Millimeter-Wave Imaging for Skin Cancer Detection", *IEEE Transactions on Biomedical Engineering*, Vol. 66, No. 1, pp. 61–71, 2018; doi:10.1109/tbme.2018.2837102.

[6] Inum R., Rana M., Shushama K. N., *et al.*, "EBG Based Microstrip Patch Antenna for Brain Tumor Detection via Scattering Parameters in Microwave Imaging System", *International Journal of Biomedical Imaging*, Vol. 2018, 2018, Article ID 8241438, 12 pages.

[7] Sohani B., Khalesi B., Ghavami N., *et al.*, "Detection of Haemorrhagic Stroke in Simulation and Realistic 3-Dhuman Head Phantom Using Microwave Imaging", *Biomedical Signal Processing and Control*, Vol. 61, 2020.

[8] Bashri M. S. and Arslan T., "Low-Cost and Compact RF Switching System for Wearable Microwave Head Imaging With Performance Verification on Artificial Head Phantom", *IET Microwave, Antennas and Propagation*, Vol. 12, No. 5, pp. 706–711, 2018.

[9] Hossain A., Islam M. T., Islam M. T., *et al.*, "A Planar Ultrawideband Patch Antenna Array for Microwave Breast Tumor Detection", *Materials*, Vol. 13, p. 4918, 2020; doi:10.3390/ma13214918.

[10] Abbosh A. M., Mohammed B., and Bialkowski K. S., "Differential Microwave Imaging of the Breast Pair", *IEEE Antennas and Wireless Propagation Letters*, Vol. 15, 2016.

[11] Rezaeieh S. A., Zamani A., Bialkowski K. S., *et al.*, "Feasibility of Using Wideband Microwave System for Non-Invasive Detection and Monitoring of Pulmonary Oedema", *Scientific Reports*, Vol. 5, p. 14047, 2015.

[12] Wang L., "Three-Dimensional Holographic Electromagnetic Imaging for Accessing Brain Stroke", *Sensors*, Vol. 18, p. 3852, 2018; doi:10.3390/s18113852.

[13] Porter E., Bahrami H., Santorelli A., *et al.*, "A Wearable Microwave Antenna Array for Time-Domain Breast Tumor Screening", *IEEE Transactions on Medical Imaging*, Vol. 35, No. 6, 2016.

[14] Subramanian S., Sundarambal B. and Nirmal D., "Investigation on Simulation-Based Specific Absorption Rate in Ultra-Wideband Antenna for Breast Cancer Detection", *IEEE Sensors Journal*, Vol. 18, No. 24, 2018.

[15] Bahramiabarghouei H., Porter E., Santorelli A., *et al.*, "Flexible 16 Antenna Array for Microwave Breast Cancer Detection", *IEEE Transactions on Biomedical Engineering*, Vol. 62, No. 10, 2015; doi:10.1109/TBME.2015.2434956.

[16] Alhawari A. R. H., "Lung Tumour Detection Using Ultra-Wideband Microwave Imaging Approach", *Journal of Fundamental and Applied Sciences*, 2018.

[17] Casu M. R., Vacca M., Tobon J. A, *et al.*, "A COTS-Based Microwave Imaging System for Breast-Cancer Detection", *IEEE Transactions on Biomedical Circuits and Systems*, Vol. 11, No. 4, 2017.

[18] Ameer W., Awan D., Bashir S., *et al.*, "Use of Directional UWB Antenna for Lung Tumor Detection", 2nd International Conference on Advancements in Computational Sciences (ICACS), 2019.

[19] Babarinde O. J., Jamlos M. F., Soh P. J., *et al.*, "Microwave Imaging Technique for Lung Tumour Detection", *GeMiC*, 2016.

[20] Elahi M. A., O'Loughlin D., Lavoie B. R., *et al.*, "Evaluation of Image Reconstruction Algorithms for Confocal Microwave Imaging: Application to Patient Data", *Sensors*, Vol. 18, p. 1678, 2018; doi:10.3390/s18061678.

[21] Wang L. and Chen H., "Design of a Wideband Antipodal Vivaldi Antenna with High Gain for Detecting Breast Cancer", *Proceedings of Computational and Experimental Simulations in Engineering (ICCES)*, 2019.

[22] Biswas B., Ghatak R. and Poddar D. R., "A Fern Fractal Leaf Inspired Wideband Antipodal Vivaldi Antenna for Microwave Imaging System", *IEEE Transactions on Antennas and Propagation*, Vol. 65, No. 11, 2017.

[23] Selvaraj V., Baskaran D., Rao P. H., *et al.*, "Breast Tissue Tumor Analysis Using Wideband Antenna and Microwave Scattering", *IETE Journal of Research*, 2018.

[24] Arayeshnia A., Amiri S., and Keshtkar A., "Miniaturized On-Body Antenna for Small and Wearable Brain Microwave Imaging Systems", *International Journal of RF and Microwave Computer-Aided Engineering*, Vol. 30, p. e22133, 2020; doi:10.1002/mmce.22133.

[25] Gabriel, C., "Compilation of the Dielectric Properties of Body Tissues at RF and Microwave Frequencies." Report N.AL/OE-TR- 1996-0037, Occupational and environmental health directorate, Radiofrequency Radiation Division, Brooks Air Force Base, Texas (USA), 1996.

[26] Gupta H. K., Sharma R. and Thakare V. V., "Design of Symmetrical Shaped DGS Pattern Rectangular Microstrip Patch Antenna for Brain Tumor Detection by Microwave Imaging", *Materials Today: Proceedings*, Vol. 29, No. Part 2, pp. 548–555, 2020; doi.org/10.1016/j.matpr.2020.07.31.

[27] Widyatama P. Z., Nugroho B. S. and Nur L. O, "Design of Circular Modified UWB Antenna Microstrip for Brain Cancer Detection", IEEE Asia Pacific Conference on Wireless and Mobile (APWiMob), 2019.

[28] Jamlos M. A., Jamlos M. F. and Ismail A. H., "High Performance Novel UWB Array Antenna For Brain Tumor Detection Via Scattering Parameters in Microwave Imaging Simulation System", 9th European Conference on Antennas and Propagation (EuCAP), Lisbon, 2015, pp. 1–5.

[29] Bashri M. S. R., Arslan T., Zhou W., *et al.*, "Wearable Device for Microwave Head Imaging", Proceedings of the 46th European Microwave Conference, UK, 2016.

[30] Rodriguez-Duarte D. O., Vasquez J. A. T., Scapaticci R., *et al.*, "Brick-Shaped Antenna Module for Microwave Brain Imaging Systems", *IEEE Antennas and Wireless Propagation Letters*, Vol. 19, No. 12, pp. 2057–2061, 2020; doi:10.1109/LAWP.2020.3022161.

[31] Abdelhamid M. M. and Allam A. M., "Detection of Lung Cancer Using Ultra Wide Band Antenna", 2016 Loughborough Antennas & Propagation Conference (LAPC), 2016.

[32] Zamani A., Rezaeieh S. A. and Abbosh A. M, "Lung Cancer Detection Using Frequency Domain Microwave Imaging", *Electronics Letters*, 2015.

[33] Tripathi A. C., Rao P. K., and Mishra R., "An AMC Inspired Wearable UWB Antenna for Skin Cancer Detection", 2020 International Conference on Electrical and Electronics Engineering (ICE3-2020), 2020.

Chapter 7

Long-term condition monitoring using wearable sensors and IoT-based applications

Mirza Mansoor Baig[1], Hamid Gholam Hosseini[2], Jairo Gutierrez[2], Ehsan Ullah[2], Maria Lindén[3] and Sandra Oldfield[1]

Long-term conditions (LTCs) such as type 2 diabetes mellitus and pre-LTCs such as prediabetes have been rising rapidly worldwide. It is evident that to prevent and/or minimize these complications, it is important to manage and maintain an active and healthy lifestyle. We aim to early detect prediabetes using integrated wearable body sensors and Internet-of-things (IoT) applications. We co-designed and developed an early detection model for prediabetes based on the individual's ranges and baseline. The study collected activity data (such as steps), vital signs (such as heart rate, breathing rate) and demographic data (e.g., age, gender, height, weight) for the prediction. The prediabetes detection was based on the best practice clinical knowledge, individualized baseline data and localized fuzzy rules. The proposed model was tested and validated using Kappa analysis and achieved an overall agreement of 91%. Moreover, we discussed the key challenges and barriers for wider adoption of wearable sensor (WS)/IoT in healthcare settings. We observed the good improvement in health outcomes for participants using mHealth, WSs and IoT applications when compared with the traditional or routine practice.

7.1 Introduction

WSs and IoT systems are emerging as an effective tool for prevention, early detection and management of pre-LTCs. As WS, IoT, smart textiles and body-worn garments become smaller, cheaper and more consumer-accessible, it is expected

[1]Health Informatics Specialist, Data Science Team, Orion Health, Auckland, New Zealand
[2]School of Engineering, Computer and Mathematical Sciences, Auckland University of Technology, Auckland, New Zealand
[3]School of Innovation Design and Engineering, Mälardalen University, Västerås, Sweden

that they will be used more extensively across a wide variety of contexts. The expansion of wearable/IoT systems for data collection offers the potential for user-engagement and self-management of age-related illness and diseases [1–4]. Exploiting IoT technologies have been studied for developing ambient assisted living systems for healthcare. However, many challenges exist for achieving reliable and effective systems with high performance. WSs have been widely used in various health areas such as fall detection, older adults' health and well-being, Parkinson's disease and more [5–12].

Accuracy, usability, real-time data access, wireless capability and interoperability were few key factors required for a success wearable/IoT solution. We conducted a market analysis for body-worn smart shirt and IoT devices and found Hexoskin smart vest [13–16] to satisfy the requirements to collect real-time vital signs and activity data. Hexoskin solution offers access to data via application programming interface (API), mobile app, web dashboard and more. These features met our criteria to early detect prediabetes. We combined activity data and vital signs from the wearable vest (Hexoskin) and combined with the participants' demographic information after obtaining ethical approvals (AUTEC: 16/412). This research aimed to design and develop a clinical decision support system to detect prediabetes. The early detection model was based on the local and national guidelines and best practice recommendation for prediabetes [8,9]. The proposed study helps to determine the prediabetes risk factor but not make an actual diagnosis.

7.2 Overview of wearable sensor and IoT systems for older adults with long-term conditions

A wrist-wearable accelerometer-based solution was presented for improving fall detection of older adults [17]. A threshold-based peak detection approach was used and extended with an optimization stage for tuning the threshold. The feature extraction stage was also extended to balance the classes of the dataset. Alternative classifiers were analyzed to optimize computation and adaptability, aiming to embed within smart wristbands/phones. Many different published datasets were applied in this study, in addition to a comprehensive comparison to analyze various solutions for fall detection. Results showed that using an SVM model could optimize the specificity and number of false alarms.

A modular decision support framework was proposed for improving independent living and aging well based on geriatric depression case study [18]. The proposed decision system consists of three main components: trend analysis, decision support core, and risk prediction and assessment. The proposed system is based on statistical process control for identifying trends and fuzzy cognitive maps learning for depression classification. The presented framework adopted the FCM-DDNHL classification method, where an estimated mean value of 78.66% was achieved for the classification accuracy.

A front-door events classification algorithm was proposed aiming to detect the forget event of older adults in smart houses [19]. A novel brief-return-and-exit (BRE) event classification was introduced targeting noninvasive detection of forgetting event using wireless binary sensors. Results demonstrated a positive correlation between the number of exits, BRE events and BRE percentage, which shows that the proposed forget event detection method could help in evaluating people with dementia.

A waist-worn detector was presented for fall detection of older adults, which utilized an attitude and heading reference system combining a 3-axis accelerometer, a 3-axis gyroscope and a 3-axis magnetometer [20]. A barometer sensor was integrated into the targeting device to improve the efficiency and performance of the system by measuring the altitude variation in a fall [20,21]. Three different experimental protocols of falls and ADLs were adopted for evaluating the developed fall detection system. The results demonstrated that better performance compared to existing conventional fall detection systems exists in the literature through using the four combined sensors with the data fusion algorithms efficiently (Table 7.1).

7.3 System overview and challenges

Figure 7.1 shows the basic building blocks of the proposed model, including model architecture with activity data, vitals data and demographic data fed to the knowledge base learning module for processing. The initial learning of the proposed model was based on the activity data, vital signs and demographic information using the self-learning interpretation engine. The main learning module consists of a medical knowledge base and individualized weighted parameters combined with the national/local diabetes guidelines. We used multiple in–out combinational cross-pattern relationship to best utilize the medical knowledge base with the baseline values for each individual. The body mass index (BMI) was considered as a contributing factor that computed from individual height and weight to train the model.

The proposed model consists of medical knowledge sources, best practice recommendation and weighted ranking based on the individual's data. The prediction model was designed for multiple input–output combinational relationship with multilayered outcomes.

The interpretation of the diagnostic values and the relationship between vital signs, activity data, demographics data and their clinical interpretation is mapped to the ANFIS *fuzzy* rules [22]. Moreover, the clinical acceptability of assessment procedures via expert agreement analysis is evaluated. The factors that affect ongoing data collection, barriers to this intervention, accuracy and the potential for person' self-management were also be measured. A multilayer concept has been introduced, as it has the potential of early detection. This mechanism is best utilized in this context by feeding multiple input–output combinational relationships in real time.

7.4 Evaluations and results

Data is collected using market available wearable vest—{Hexoskin (www.hexoskin.com), *Montreal, Canada*} [23] as Hexoskin satisfies the project requirements and allows users to download the raw data in machine-readable format. Moreover, the

Table 7.1 Summary of the selected papers related to the WS and IoT-based systems

Author and references	**Target area or population**	**Study aims**	**Platform/sensors used**	**Outcomes/findings**
Pierleoni *et al.* [20,21]	A waist-worn fall detector of older adults	To develop a wearable device based on barometric sensor to detect all kinds of falls	Fall detector of ATmega328 MCU with a 3-axis accelerometer, a 3-axis gyroscope, a 3-axis magnetometer and a barometric sensor	The developed system is extremely efficient for fall detection with 100% sensitivity
Billis *et al.* [18]	Evaluating the progression of depressive symptoms (geriatric depression case study)	To develop a modular decision support framework for the promotion of independent living and aging well	Decision support framework using statistical process control and an FCM-DDNHL method	The proposed framework will detect elders either suffering from depressive systems or being at high risk in the future
Tan *et al.* [19]	Front-door events classification algorithm to detect the forget event of older adults in smart houses	To develop a novel device-free noninvasive front-door events classification algorithm for the forget event detection using wireless binary sensors	Testbeds with ZigBee wireless module-based binary sensors	The proposed algorithm is a useful tool for the forget event detection to evaluate people with dementia
Khojasteh *et al.* [17]	Improving fall detection of older adults using an on-wrist wearable accelerometer	To develop a wrist wearable solution for improving fall detection by adding optimization stages	A 3D-axis accelerometer-based wrist-worn on a smart wristband with a peak detection optimization stage, dataset balancing stage and alternative machine learning methods	The rule-based systems represent a promising research line like neural networks while reducing computational cost. support vector machine achieved a high specificity

Hexoskin provides users with raw, processed and/or meaningful data. The access to the APIs and raw data in machine-readable format enables the healthcare professionals, researchers and developers to leverage the existing open platform for data mining, machine learning for various clinical, social, behavioral and physical (activity related) use-cases and explore the data further for enormous healthcare benefits. Hexoskin vest captures heart rate, HRV (allowing to estimate stress and fatigue), heart rate recovery, ECG, breathing rate (RPM), minute ventilation (L/min), activity intensity, peak acceleration, steps and cadence. The proposed model was trained and fine-tuned using 36 participant data, containing age, gender, BMI and any significant medical condition from PhysioNet [24]. For the real-time testing, longitudinal data was collected from two participants over multiple times, activities and durations after obtaining appropriate ethics approvals (AUTEC: 16/412).

Sensors details: analog 256-Hz ECG data; analog dual-channel 128-Hz breathing sensors and analog 3D 64-Hz acceleration. We found that participants' statistical information of average heart rate was between 104 and 115 bpm, 58.5 average age (range of 55–62 years), breathing rate of 21–23 bpm and HbA1c of 75.7 mmol/mol for our participants.

The study collected over 430 min of data (approximately 7–8 of data) during multiple settings and combinations for sensors and applications. The outcomes

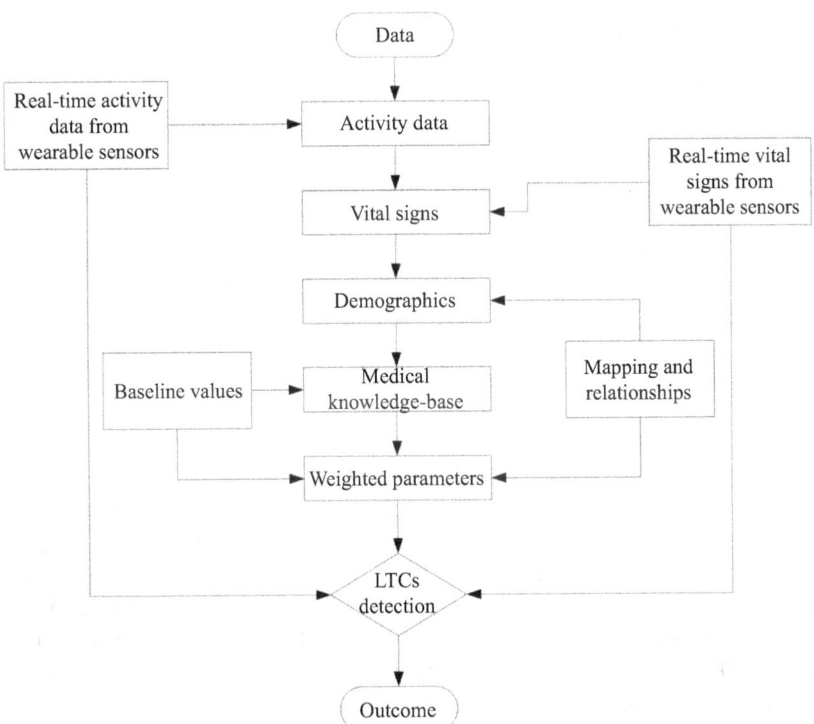

Figure 7.1 The basic building blocks of the proposed model [22]

Table 7.2 Kappa analysis values for the collected data

	Expert (+ve)	Expert (−ve)	Total
System (+ve)	82 (TP)	32 (FP)	114
System (−ve)	5 (FN)	316 (TN)	321
Total	87	348	435

Table 7.3 Kappa analysis of the whole dataset

Overall agreement	Positive agreement	Negative agreement	Agreement by chance	Standard error	95% Confidence intervals for κ
P_o	P_{pos}	P_{neg}	P_e	SE	$CI_{95\%}$
0.91	0.82	0.94	0.64	0.038	0.82 and 0.67

were classified into true positive and negative and false positive and negative. We used kappa analysis, which measures and allows the agreement between the human expert and the electronic/computer system using the abovementioned classification measures. The importance of observer reliability lies in the fact that it represents the extent to which the data collected in the study are correct representations of the variables measured.

Table 7.2 shows the true positive and negative and false positive and negative classifications derived from the expert analysis. Table 7.3 shows the kappa analysis of the whole dataset. The overall kappa value was κ=0.75, shows the κ-values expressed as the strength of agreement. The detection model has an accuracy of 91%, sensitivity of 94%, specificity of 90% and predictability of 72%. The accuracy was calculated using ((TP+TN)/(sum of TP, TN, FP and FN)), sensitivity as ((TP)/(TP+FN)), specificity as ((TN)/(TN/FP)) and predictability as ((TP)/(TP+FP)).

7.5 Discussion, challenges and conclusions

One of the most common issues with wearable systems is the delay in providing results and generating alerts due to data loss, buffering, network communication, monitoring or processing [25–27]. These systems were developed for specific setup and care settings to assist patients' specific needs. Wearable systems using 3G/4G data suffer connectivity issues due to the remote network, low signal strength in remote places, low battery lifetime, low transmission speed, thus resulting in delay or low-quality data for periods of short time [25,28]. To address these issues, a cross-layer framework has been developed based on unequal resource allocation to support secure wireless wearable data encryption and transmission [29,30]. The low battery life issue occurs due to continued connectivity of device/sensor with the Bluetooth, Wi-Fi or 3G/4G networks [31–33]. Moreover, if the power supply is not an issue, then the mobility of the device may become problematic, especially for older adults [6–8,11,34].

A portable ECG-monitoring device developed by Lee *et al.* [32] can easily measure the ECG by connecting the measuring module to a patch with a minimized electrode array using a snap button. The measuring module is small (38 mm wide, 38 mm long and 7 mm thick). The weight of the module, including the battery, is 10 g. The study reported that an ECG signal was collated using a commercial device that was similar to the conventional Holter monitor [32].

The current state of wearable monitoring systems can be further enhanced with the integration of such techniques into the hardware or in the cloud computing platforms for real-time processing. From a software point-of-view, processing big data is usually linked with programming paradigms [35]. Several open-source frameworks such as Hadoop [36] are being used to set up distributed database environments via a scalable architecture. This provides a basis for further usage via other tools (such as Cascading, Pig, Hive) [36] that enable developing applications to process vast amounts of data (by order of terabytes) on commodity clusters. However, when combined with continuous streams of pervasive health monitoring, this also requires capacities for iterative and low-latency computations, which depends on sophisticated models of data caching and in-memory computation. Thus, other frameworks such as Storm and Spark have been created to fulfill this gap [36].

There are very few existing studies that address usability and acceptability challenges for health monitoring. Usability and acceptability performance is evaluated based on different measurements of willingness to use and keep, simplicity, reliability, wearable time, satisfaction level and ADLs interference [37]. The existing WS and IoT devices need modifications in terms of manufacturing and technical capabilities to address critical issues such as battery/power consumption, restricting the user's movements within a confined area/space and high cost. Interoperability is required for IoT applications to support the electronic health record of the user and also to maintain the large health data, especially related to LTC or chronic care conditions [38,39].

Future improvements could be made to the prediction of prediabetes model by adding localized information such as ethnicity, family history and social variants such as living status, socioeconomic status and more. A paradigm shift in healthcare delivery is occurring, which has been made possible by the technological revolution in wearables, advanced sensors, the IoT devices and the potential of employing machine learning, deep learning and artificial intelligence [28] to gain rich insights from the collected data. The treatment of many medical conditions is guaranteed to benefit from the use of wearable and IoT technology [28]. Consequently, WS and IoT applications are showing some potential for low-cost remote monitoring, supporting independent living, reducing falls among older adults, early detection of various LTCs and more. However, the presented technical challenges need to be fully understood and resolved before the WS, and IoT-based wearable sensing and IoT-based monitoring applications can be successfully used to support older people at home.

Acknowledgments

The authors thank Hexoskin for providing the advanced wearable vest (smart shirt) used in this study for the data collection. Also, the authors thank clinicians at Auckland District Health Board and Waitematā District Health Board for their clinical advice and support.

Conflict of interest statement

Authors declare no conflict of interest.

References

[1] Kaiser, L.H. and W.S. Saunders, Vision Mātauranga research directions: opportunities for iwi and hapū management plans. *Kōtuitui: New Zealand Journal of Social Sciences Online*, 2021: p. 1–13.

[2] Hamley, L. and J.L. Grice, He kākano ahau – identity, Indigeneity and wellbeing for young Māori (Indigenous) men in Aotearoa/New Zealand. *Feminism & Psychology*, 2021. 31(1): p. 62–80.

[3] Dobson, R., R. Whittaker, Y. Jiang, *et al.*, Long-term follow-up of a randomized controlled trial of a text-message diabetes self-management support programme, SMS4BG. *Diabetic Medicine*, 2020. 37(2): p. 311–318.

[4] Malik, S., C. Moloney, E. Koledova, J. Reston, and J. Weinman, Designing a personalized digital patient support program for patients treated with growth hormone: key design considerations. *Journal of Medical Internet Research*, 2020. 22(7): p. e18157.

[5] Hosseini, H.G., M.M. Baig, and M. Lind, A smartphone-based obesity risk assessment application using wearable technology with personalized activity, calorie expenditure and health profile. *European Journal of Biomedical Informatics*, 2020.

[6] Baig, M.M., H. Gholamhosseini, S. Afifi, and F. Mirza, Current challenges and barriers to the wider adoption of wearable sensor applications and Internet-of-things in health and well-being, in *International Conference on Information Resources Management (CONF-IRM)*. 2019. AIS: Auckland, New Zealand. Available from: https://aisel.aisnet.org/confirm2019/20/.

[7] Baig, M.M., S. Afifi, H. GholamHosseini, and F. Mirza, A systematic review of wearable sensors and IoT-based monitoring applications for older adults – a focus on ageing population and independent living. *Journal of Medical Systems*, 2019. 43(8): p. 233. doi: 10.1007/s10916-019-1365-7.

[8] Baig, M.M., S. Afifi, H. GholamHosseini, and F. Mirza, Managing long-term conditions: wearable sensors and IoT-based monitoring applications, in *Encyclopedia of Gerontology and Population Aging*, D. Gu and M.E. Dupre, Editors. 2019, Springer International Publishing: Cham. p. 1–5.

[9] Baig, M.M., F. Mirza, H. GholamHosseini, J. Gutierrez, and E. Ullah, Automated and early detection of long-term conditions using a real-time

wearable patient monitoring system. in *35th International Conference of International Society for Quality in Health Care (ISQua)*. 2018. ISQua: Kuala Lumpur, Malaysia. Available from: https://epostersonline.com/isqua2018/node/2324.

[10] Nguyen, H., F. Mirza, M.A. Naeem, and M.M. Baig, Detecting falls using a wearable accelerometer motion sensor. in *Proceedings of the 14th EAI International Conference on Mobile and Ubiquitous Systems: Computing, Networking and Services*. 2017. ACM, p. 422–431.

[11] Baig, M.M., H. GholamHosseini, A.A. Moqeem, F. Mirza, and M. Lindén, A systematic review of wearable patient monitoring systems–current challenges and opportunities for clinical adoption. *Journal of Medical Systems*, 2017. 41(7): p. 115.

[12] Baig, M.M., H. Gholamhosseini, and M.J. Connolly, A comprehensive survey of wearable and wireless ECG monitoring systems for older adults. *Medical & Biological Engineering & Computing*, 2013. 51(5): p. 485–495.

[13] Hexoskin. Hexoskin Smart Vest. [cited 2019 2019]; Available from: https://www.hexoskin.com/.

[14] Smith, C.M., S.N. Chillrud, D.W. Jack, P. Kinney, Q. Yang, and A.M. Layton, Laboratory validation of Hexoskin biometric shirt at rest, submaximal exercise, and maximal exercise while riding a stationary bicycle. *Journal of Occupational and Environmental Medicine*, 2019. 61(4): p. e104–e111.

[15] Elliot, C.A., M.J. Hamlin, and C.A. Lizamore, Validity and reliability of the Hexoskin wearable biometric vest during maximal aerobic power testing in elite cyclists. *The Journal of Strength & Conditioning Research*, 2019. 33 (5): p. 1437–1444.

[16] Moriarty, T.A., Y. Feito, J. Monahan, and C. Williamson, Using the Hexoskin smart garment to measure cardiorespiratory variables during high intensity functional training: 2760 Board# 43 June 1 200 PM-330 PM. *Medicine & Science in Sports & Exercise*, 2018. 50(5S): p. 673.

[17] Khojasteh, S.B., J.R. Villar, C. Chira, V.M. González, and E. de la Cal, Improving fall detection using an on-wrist wearable accelerometer. *Sensors (Basel, Switzerland)*, 2018. 18(5): p. 1350.

[18] Billis, A.S., E.I. Papageorgiou, C.A. Frantzidis, M.S. Tsatali, A.C. Tsolaki, and P.D. Bamidis, A decision-support framework for promoting independent living and ageing well. *IEEE Journal of Biomedical and Health Informatics*, 2015. 19(1): p. 199–209.

[19] Tan, T.-H., M. Gochoo, F.-R. Jean, S.-C. Huang, and S.-Y. Kuo, Front-door event classification algorithm for elderly people living alone in smart house using wireless binary sensors. *IEEE Access*, 2017. 5: p. 10734–10743.

[20] Pierleoni, P., A. Belli, L. Palma, M. Pellegrini, L. Pernini, and S. Valenti, A high reliability wearable device for elderly fall detection. *IEEE Sensors Journal*, 2015. 15(8): p. 4544–4553.

[21] Pierleoni, P., A. Belli, L. Maurizi, *et al.*, A wearable fall detector for elderly people based on AHRS and barometric sensor. *IEEE Sensors Journal*, 2016. 16(17): p. 6733–6744.

[22] Baig, M.M., H. GholamHosseini, J. Gutierrez, E. Ullah, and M. Lindén, Early detection of prediabetes and T2DM using wearable sensors and Internet-of-things-based monitoring applications. *Applied Clinical Informatics*, 2021. 12(01): p. 001–009.

[23] Villar, R., T. Beltrame, and R.L. Hughson, Validation of the Hexoskin wearable vest during lying, sitting, standing, and walking activities. *Applied Physiology, Nutrition, and Metabolism*, 2015. 40(10): p. 1019–1024.

[24] Goldberger, A.L., L.A. Amaral, L. Glass, *et al.*, PhysioBank, PhysioToolkit, and PhysioNet: components of a new research resource for complex physiologic signals. *Circulation*, 2000. 101(23): p. e215–e220.

[25] Rault, T., A. Bouabdallah, Y. Challal, and F. Marin, A survey of energy-efficient context recognition systems using wearable sensors for healthcare applications. *Pervasive and Mobile Computing*, 2017. 37: p. 23–44.

[26] Wu, J., H. Li, S. Cheng, and Z. Lin, The promising future of healthcare services: when big data analytics meets wearable technology. *Information & Management*, 2016.

[27] Thomas, S.S., V. Nathan, C. Zong, K. Soundarapandian, X. Shi, and R. Jafari, BioWatch: a noninvasive wrist-based blood pressure monitor that incorporates training techniques for posture and subject variability. *IEEE Journal of Biomedical and Health Informatics*, 2016. 20(5): p. 1291–1300. doi: 10.1109/JBHI.2015.2458779.

[28] Ribeiro, J., Wearable technology spending: a strategic approach to decision-making, in *Wearable Technology and Mobile Innovations for Next-Generation Education*. 2016. IGI Global, p. 517–537.

[29] Balamurugan, S., R. Madhukanth, V. Prabhakaran, and R.G. K. Shanker, Internet of health: applying IoT and big data to manage healthcare systems. *International Research Journal of Engineering and Technology*, 2016. 310: p. 732–735.

[30] Ghosh, A.M., D. Halder, and S.A. Hossain, Remote health monitoring system through IoT. in *2016 International Conference on Informatics, Electronics and Vision (ICIEV)*. 2016. IEEE, p. 921–926.

[31] Michard, F., A sneak peek into digital innovations and wearable sensors for cardiac monitoring. *Journal of Clinical Monitoring and Computing*, 2016: p. 1–7.

[32] Lee, W., H. Yoon, and K. Park, Smart ECG monitoring patch with built-in R-peak detection for long-term HRV analysis. *Annals of Biomedical Engineering*, 2016: p. 1–10.

[33] Iqbal, M.H., A. Aydin, O. Brunckhorst, P. Dasgupta, and K. Ahmed, A review of wearable technology in medicine. *Journal of the Royal Society of Medicine*, 2016. 109(10): p. 372–380.

[34] Baig, M. M., F. Mirza, H. GholamHosseini, J. Gutierrez, and E. Ullah, Clinical decision support for early detection of prediabetes and type 2 diabetes mellitus using wearable technology. in *2018 40th Annual International Conference of the IEEE Engineering in Medicine and Biology Society (EMBC)*. 2018. IEEE, p. 4456–4459.

[35] Araújo, F.H., A.M. Santana, and P.d.A.S. Neto, Using machine learning to support healthcare professionals in making preauthorisation decisions. *International Journal of Medical Informatics*, 2016. 94: p. 1–7.

[36] Elsebakhi, E., F. Lee, E. Schendel, *et al.*, Large-scale machine learning based on functional networks for biomedical big data with high performance computing platforms. *Journal of Computational Science*, 2015. 11: p. 69–81.

[37] Klaassen, B., B.J. van Beijnum, and H.J. Hermens, Usability in telemedicine systems—a literature survey. *International Journal of Medical Informatics*, 2016. 93: p. 57–69.

[38] Ullah, F., M.A. Habib, M. Farhan, S. Khalid, M.Y. Durrani, and S. Jabbar, Semantic interoperability for big-data in heterogeneous IoT infrastructure for healthcare. *Sustainable Cities and Society*, 2017. 34: p. 90–96.

[39] Kovacs, E., M. Bauer, J. Kim, J. Yun, F. Le Gall, and M. Zhao, Standards-based worldwide semantic interoperability for IoT. *IEEE Communications Magazine*, 2016. 54(12): p. 40–46.

Chapter 8

Magnetic nanoparticle hyperthermia for cancer treatment

Saeed Tiari[1], Kassianne Tofani[1], Julia Baumgarner[1] and Davide Piovesan[1]

Targeted hyperthermia (TH) has recently been explored as a potential new cancer treatment technique. Cancerous cells and tumors are beset using the activation of magnetic nanoparticles in an alternating magnetic field. Various types of magnetic nanoparticles have been examined for this purpose, focusing on different concentrations and surface properties. This chapter provides a brief overview of the recent studies conducted in this area.

8.1 Cancer treatment

Cancer leads to the death of more than half a million people in the United States annually, which makes it the second cause of mortality in the country [1]. Chemotherapy, surgery, and radiation therapy are currently the most common cancer treatment methods. However, each of these methods is associated with severe side effects in healthy tissues [2]. Chronic side effects are of great concern, especially as the survival rate increases and the number of treated individuals is significant, such as for breast cancer survivors [3]. When considering prostate cancer, the 5-year survival rate is 95%, and most prostate cancer survivors die from non-cancer causes [4]. Thus, the long-lasting side effect of treatment must be minimal. The most common modes of treatment for patients with prostate cancer, besides surgery, include radiotherapy, hormone therapy, and active surveillance, and each is associated with its own set of side effects [4].

The most common postsurgical treatments for many types of cancer are still radiotherapy and chemotherapy [5]. Radiotherapy is often complementary to chemotherapy treatment. Both treatments have been proven effective to reduce local relapses and extend overall survival in patients with breast cancer [3]. Hofman *et al.* [6] have suggested that the majority of the cancer patients had an expectation of developing either severe or long-lasting side effects, with fatigue (90.6%) and

[1]Biomedical, Industrial and Systems Engineering Department, Gannon University, Erie, USA

nausea (78%) on the top of the list [7]. The behavioral disturbances experienced by breast cancer patients receiving radiotherapy are several, including sleep problems, depression, and cognitive disturbance [8]. In focused studies, cervical cancer survivors who received radiation therapy developed a recurrent number of systemic problems such as "*diarrhea, dietary changes, precocious menopause, and moderate nausea arose*," as well as specific localized problems such as "*vaginal shortening, rectal bleeding, sexual dysfunction, and urinary self-catheterization*" [9].

Radiotherapy also remains a major therapeutic option for patients with advanced lung cancer. However, in this particular type of cancer, radiation promotes tumor migration, distant metastasis, and the invasive potential of cancer cells in other tissues [10]. In patients with lung cancer, radiotherapy is almost always associated with chemotherapy. The top three side effects concerning the survivor were shortness of breath, bleeding, and fatigue [11]. "*The side-effects and long-term sequelae of anticancer chemotherapy remain a major source of concern for both patients and clinicians despite the improved efficacy and enhanced survival offered by modern treatments*," Nurgali *et al.* have reported [5]. Agrawal [3] has recently reported that chemotherapy can induce cardiovascular toxicity which "*may include cardiomyopathy with or without overt congestive heart failure (CHF), endothelial dysfunction, and arrhythmias. RT-induced cardiovascular toxicity may include coronary artery disease (CAD), valvular disease, chronic pericardial disease, arrhythmias and conduction disturbances, cardiomyopathy, or carotid artery stenosis.*"

Many anticancer drugs can also induce neurological side effects, i.e., induced peripheral neuropathy. Comorbidity associated with peripheral neurological damage includes some of the aforementioned behavioral complications such as depression, insomnia, as well as more severe cases of moto-neural problems such as ataxia [5]. Recent studies on the side effects of chemotherapy regimen have taken into consideration several confounding factors such as cancer type and stage of the disease identifying the following as the most common self-reported side effects: (A) chest pain, (B) constipation, (C) diarrhea, (D) dyspnea, (E) fatigue, (F) mucositis, (G) pain, (H) rash, (I) vomiting, where fatigue is the most commonly reported (73%) and chest pain the least reported (4%) [12].

Over the last six decades, several discoveries in immunology, molecular biology, and virology have allowed for the development of novel cancer treatments to complement radiotherapy and chemotherapy [13]. Molecular targeted therapy allows for improved selectivity of attacking cancer cells, rather than using a broad-spectrum approach. Given the improved targeted action, the treatment was posited to have a decreased toxicity when compared to traditional chemotherapy. Conversely, while the pathways of the cancer treatment are different, they can still produce a reduced quality of life for oncology patients [14].

Hyperthermia can be an alternative treatment in which cancer cells are exposed to a temperature higher than the normal body temperature. TH is not immune to side effect. TH is carefully planned not to damage surrounding tissues that are preserved if the temperature remains under 43°C [15,16]. On the other hand, given the specific characteristics of tissues in different areas of the body, this temperature threshold could be exceeded. As a consequence, pain at the target site, swelling, burns, and blistering could manifest [17]. Techniques based on perfusion, where the blood on the area of interest is warmed, could induce tissue swelling, blood clots, bleeding in the perfused area. On the other hand, most of these side effects are temporary.

8.2 Therapeutic hyperthermia

Hyperthermia has been used in medical treatment dating back to ancient Egyptian times. While this practice of using heat to treat diseases is not new, it is still extremely relevant and rapidly expanding today [18]. According to the Society for Thermal Medicine, hyperthermia can be used to treat a variety of problems, including cardiac arrhythmias, endometrial bleeding, varicose veins, excess fat to help treat obesity and metabolic disorders, and the most commonly known use for hyperthermia—cancer treatment [19]. Hyperthermia kills cancer cells by increasing the temperature above that at which they can function. These high temperatures destroy the structures of the cells and their proteins [17]. Currently, hyperthermia is rarely used alone—more often it is used alongside other cancer treatment methods such as chemotherapy, radiation, surgery, gene therapy, or immunotherapy [20].

Three main types of hyperthermia exist: local, regional, and whole-body hyperthermia. Local targets only the tumor, regional targets a whole area of the body, and whole-body hyperthermia is used for cancer that is spread throughout the body [17]. These can be achieved through heating a patient's blood, the use of heating blankets, heating up the room, infrared technology, microwaves, and ultrasounds [18]. Local hyperthermia has a few different methods depending on the location of the tumor that is being targeted. For tumors that are close to the surface of the skin, external heat applicators can be applied. Endocavitary hyperthermia is used when the tumor is in a body cavity such as the esophagus; in this method, probes are inserted into the body cavity to heat up the tumor. The third method for local hyperthermia is interstitial, which is used when tumors are in less accessible parts of the body. Probes are inserted to heat the tumor, while external measurements, such as ultrasound, are used to determine that the probes are in the right place [17]. Regional hyperthermia is more often used for these deeper tumors and covers a larger area. It can be done through methods such as heating of the blood, radiofrequency, or body cavity irrigation [18]. Whole-body hyperthermia is performed with the help of anesthesia, and it is still a difficult procedure (Figure 8.1). Safe intubation methods have not yet been confirmed, and the side effects are more severe than with the other two methods. The stresses on the body from the anesthetic combined with the hyperthermia can be toxic. Though rarely, it can lead to issues with the heart or other organs [17].

8.3 Magnetic nanoparticle hyperthermia

In addition to their side effects, these methods often do not target only the tumor area or evenly distribute heat. A developing method for local hyperthermia that uses magnetic nanoparticles to heat tumors promises to resolve these problems

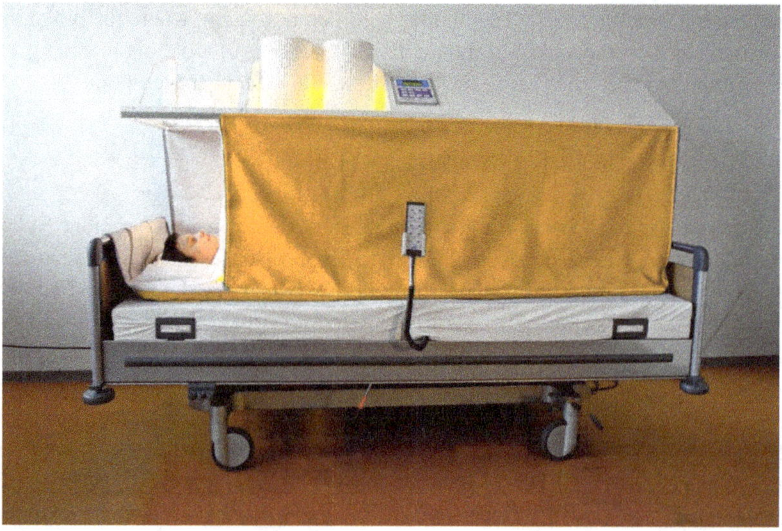

Figure 8.1 Whole-body hyperthermia device [21]

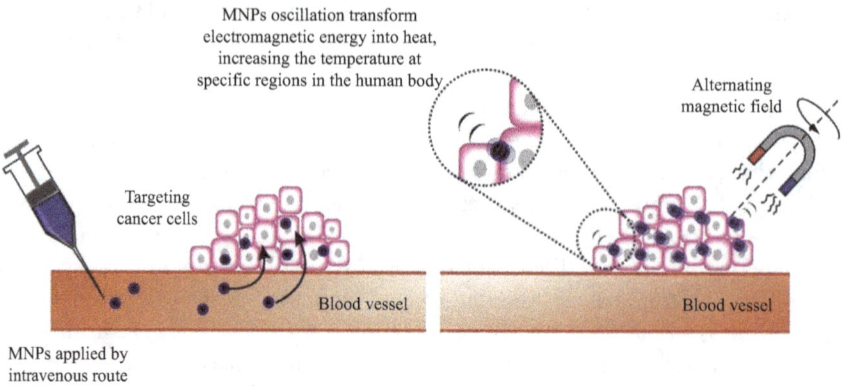

Figure 8.2 Schematic showing how magnetic nanoparticle hyperthermia works [22]

(Figure 8.2). In this method, magnetic nanoparticles, such as iron oxide, are deposited into the target tissue, and an alternating magnetic field is used to heat the particles [20]. The heat generated by the magnetic nanoparticles increases the tumor temperature. This leads to the enhancement of tumor oxygenation and eventually shrinking of the tumor. Magnetic nanoparticles are very susceptible to being controlled by a magnetic field and are often coated in polymers such as polylactic acid, polycaprolactone, and poly(lactic-*co*-glycolic acid) to achieve great biocompatibility [22]. Since nanoparticles are so small relative to the region of interest, they can target the area of the tumor, theoretically without damaging the surrounding tissue. Still, magnetic nanoparticle hyperthermia treatment has not been used broadly, yet. This is mostly due to the limitation in accurate temperature determination and control as the treatment is given. This may cause organ damage due to exposure to high temperature and overheating during the treatment. These nanoparticles can also be used to target drug delivery to the tumors and aid in diagnosis with the help of magnetic resonance imaging [22]. Nevertheless, the latter method has not yet been perfected.

8.4 Types of particles and delivery methods

Many different types of nanoparticles exist, along with various forms of encapsulation. There is much promise in the variety of particles that have been tested. One popular element used in nanoparticles is iron (Fe) that is usually combined with gold or made into iron oxide, then combined with a coating, encapsulated, or attached to another molecule in order to increase biocompatibility and targeting properties for the therapeutic hyperthermia purpose.

In a study by Hsu *et al.* [23], a cell-penetrating peptide was attached to iron–gold alloy nanoparticles to target glioma. These brain tumors can be difficult to treat due to the blood brain barrier, a highly selective semipermeable border of endothelial cells that prevents solutes in the circulating blood from nonselectively crossing into the extracellular fluid of the central nervous system where neurons reside. A low-density lipoprotein receptor-related protein (LRP1) that is present on both the blood brain barrier and gliomas can be targeted by a peptide called Angiopep-2. The team in [23] synthesized iron–gold alloy nanoparticles then bonded the gold to the cysteine in Angiopep-2, shown in Figure 8.3. Their ability to generate heat when exposed to an alternating magnetic field was analyzed by dispersing various concentrations of the nanoparticles in distilled water, applying the magnetic field, and measuring the increase in temperature over time. The results showed a direct correlation between nanoparticle concentration and heat generation rate. The nanoparticles magnetic properties were tested using a superconducting quantum interference device (SQUID) magnetometer. The particles were found to be superparamagnetic [24] at and below room temperature. These nanoparticles proved effective, killing 95% of the glioma cells in only 15 min. When studied in vivo, they also showed to limit tumor growth and increase the lifespan of the rats as opposed to no treatment.

Other studies tested iron oxide with various modifications. One such study encapsulated the nanoparticles in a polyaspartamide (PA) biopolymer, conjugated with biotin, to increase cellular uptake [25]. The PA coating was used to increase the hydrophilicity, biocompatibility, and biodegradability of these nanoparticles. These superparamagnetic iron-oxide nanoparticles (SPIONS) were synthesized by thermal decomposition and tested with SQUID for magnetic properties and heating abilities, similar to the previous study. Samples of different concentrations were exposed to an alternating magnetic field, and their temperature was recorded over time with a fiber-optic thermometer. Although the magnetic properties of the

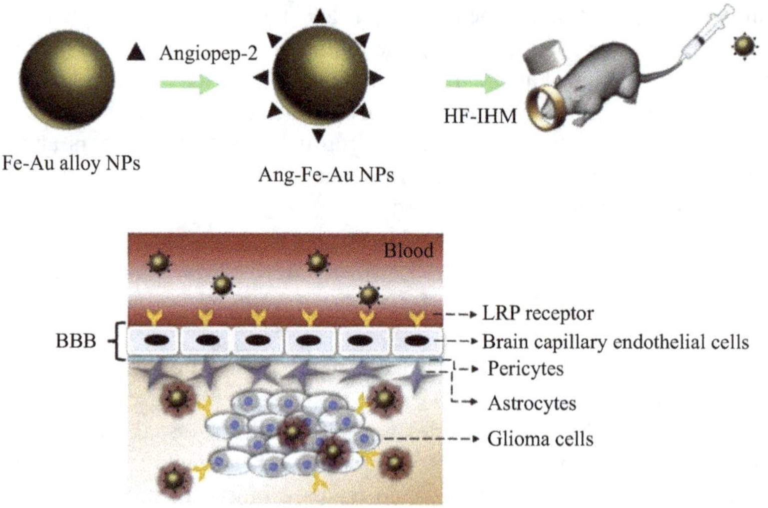

Figure 8.3 Iron–gold alloy nanoparticles conjugated with Angiopep-2 were developed for glioma treatment by Hsu et al. [23]

nanoparticles were not as strong once encapsulated, as shown in Figure 8.4, they are still stronger than the nanoparticles from the previously discussed study. The nanoparticles had good heating ability at low in vitro concentrations despite not being as strong as their unencapsulated counterparts. Mice were used to test the SPIONS in vivo, and the treatment greatly inhibited cancer growth when compared to the control, with a volume less than 1,000 mm^3 after 28 days, while the control tumors were 3,000 mm^3.

Another study [26] using iron-oxide nanoparticles coated them in citric acid. The nanoparticles were synthesized using spray-flame synthesis [27]. The magnetic properties of these particles were analyzed with Physical Property Measurement System DynaCool by Quantum Design, and the heating properties were assessed with a custom setup made from a direct current generator, an alternate current resonant oscillator and a copper coil. Figure 8.5 shows that the nanoparticles coated in citric acid had better magnetization than plain iron-oxide nanoparticles. The nanoparticles also had better specific absorption rate (SAR) values and heat performance than those of iron oxide currently being used in other experiments. This experiment successfully developed a standardized method of synthesizing these magnetic nanoparticles [26].

Chalkidou *et al.* [28] studied iron nanoparticles with a magnesium oxide shell for magnetic hyperthermia on cancer cells. The nanoparticles' magnetic characteristics were studied using vibrating sample magnetometry, and heating efficiency was found by subjecting various concentrations of the nanoparticles to an alternating magnetic field and recording heat generation. This data was used to calculate the SAR. The nanoparticles used in this study showed great uptake, high

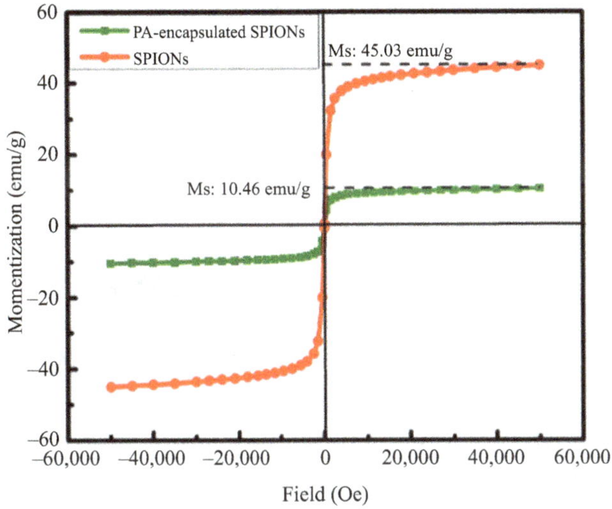

Figure 8.4 SQUID measurements of the superparamagnetic iron-oxide nanoparticles with and without PA encapsulation [25]

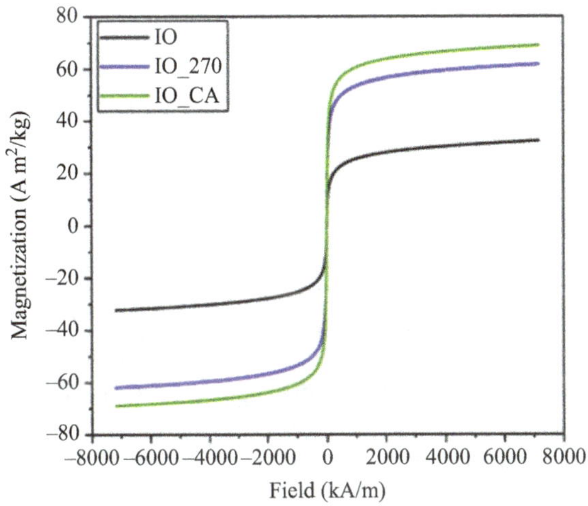

Figure 8.5 Hysteresis loops for pristine iron-oxide (IO), heated iron-oxide (IO_270), and citric acid-coated iron-oxide (IO_CA) nanoparticles at room temperature [26]

SARs, as well as great cytotoxicity. Various cell types, including breast cancer cells, were used to test these nanoparticles. The nanoparticles were ferromagnetic at room temperature, which can be seen by the results shown in Figure 8.6. They showed high thermal efficiency and short treatment duration. However, more in vitro testing of these nanoparticles is needed before they can be tested in vivo.

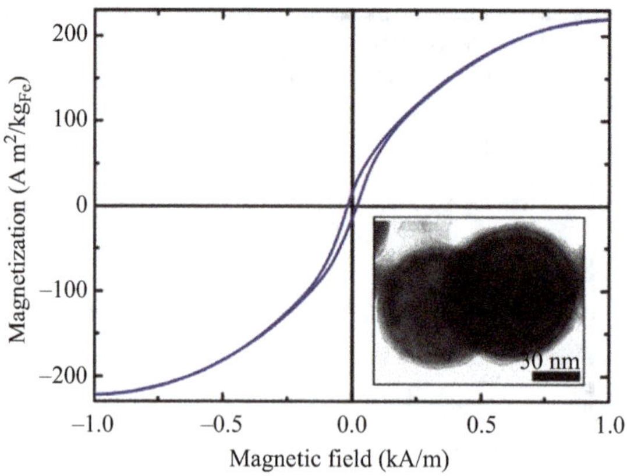

Figure 8.6 Hysteresis loop of the iron nanoparticles with magnesium-oxide shell recorded at room temperature [28]

8.5 Bioheat transfer studies

A few numerical studies have been conducted to study the impact of magnetic nanoparticle hyperthermia treatment on tumor and healthy tissues thermal behavior. Most of these studies used the well-known Pennes bioheat transfer equation [29]. This equation is used as a balance equation in bioheat transfer models and can describe the thermal behavior of living tissue as follows:

$$\rho c \frac{\partial T}{\partial t} = \frac{\partial}{\partial x}\left(k \frac{\partial T}{\partial x}\right) + \omega_b \rho_b c_b (T_b - T) + q_m + q_s$$

where on the left-hand side of the equation, ρ, c, T, and t are the tissue density, the specific heat for the tissue, the temperature of the tissue, and time, respectively. On the right-hand side of the equation, x is the spatial coordinate, k the thermal conductivity of the tissue, ω_b the blood perfusion rate, ρ_b the blood density, c_b the blood specific heat, T_b the blood temperature, q_m the metabolic heat generation within the tissue, and q_s the external heat source, respectively.

Boroon *et al.* [30] used the Pennes equation to estimate the optimum number and location of magnetic nanoparticle injections and the specific power loss for ideal hyperthermia treatment. They evaluated three-point injection, four-point injection, and five-point injection to reach the desired conditions, which was the uniform temperature of 43°C for the tumor. It was shown that three-point injection and four-point injection could not meet the criteria; however, five-point injection gained the desired uniform temperature. Reis *et al.* [31] developed a two-dimensional numerical model to investigate the influences of the number and location of magnetic nanoparticles injection during the hyperthermia treatment. In their two-dimensional model, they considered a square domain with a length of 10 cm and a square tumor with a length of 2 cm located at the center of the domain.

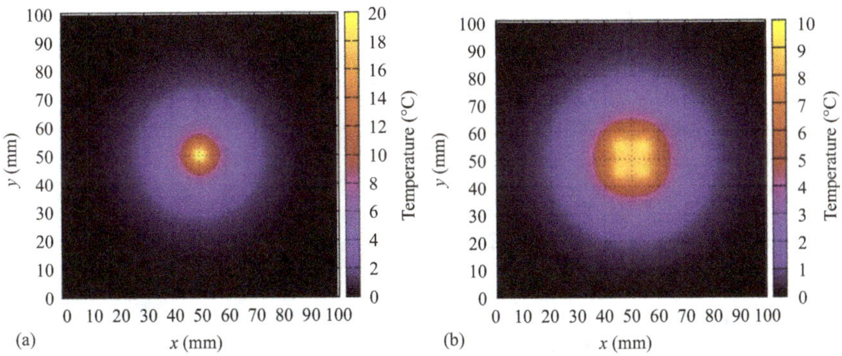

Figure 8.7 Temperature distributions for (a) one injection and (b) four injection sites by Reis et al. [31]

Two cases one with a single injection and the other one with four injection sites were investigated in this study, shown in Figure 8.7.

Lin and Liu [32] predicted the thermal behavior of biological tissues during magnetic nanoparticle hyperthermia using a transient bilayer bioheat transfer model. In their model, a small spherical tumor was surrounded by the normal tissue, and a spherical heat source with a constant power density was generated by an alternating magnetic field as magnetic nanoparticles were injected into the tumor. Chauhan *et al.* [33] developed a transient three-dimensional numerical model to study the thermal behavior of a tumor surrounded by multiple layers of healthy tissues such as fat, muscle, dermis, and epidermis during the magnetic nanoparticle hyperthermia treatment. The effect of two different therapeutic heat generation rates (1.95×10^5 and 3.97×10^5 W/m^3) inside the tumor was compared. It was shown that in the case with the lower therapeutic heat generation rate (1.95×10^5 W/m^3), it took 5 min for the tumor to reach the desired temperature of 43°C while in the case with the higher therapeutic heat generation rate (3.97×10^5 W/m^3), this time was close to 2 min. Mohajer *et al.* [34] developed a one-dimensional model based on the Pennes bioheat transfer equation to investigate the thermal response of the tumor and the normal tissue around it. The results indicated that the thermal diffusivity of the tissues as well as the geometry plays an essential role on the thermal response of the tissue. Adhikary and Banerjee [35] employed a three-dimensional model with two different types of tumor model to study the temperature distribution of tissues during the magnetic hyperthermia treatment. In the first model, they considered a single artery transiting the tumor, while in the second model, countercurrent flow vessels transiting the tumor (CVTT), two different blood vessels of countercurrent flow were considered, and both shown in Figure 8.8. They also studied the influence of different volumetric distribution patterns of magnetic nanoparticles within the tumor such as homogenous, parabolic, and liner distribution. Based on the obtained results, the CVTT model provides stronger cooling effect compared to the other model. It was also shown that the linear distribution pattern of

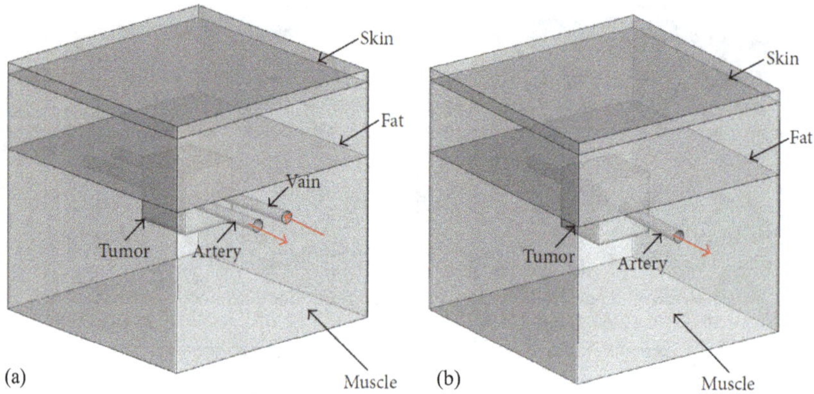

Figure 8.8 Two different tumor models (a) counter current flow vessels with both artery and vain and (b) single artery passing through the center of the tumor used by Adhikary and Banerjee [35]

magnetic nanoparticle distribution is associated with a high value of temperature within the tumor, which favors the tumor necrosis instead of healthy tissue necrosis.

Using a transient thermo-viscoelastic model based on the Pennes bioheat transfer equation, Ezzat [36] performed a numerical study to investigate the impact of thermal and mechanical material properties on tumorous tissue during hyperthermia treatment. It was shown that the thermal conductivity and volume relaxation parameters play a key role in temperature distribution. It was also concluded that the quality of hyperthermia treatment is significantly affected by the method of temperature control that highly depends on the thermal and mechanical properties of the living tissue.

8.6 Case study: effect of cooling during hyperthermia

As was mentioned before, hyperthermia treatment has not been used broadly because of the limitation in accurate temperature control during the treatment, specifically in healthy tissues, which can cause serious damage. One of the possible solutions for this issue are using a cooling method along with the hyperthermia treatment to minimize the damage to healthy tissues around the tumor. In a numerical study, Tiari *et al.* [37] studied the effect of different cooling methods on temperature distribution within healthy and cancerous tissues during the magnetic hyperthermia treatment. In their study, a transient multilayer two-dimensional numerical model was employed to simulate the thermal behavior of the tumor and healthy tissues during the magnetic nanoparticle hyperthermia treatment. The governing equations, including the famous Pennes bioheat transfer equation, were solved using ANSYS-FLUENT18.1. The model consists of a cylindrical tumor with the radius of 2 cm located at the center of cubic healthy tissues. The surrounding healthy tissues are composed of different layers such as epidermis,

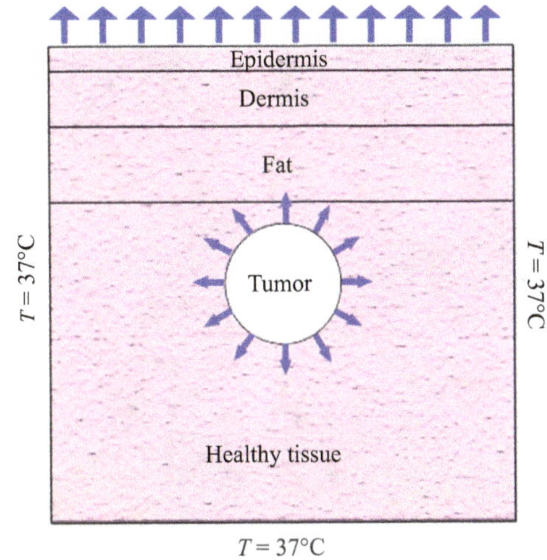

Figure 8.9 Schematic of the model developed by Tiari et al. [37]

dermis, and fat layer and a layer of healthy muscle tissues. A schematic of the model, along with the boundary conditions, is displayed in Figure 8.9.

To account for the therapeutic heat generated by the magnetic nanoparticles during hyperthermia treatment, a constant volumetric heat generation rate was added to the tumor. The top boundary, which corresponds to the external layer of the skin, was in contact with different coolants at various conditions that included air at ambient temperature (17°C), ice pack (0°C), and stagnant water at 17°C. For the cooling with the ice pack, the boundary condition of constant temperature of 0°C was considered for the skin while, empirical correlations were used to calculate the convection heat-transfer coefficients for cooling with air and water. It was also assumed that all the other surfaces are at the normal body core temperature of 37°C. In addition, it was assumed that the considered tissue section does not contain any blood vessel; hence the blood flow impact on thermal characteristics of the tissue could be ignored. The entire model, including the tumor and different layers of other tissues, was initially at the temperature of 37°C. The effects of different concentrations of magnetic nanoparticle were considered by applying three different therapeutic heat generation rates of 50, 100, and 150 kW/m^3.

To study the effect of concentrations of magnetic nanoparticles (therapeutic heat generation rate), the case with the skin subjected to air at the temperature of 17°C was considered. To attain a successful hyperthermia treatment and destroy the cancerous cells, the tumor temperature should be increased to a desired range of 42°C –45°C without damaging the surrounding healthy tissues. Their results, as shown in Figure 8.10, indicated that the desired temperature range was achieved after 10 min in the case with the therapeutic heat generation rate of 150 kW/m^3, while the tumor temperature was significantly lower than the desired range in the other two cases (50 kW/m^3, 100 kW/m^3) at the same time. For the case with the

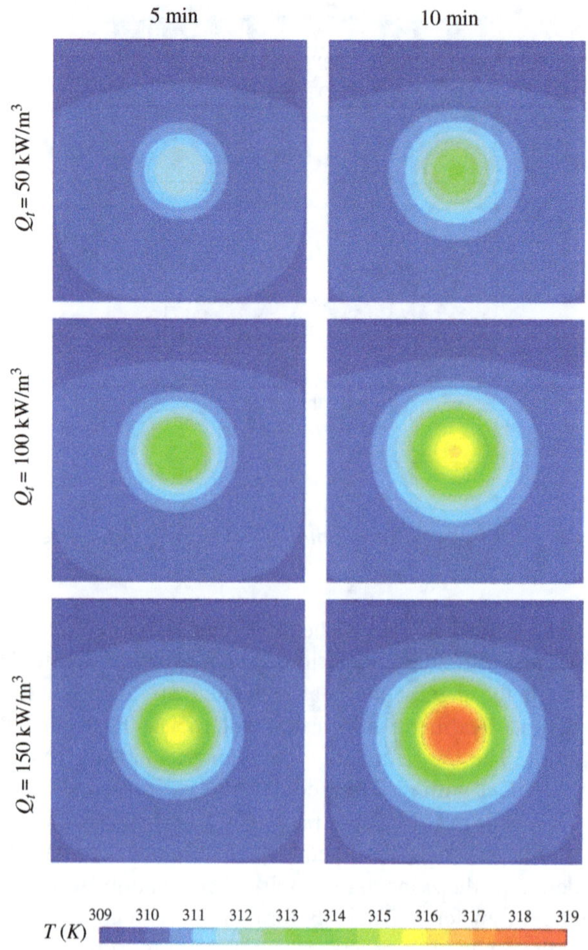

Figure 8.10 Tumor and normal tissue temperature distribution for different heat generation rates [37]

therapeutic heat generation rate of 150 kW/m^3, it was also shown that the temperature of the healthy tissues around the tumor is considerably high and in the range of 40°C–43°C, which can cause serious damage.

To avoid the possible damages to the healthy tissues, two other cooling conditions with ice cooling and water cooling were tested on top of the air cooling for different therapeutic heat generation rates. Figure 8.11 shows the tissue temperature along the vertical symmetry line starting from the center of the tumor to the surface of the skin for various cooling methods and therapeutic heat generation rates. The results indicated that for all three therapeutic heat generation rates, the tumor temperature has not been affected as different cooling conditions are applied. In the tissues located far away from the tumor, the effect of cooling methods becomes more notable. The

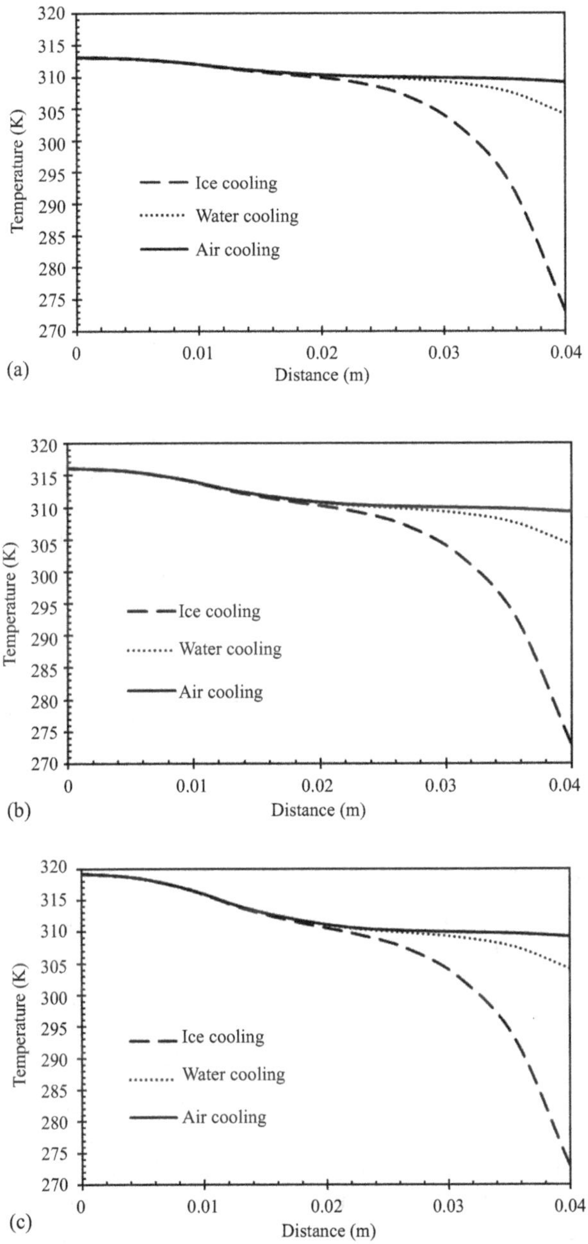

Figure 8.11 Temperatures for the cases with the therapeutic heat generation rates of (a) 50, (b) 100, and (c) 150 kW/m^3 and different cooling methods

temperatures of the healthy tissues in the cases with ice pack cooling are noticeably lower comparing to those resulted in the cases with air and water cooling.

8.7 Conclusion

In this review, we addressed the type of side effects that anticancer treatments could produce, given different types of neoplasms. It is found that the use of TH provides the least amount of side effects when compared to less localized, wide-spectrum treatments. TH is based on the injection of nanoparticles into the site to be treated, which is possible with extreme precision. The nanoparticles are made of ferromagnetic alloys and coated with biocompatible materials. The alloys' nature allows for supermagnetism in the particles, a property that is often thwarted by the biocompatible coating. On the other hand, new research has found that a coating of citric acid preserves the biocompatibility and even enhances the particles' supermagnetic properties. Exposing a neoplasm infiltrated with such nanoparticles to a magnetic field increases the nanoparticles' temperature via hysteresis, and consequentially the internal temperature of the tumor causing necrosis of the tissues. A number of simulation studies have been performed considering the heat-transfer properties of the tumor, due to internal vascularization, as well as considering the properties of the surrounding tissues. The treatment can optimize the temperature of the tumor to be above the necrosis inducing the threshold of 43°C while limiting the temperature increase in the surrounding healthy tissues. Simulations can guide the best choice for the number of injection sites, the spatial distribution of the nanoparticles, and the choice of cooling methods for the surrounding tissues, so to optimize the kill zone while preserving healthy tissues.

References

[1] Nicholos, H., *What Are the Leading Causes of Death in the Us?* Available from: medicalnewstoday.com/articles/282929.

[2] Bañobre-López, M., Teijeiro, A., and Rivas, J., 'Magnetic Nanoparticle-Based Hyperthermia for Cancer Treatment', *Reports of Practical Oncology & Radiotherapy*, 2013, 18, (6), pp. 397–400.

[3] Agrawal, S., 'Late Effects of Cancer Treatment in Breast Cancer Survivors', *South Asian Journal of Cancer*, 2014, 3, (2), pp. 112–115.

[4] Gegechkori, N., Haines, L., and Lin, J.J., 'Long-Term and Latent Side Effects of Specific Cancer Types', *The Medical Clinics of North America*, 2017, 101, (6), pp. 1053–1073.

[5] Nurgali, K., Jagoe, R.T., and Abalo, R., 'Editorial: Adverse Effects of Cancer Chemotherapy: Anything New to Improve Tolerance and Reduce Sequelae?', *Frontiers in Pharmacology*, 2018, 9, pp. 245–245.

[6] Hofman, M., Morrow, G.R., Roscoe, J.A., *et al.*, 'Cancer Patients' Expectations of Experiencing Treatment-Related Side Effects: A University of Rochester Cancer Center–Community Clinical Oncology Program Study of 938 Patients from Community Practices', *Cancer*, 2004, 101, (4), pp. 851–857.

[7] Quidde, J., Pan, Y., Salm, M., *et al.*, 'Preventing Adverse Events of Chemotherapy by Educating Patients About the Nocebo Effect (RENNO

Study) – Study Protocol of a Randomized Controlled Trial with Gastrointestinal Cancer Patients', *BMC Cancer*, 2018, 18, (1), pp. 916–916.

[8] Bower, J.E., 'Behavioral Symptoms in Patients with Breast Cancer and Survivors', *Journal of Clinical Oncology: Official Journal of the American Society of Clinical Oncology*, 2008, 26, (5), pp. 768–777.

[9] Sun, C., Brown, A.J., Jhingran, A., Frumovitz, M., Ramondetta, L., and Bodurka, D.C., 'Patient Preferences for Side Effects Associated with Cervical Cancer Treatment', *International Journal of Gynecological Cancer: Official Journal of the International Gynecological Cancer Society*, 2014, 24, (6), pp. 1077–1084.

[10] Huang, C.-Y., Ju, D.-T., Chang, C.-F., Muralidhar Reddy, P., and Velmurugan, B.K., 'A Review on the Effects of Current Chemotherapy Drugs and Natural Agents in Treating Non-Small Cell Lung Cancer', *BioMedicine*, 2017, 7, (4), pp. 23–23.

[11] Islam, K.M., Anggondowati, T., Deviany, P.E., *et al.*, 'Patient Preferences of Chemotherapy Treatment Options and Tolerance of Chemotherapy Side Effects in Advanced Stage Lung Cancer', *BMC Cancer*, 2019, 19, (1), pp. 835–835.

[12] Pearce, A., Haas, M., Viney, R., *et al.*, 'Incidence and Severity of Self-Reported Chemotherapy Side Effects in Routine Care: A Prospective Cohort Study', *PLoS One*, 2017, 12, (10), p. e0184360.

[13] Schirrmacher, V., 'From Chemotherapy to Biological Therapy: A Review of Novel Concepts to Reduce the Side Effects of Systemic Cancer Treatment (Review)', *International Journal of Oncology*, 2019, 54, (2), pp. 407–419.

[14] De Angelis, C., 'Side Effects Related to Systemic Cancer Treatment: Are We Changing the Promethean Experience With Molecularly Targeted Therapies?', *Current Oncology (Toronto, Ont.)*, 2008, 15, (4), pp. 198–199.

[15] Falk, M.H. and Issels, R.D., 'Hyperthermia in Oncology', *International Journal of Hyperthermia*, 2001, 17, (1), pp. 1–18.

[16] van der Zee, J., 'Heating the Patient: A Promising Approach?', *Annals of Oncology*, 2002, 13, (8), pp. 1173–1184.

[17] Jha, S., Sharma, P.K., and Malviya, R., 'Hyperthermia: Role and Risk Factor for Cancer Treatment', *Achievements in the Life Sciences*, 2016, 10, (2), pp. 161–167.

[18] Mallory, M., Gogineni, E., Jones, G.C., Greer, L., and Simone, II, C.B., 'Therapeutic Hyperthermia: The Old, the New, and the Upcoming', *Critical Reviews in Oncology/Hematology*, 2016, 97, pp. 56–64.

[19] Society for Thermal Medicine, 2020, 'What is Thermal Medicine?', The Society for Thermal Medicine. Available from: https://www.thermaltherapy.org/ebusSFTM/SOCIETYINFO/WhatisThermalMedicine.aspx [Accessed 19 September 2021].

[20] Behrouzkia, Z., Joveini, Z., Keshavarzi, B., Eyvazzadeh, N., and Aghdam, R.Z., 'Hyperthermia: How Can It Be Used?', *Oman Medical Journal*, 2016, 31, (2), pp. 89–97.

[21] Sulyok, I., Fleischmann, E., Stift, A., *et al.*, 'Effect of Preoperative Fever-Range Whole-Body Hyperthermia on Immunological Markers in Patients Undergoing Colorectal Cancer Surgery', *British Journal of Anaesthesia*, 2012, 109, (5), pp. 754–761.

[22] Lima-Tenorio, M.K., Pineda, E.A.G., Ahmad, N.M., Fessi, H., and Elaissari, A., 'Magnetic Nanoparticles: In Vivo Cancer Diagnosis and Therapy', *International Journal of Pharmaceutics*, 2015, 493, (1–2), pp. 313–327.

[23] Hsu, S.P., Dhawan, U., Tseng, Y.-Y., *et al.*, 'Glioma-Sensitive Delivery of Angiopep-2 Conjugated Iron Gold Alloy Nanoparticles Ensuring Simultaneous Tumor Imaging and Hyperthermia Mediated Cancer Theranostics', *Applied Materials Today*, 2020, 18, p. 100510.

[24] Bedanta, S., Petracic, O., and Kleemann, W., Chapter 1 – Supermagnetism, in Buschow, K.H.J. (ed.), *Handbook of Magnetic Materials*, 2015. Amsterdam, The Netherlands: Elsevier.

[25] Nguyen, M.P., Nguyen, M.H., Kim, J., and Kim, D., 'Encapsulation of Superparamagnetic Iron Oxide Nanoparticles with Polyaspartamide Biopolymer for Hyperthermia Therapy', *European Polymer Journal*, 2020, 122, p. 109396.

[26] Hammad, M., Hardt, S., Mues, B., *et al.*, 'Gas-Phase Synthesis of Iron Oxide Nanoparticles for Improved Magnetic Hyperthermia Performance', *Journal of Alloys and Compounds*, 2020, 824, p. 153814.

[27] Nunes, D., Pimentel, A., Santos, L., *et al.*, 2 – Synthesis, Design, and Morphology of Metal Oxide Nanostructures, in Nunes, D., Pimentel, A., Santos, L., *et al.* (eds.), *Metal Oxide Nanostructures*, 2019. Amsterdam, The Netherlands: Elsevier.

[28] Chalkidou, A., Simeonidis, K., Angelakeris, M., *et al.*, 'In Vitro Application of Fe/MgO Nanoparticles as Magnetically Mediated Hyperthermia Agents for Cancer Treatment', *Journal of Magnetism and Magnetic Materials*, 2011, 323, (6), pp. 775–780.

[29] Pennes, H.H., 'Analysis of Tissue and Arterial Blood Temperatures in the Resting Human Forearm', *Journal of Applied Physiology*, 1948, 1, (2), pp. 93–122.

[30] Boroon, M.P., Ayani, M.-B., and Bazaz, S.R., 'Estimation of the Optimum Number and Location of Nanoparticle Injections and the Specific Loss Power for Ideal Hyperthermia', *Journal of Thermal Biology*, 2018, 72, pp. 127–136.

[31] Reis, R.F., Loureiro, F.S., and Lobosco, M., 'A Parallel 2D Numerical Simulation of Tumor Cells Necrosis by Local Hyperthermia', *Journal of Physics: Conference Series*, 2014, 490, p. 012138.

[32] Lin, C.-T. and Liu, K.-C., 'Estimation for the Heating Effect of Magnetic Nanoparticles in Perfused Tissues', *International Communications in Heat and Mass Transfer*, 2009, 36, (3), pp. 241–244.

[33] Chauhan, K., Tiari, S., and Mahdavi, M., 'Numerical Study of Heat Transfer in Living Tissues During Hyperthermia Treatment of Cancer', in, *ASTFE Digital Library*, 2018. Fort Lauderdale, FL, USA: Begell House Inc.

[34] Mohajer, M., Ayani, M.B., and Tabrizi, H.B., 'Numerical Study of Non-Fourier Heat Conduction in a Biolayer Spherical Living Tissue During Hyperthermia', *Journal of Thermal Biology*, 2016, 62, pp. 181–188.

[35] Adhikary, K. and Banerjee, M., 'A Thermofluid Analysis of the Magnetic Nanoparticles Enhanced Heating Effects in Tissues Embedded with Large Blood Vessel During Magnetic Fluid Hyperthermia', *Journal of Nanoparticles*, 2016, 2016.

[36] Ezzat, M.A., 'The Effects of Thermal and Mechanical Material Properties on Tumorous Tissue During Hyperthermia Treatment', *Journal of Thermal Biology*, 2020, 92, p. 102649.

[37] Tiari, S., Mahdavi, M., Chauhan, K., and Piovesan, D., 'Numerical Investigation of Heat Transfer in Tissues During Therapeutic Hyperthermia', in *ASME 2018 International Mechanical Engineering Congress and Exposition*, (2018).

Chapter 9
Hyperpolarized 3He MRI in lung

Shuhao Pan[1]

Compared to traditional imaging methods (chest radiographs (CXRs), computed tomography (CT), and positron emission tomography (PET)), noble gas imaging has opened the new field of direct imaging of pulmonary ventilation by magnetic resonance imaging (MRI). It has great potential in the early diagnosis of lung cancer. The use of hyperpolarized (HP) 3He gas for MRI of the lung has been pioneered by a number of groups worldwide. Due to the enormous progress in the fields of hyperpolarization technology, administration of HP 3He, MR hardware, and MR pulse sequences, significant progress has been made and the translation into the clinical arena has been accomplished. This chapter gives an overview of the technical methods for HP 3He MRI for human lung imaging, which consists of three parts: focusing on gas polarization physical methods—spin-exchanged optical pumping (SEOP), MRI considerations; how 3He noble gas images can be used to probe lung function; clinical applications that can be carried out such as HP 3He gas MRI studies for pulmonary disease, radiation-induced lung injury (RILI), and radiomics in lung cancer.

9.1 Introduction

9.1.1 Epidemiology of lung cancer

Lung cancer has been the most common cancer in the world for several decades. The International Agency for Research on Cancer released on December 14 the updated GLOBOCAN 2020 with new estimates on the global cancer burden, indicating that lung cancer accounted for approximately 2.2 million new cases worldwide (1.44 million men and 0.77 million women), representing approximately 11.4% of all new cancer cases [1]. Worldwide, lung cancer is the leading cause of cancer death in men and the second leading cause of cancer death in women, with about 1.8 million individuals dying from the disease in 2020, that is, 18.4% of all cancer deaths.

[1]Department of Radiation Oncology, The First Affiliated Hospital of Anhui Medical University, Hefei, China

Worldwide, lung cancer incidence is generally higher in men than in women, and the magnitude of the difference varies between 2- and 9-fold. Among men, lung cancer was the most common cancer in the world in 2020, with the highest incidence rates in Micronesia/Polynesia, Eastern and Western Europe, and Eastern Asia [1]. In addition, worldwide, lung cancer is the third most frequent cancer in women; the highest lung cancer incidence rates, over 24.0 per 100 000 per year, are observed in North America, Northern and Western Europe, and Australia/New Zealand [1,2]. In many developed countries, the age-standardized incidence of lung cancer has decreased steeply in men compared to a rising trend in incidence among women over the past three decades [1]. Given the variations of trend by gender, lung cancer incidence rates are converging in men and women in the United States (US) and several European countries. In the US, the lung cancer incidence rate is higher among young women (less than 50 years old) than among young men, particularly among non-Hispanic whites and Hispanics [3], and this cannot be fully explained by gender differences in smoking behavior.

The geographical and temporal variations in the incidence of lung cancer are to a large extent determined by past exposure to tobacco smoking and the relative maturity of the tobacco epidemic in a given country [4–7]. An increase in tobacco consumption is paralleled several decades later by an increase in the incidence of lung cancer; similarly, a decrease in consumption is followed by a decrease in incidence. In populations that are not exposed to tobacco smoke or industrial lung carcinogens, the age-adjusted incidence rate of lung cancer is generally low (less than 5 per 100 000 per year) [2,8].

Many developing countries have still not experienced the worst consequences of the tobacco epidemic, as cigarette smoking became widespread only during the last 30 years. China has a 1.41178 billion population, which is inhabited by one-fifth of the world's population, and thus determines to a great extent the cancer burden at a global level. From the GLOBOCAN 2020, the number of new cancer cases in China is 4.57 million, and the death of cancer is 3 million, for lung cancer, the number is 0.8 and 0.71 million.

It was estimated that the lung cancer incidence in China would increase by 27% in men and 38% in women from the year 2000 to 2005, due mostly to changes in cancer risk (cigarette smoking), as well as to some degree alterations of population size and age structure [9]. If current incidence rates and trends prevail, it is estimated that the number of new lung cancer cases in China will increase to 1 million by 2030 [10]. The full effects of increased tobacco consumption are expected to occur in the next few decades. It has been estimated that worldwide smoking caused 11.5% (6.4 million) of global deaths from all causes in 2015 [11], while by around 2030, worldwide deaths from tobacco will most likely increase to approximately 10 million of 60 million deaths from all causes, with the majority of the increase taking place in Asia, Africa, and South America [12]. The main histological types of lung cancer are squamous cell carcinoma, small cell carcinoma, adenocarcinoma, and large cell carcinoma. Over the last 20 years, the distribution of the histological types of lung cancer has been changing. The proportion of squamous cell carcinoma, the previously predominant type, has declined for both sexes in many countries since the 1970s, whereas during the same period of time the incidence rates of adenocarcinoma have been increasing, particularly in women [13–15]. The possible explanations for the increase of lung adenocarcinoma include changes in the composition and patterns of tobacco consumption (deeper inhalation of low-nicotine and tar tobacco smoke), air pollution, and improvements of diagnostic techniques [14,16].

Largely due to improvements in the diagnosis and treatment of lung cancer, the 1-year relative survival of lung cancer patients has been improved in some countries. In the US, the 1-year lung cancer survival rate increased from 37% in 1975–79 to 45% in 2008–11 [17]. However, lung cancer continues to have one of the lowest 5-year survival rates among all malignancies around the world. The 5-year survival of lung cancer ranged from 10% to 20% for most geographical areas, both in the developed and developing countries [18,19]. Because the early disease is typically asymptomatic, only 16% of lung cancers are diagnosed at the local stage, for which the 5-year survival rate is 56% [18]. Data from these reports suggested the importance of early diagnosis and adequate treatment procedures for lung cancer survival and prognosis.

9.1.2 Pulmonary diagnosis

Due to climate change and atmospheric pollution, the number of patients with chronic obstructive pneumonia, cystic pulmonary fibrosis, asthma, emphysema, and other lung diseases is increasing year by year, and these chronic lung diseases could induce lung cancer. The most effective way to prevent cancer is early diagnosis.

The diagnosis of lung cancer has relied on findings on CXRs [19] and the detection of cells in sputum or biopsy specimens. Perhaps even more important, however, are specific findings on chest CT [20] and PET integrated with CT (PET/CT) [21]. Moreover, the staging and follow-up of lung cancer have relied more on CT, PET/CT than on CXRs. The goal of diagnosis and management of pulmonary nodules is to bring promptly to surgery all patients with operable malignant nodules while avoiding unnecessary thoracotomy for patients with benign lesions.

Currently, CT is considered to be the most widely applicable modality for the evaluation of lung cancer. In addition, PET/CT qualifies as another important innovation in lung cancer imaging. Standard imaging techniques are based on differences in the structure of tissues, whereas PET/CT can show the enhanced glucose metabolism of lung cancer cells. For these reasons, MRI has been utilized for only a few cases, such as superior sulcus tumor, mediastinal invasion, and chest wall invasion since 1991, when the Radiologic Diagnostic Oncology Group reported no significant difference in the diagnostic capability of CT and conventional T_1-weighted imaging for the staging of lung cancer except for mediastinal invasion. However, recent advances in MRI techniques and utilization of contrast media have resulted in further improvement of the image quality and diagnostic capability of MRI for lung cancer patients. However, CT and PET scans are the most widely used modalities for the diagnosis and staging of lung cancer. Such radiation-based imaging diagnostic methods have the following characteristics: (1) high radioactivity. In general, the radiation dose of a single examination is 0.02 mSv for X-ray, 8 mSv for CT, and 10.5 mSv for PET. According to the International Regulations on Ionizing Radiation Protection, the annual effective public exposure dose of human should be controlled below 1 mSv, so those kinds of radiation diagnosis methods are not suitable for getting repeated in a short period of time. (2) It has a poor effect to diagnose the early lesions such as chronic obstruction disease and emphysema, generally, only lumpy and high-density lesions can be diagnosed easily.

MRI has been widely used in medical diagnosis. Unfortunately, the process of pulmonary MR diagnosis is quite difficult, traditional MR uses the hydrogen nucleus (1H) spin in water to image; however, the physiological structure of the lung limits the use of MRI.

In the 1980s, a group of physicists and radiologists began trying to use MRI to diagnose different lung diseases; unfortunately, they failed to capture clear lung MR images. So most people would choose high-resolution CT to obtain lung characteristic information and determine the type of lung disease. At the same time, CT is more advantageous than MRI in the diagnosis of pulmonary angiography and pulmonary embolism, so the idea of introducing MRI into lung diagnosis has been put on hold for a while. At that time, scientists, medical workers, and instrument manufacturers all lost interest in lung MRI. In the 1990s, two very different groups revived lung MRI research. The first team was a group of medical workers: radiologists found that cardiopulmonary interaction was important when performed heart MRI. So in analyzing right ventricular function, they used MRI to study pulmonary arteries and veins. The second group, a group of physicists who work on basic physics and lasers, they thought it would be a good idea to use polarized inert gas to perform lung MRI, which would "light up" the lung [22]. Based on the importance of lung MRI and the breakthrough of new methods, people's enthusiasm for lung MRI has been rekindled, and more and more teams are involved in this research. With the further development, it has been found that MRI has a high spatial resolution in lung imaging, and its ability in lung structure visualization and lung disease diagnosis is second only to CT. One of the most attractive aspects of lung MRI is that it can be used to achieve lung function imaging. With the development of hardware, MRI has overcome the problem of motion artifacts caused by breathing movement, cardiac contraction, and blood vessel pulsation in imaging. The changes of lung microstructure can be observed by MRI. Imaging of different lung functions, such as perfusion, respiratory movement, ventilation, and gas exchange, allows physicians to analyze the patient's lung function quantitatively.

With the development of technology, MRI has been widely used in the diagnosis of lung diseases, such as pulmonary hypertension, congenital vascular malformation, and cystic fibrosis in the early clinical diagnosis; discriminating lung cancer and malignant pleural mesothelioma in which stage; description of features of mediastinal pleural neoplasm. These all reveal that MRI plays a significant role in the diagnosis of lung diseases. However, lung MRI has not received enough attention, because (1) CXRs, CT, PET/CT, and other radiological imaging methods

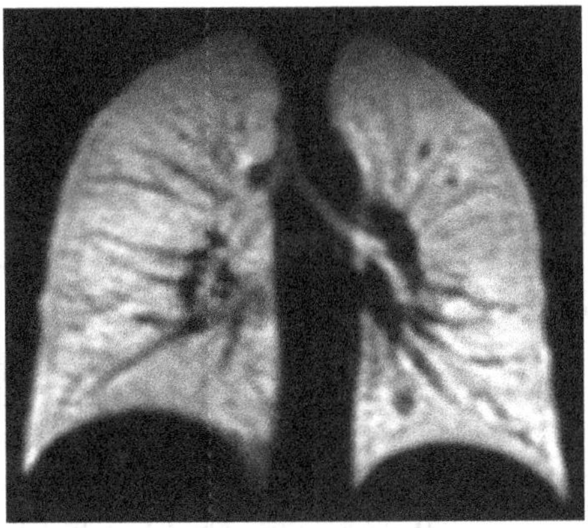

Figure 9.1 MRI of the lungs using hyperpolarized noble gases

are quite mature, which can meet the routine diagnosis of lung disease; (2) in order to meet the requirements of lung diagnosis, lung MR images need to have sufficient resolution. However, the technology to achieve high-resolution lung MRI has not been widely promoted.

It has been 25 years since the birth of the first polarized 3He-based MR image of human lung [23]. The currently, with the rapid development of gas polarization technology and MRI technology, for the most lung dysfunction (physiological changes caused by lung disease), MRI based on polarized gas can give clear lung images [24] (see Figure 9.1). Although MRI based on polarized gas has unique advantages in lung function examination, it was not the mainstream method in clinical diagnosis of the lung due to various reasons.

9.1.3 Hyperpolarized gas MRI

Because of the lack of water in the lungs, it is difficult for conventional lung MRI. However, due to the introduction of polarized gas, it is easy to get the clear lung MR images.

So, what kind of gas we need?

The gas selected must be inert, nontoxic, and have an odd number of nucleons. Helium isotopes 3He, xenon isotopes 129Xe, and krypton (83Kr) are qualified. At present, MRI studies based on HP inert gases mainly focus on 3He and 129Xe gases. Meanwhile, the polarization studies of new substances such as 13C, 19F [25,26] and 83Kr have begun to attract people's attention. For 3He and 129Xe, each has its merits. In fact, 3He HP gas has unique advantages in lung tissue microstructure imaging, so we will focus on polarized 3He in this chapter. 3He gas is an isotope of the inert gas 4He. On earth, the natural abundance of 3He is extremely low, about 0.000137%. Most of the 3He used comes from the decay of tritium in nuclear reactions. The atomic spin number of 3He is 1/2 and the rotational magnetic ratio is 32.3 MHz T^{-1}, so it has a very high sensitivity in MRI. Due to the small atomic radius, 3He has a strong diffusivity, with a diffusivity of 2 cm^2 s^{-1} in vacuum and 0.9 $cm^2\ s^{-1}$ in air. Porous media can be detected by measuring the apparent diffusion coefficient (ADC) of 3He, because the ADC of 3He is spatially correlated, which enables the diagnosis of lung tissue at the alveolar level. As an inert gas, the longitudinal relaxation time T_1 of 3He is theoretically very long, and the relaxation time can reach several days when stored in a uniform magnetic field.

How to polarize the gas?

About 60 years ago, it was discovered that the electron spin number distribution of a specific atom can be changed by circularly polarized light with a specific wavelength, then achieving electron spin polarization, this process is called laser pumping process [27]. In 1997, Walker and Happer [28] in Princeton polarized 3He nucleus by using polarized electrons and this process of spin state transfer is called spin-exchange process. This method of using a laser to eventually polarize the 3He nuclear is called the SEOP process. Subsequently, they formed a commercial company specializing in the production of SEOP polarizers, which was soon acquired by GE, and SEOP polarizers were never commercialized. It can also use metastable spin-exchange pump light [29] (metastable spin-exchange optical pumping, MEOP) method to polarize 3He.

How to use polarized gas for MRI?

Spin-polarized gas was used for MRI in the early 1990s. In 1994, Albert *et al.* obtained 129Xe images of rat lungs for the first time [30], whose signal intensity and spatial resolution were both higher than traditional 1H imaging. In 1996, MacFall *et al.* [31] and Kauczor *et al.* [32] obtained 3He images of human lungs. In 1997, Mugler *et al.* reported the 129Xe image of the human lung [33]. In December 2000, Europe began the PHIL plan [34] (Polarized Helium for Imaging the Lungs project), exploring the method of MRI using HP 3He, and applied in some of the lung pathology that was selected carefully. In terms of medical diagnosis, currently, more and more people begin to use polarized inert gas to explore lung diseases, including asthma, cystic fibrosis, emphysema (chronic obstructive pulmonary disease (COPD)), lung transplantation, and lung cancer [35–40], but most of these works are based on a high magnetic field. In 1998, in order to conduct surface flaw detection of mechanical components (nonmetallic) materials, low-field MRI of 3He-polarized gas has been studied [41]. Currently, researchers in this field include Harvard University, University of Virginia, Simon Fraser University in Canada, University Paris-VI in France.

9.2 Hyperpolarized gas production and polarimetry

9.2.1 Background

There are two optical pumping methods for polarizing 3He: SEOP and metastable exchange pumping (MEOP). MEOP uses a laser to polarize 3He gas directly, the pumping process is as follows: first, the electron in the 1^1S_0 state of the 3He atom is excited to the metastable state of 2^3S_1 by the weak ultraviolet light. Then, the electrons are excited from the metastable state 2^3S_1 to the metastable state 2^3P_0 by circularly polarized light with a wavelength of 1 083 nm. Finally, the electrons are de-excited from 2^3P_0 to the metastable state 2^3S_1. Due to the hyper fine structure, metastable 2^3S_1 splits into two sublevels $F=1/2$ and 3/2, so the electron is de-excited to these two sublevels with equal probability. Under the restriction of the circular polarization of the laser and the selection rule of electron transition, only electrons at metastable 2^3S_1 where the Zeeman energy level is ($F=1/2$, $m_F=-3/2$) or ($F=3/2$, $m_F=-1/2$) can absorb σ photons and be transited to the 2^3P_0 state. As time accumulates, eventually, the number of electros at metastable 2^3S_1 with $m_F=-3/2$ or $-1/2$ reduced, and the number of electros with $m_F=+3/2$ or $+1/2$ increased, then the electron has been spin-polarized. By the action of the fine structure, the electron transfers its spin polarization state to the 3He nucleus, and then the 3He nucleus has been polarized. The MEOP can quickly polarize 3He nuclear, and the extraction process of polarization gas is easier relatively. However, the main experimental research of MEOP was done by the Mainz laboratory in Germany [42,43]. They have conducted such research for 25 years [44], and currently, there is a stable process line for the production of 3He polarized gas. However, the MEOP method is not suitable for high-density 3He gas polarizing, such as the neutron physics experiment that needs about 10-atm pressure polarized cavity. In MEOP, the radio-frequency (RF) field excites the electrons to 2^3S_1 metastable directly; therefore, the air pressure of 3He in the polarization cavity can only be on the order of Torr.

Compared with MEOP method, in SEOP, the spin-exchange cross-section between the valence electron of alkali metal and the nucleus of 3He is smaller; however, the characteristics of a high density of alkali metal vapor and nearly complete polarization of valence electrons just make up for this deficiency; therefore, high density and high polarization 3He gas can be obtained by SEOP. By using pure rubidium, 3He-polarized gas with a polarization of about 50% can be obtained in dozens of hours. Above those, the SEOP is more popular. The following section will focus on SEOP.

HP gases may be generated via either SEOP, metastability exchange optical pumping (MEOP), "brute-force" polarization, dynamic nuclear polarization, and/or parahydrogen-induced polarization. Each of these approaches has advantages and limitations, and understanding how they work to produce and deliver a given HP gas is thus necessary for integration with a desired biomedical application. The following sections will focus on SEOP.

9.2.2 Hyperpolarized gas by SEOP

9.2.2.1 Theoretical background

The SEOP method polarizing 3He indirectly, which can be divided into two parts according to the time sequence: (1) the alkali metal atoms are pumped to polarize the extra-nuclear valence electrons by the laser; (2) by the collision, the polarized alkali metal atoms transfer spin-polarized state to 3He atom nuclear. The whole SEOP process can be attributed to the following four equations [45]:

$$P_A = \frac{R(z)}{R(z) + \Gamma_A} \tag{9.1}$$

$$\frac{R_z}{dz} = [A]\sigma_L \Gamma_A P_A \tag{9.2}$$

$$\Gamma_A = (k_{\mathrm{SE}} + k_{\mathrm{SR}})[3\mathrm{He}] + \Gamma_0 \tag{9.3}$$

$$\frac{dP_{\mathrm{He}}}{dt} = k_{\mathrm{SE}}[A](P_A - P_{\mathrm{He}}) - \Gamma_{\mathrm{He}} P_{\mathrm{He}} \tag{9.4}$$

These formulas, in turn, describe the hyperpolarization of alkali metals by the laser pumping, where P_A refers to saturation polarization of alkali metals, $R(z)$ and Γ_A are the optical pumping rate and depolarization rate of alkali metals, $[A]$ is alkali metal gas number density; the relationship between optical pumping rate and laser incidence depth, [3He] is 3He gas number density; the depolarization process of alkali metals, k_{SR} is relaxation coefficient, k_{SE} is the spin-exchange rate coefficient and Γ_0 is a constant; the polarizing process of 3He atom, where P_{He} is the 3He hyperpolarization.

9.2.2.2 Alkali polarization and relaxation

In the SEOP process, all alkali metals could polarize 3He atoms, the pure rubidium or rubidium potassium mixed medium usually be selected to polarize 3He atoms. The main reasons are as follows: first, theoretically, alkali metals with low atomic coefficient are more likely to have spin exchange with 3He; second, polarizing alkali metal valence electrons requires a specific wavelength of laser, at present, only the high-power laser with matched rubidium is relatively mature in the market. Therefore, pure rubidium or rubidium potassium mixed media are often chosen to polarize 3He in the SEOP process.

In nature, rubidium (Rb) includes 85Rb and 87Rb, with the abundance of 72.2% and 27.8%, respectively. For 85Rb, the nuclear spin **I**=5/2, and coupled with the total angular momentum **J** of valence electrons, the quantum state **F** of the hyper-fine structure in the ground state ($5^2S_{1/2}$), and the first excited state ($5^2P_{1/2}$) would be changed to **F**=**I**±**J**, which can be 2 or 3. When the magnetic field is applied, the hyper-fine level of 85Rb will split into $2F+1$ Zeeman sublevel; the energy level width is much larger than the splitting width, so the Zeeman sublevel cannot be resolved by atomic absorption spectrum. The energy level of 87Rb is consistent with that of 85Rb except that its nuclear spin is 3/2 (where F is 1 or 2). For 85Rb and 87Rb, ignoring nuclear spin [46], because the width of hyper precision energy level generated by nuclear spin coupling is 3.04 and 6.87 GHz, respectively, which is far smaller than the laser line-widths used in the SEOP.

With an external magnetic field, the ground state $S_{1/2}$ splits the Zeeman into two sublevels $m_s=\pm 1/2$. When the Rb atom reaches thermal equilibrium, the number of Rb atoms on the two sublevels will obey the Boltzmann distribution. The ratio of the number of Rb atoms in the two sublevels is $n_+/n_- = \exp\{2\mu_e B/(k_B T)\}$. At room temperature T~300 K and the magnetic field strength B~30 Gs, the ratio is about 1.00001, the number of Rb atoms in the two sublevels is roughly the same. In order to achieve the polarization of valence electrons in alkali metals [47], the ratio of the number of particles in the two sublevels should be changed. The angular momentum selection rule between states $S_{1/2}$ and $P_{1/2}$ of Rb atom is $\Delta l=1$; $\Delta m_s=+1$, so only Rb atoms with $m_s=-1/2$ in the $S_{1/2}$ state can absorb σ^+ photon then get excited to the $P_{1/2}$ state with $m_s=+1/2$. Due to the instability, Rb atoms in the P state will be deexcited to the ground state (S state) in a very short time: some atoms will be deexcited to the $m_s=+1/2$ level in the ground state with unpolarized photons σ^0, in a probability of 1/3; some atoms are deexcited to the $m_s=-1/2$ level in the ground state with releasing left-handed circular-polarized light σ^+, in a probability of 2/3. In practice, due to the interaction between excited Rb atoms and other particles, Rb atoms in the two substates of $m_s=+1/2$ and $m_s=-1/2$ in $P_{1/2}$ state are nearly identical, so the two deexcitation processes in $P_{1/2}$ state occur with equal probability, both are 1/2 [48]. In addition, only the Rb atoms with m_s in the S state$=-1/2$ can absorb σ^+ photons, so the number of Rb atoms with $m_s=+1/2$ in the S state will keep increasing, while the number of Rb atoms with $m_s=-1/2$ in the S state will decrease continuously. After repeated transporting for a long time, approximately all Rb atoms will be in the S state with $m_s=+1/2$. The excited state Rb atom is deexcited to the ground state by emitting unpolarized photons σ^0, the Rb atoms in the S state with $m_s=+1/2$ would absorb such photons and depolarize. This process will limit the final polarization of Rb, then the final polarization of 3He will be limited. To overcome this problem, N_2 gas (about 0.1 amagat) is filled into the polarized cavity generally. Thus, when Rb atoms in the excited state are deexcited, 95% of Rb atoms will collide with N_2, then they will transfer their excitation energy to N_2 [49]. Based on this, the probability that polarized Rb atoms absorbing such deexcited unpolarized photons will be greatly reduced [50], thus inhibiting the depolarization effect caused by the deexcited Rb atom radiation. In the optical pumping transport process, the spin-polarized process of alkali metal Rb is shown in Figure 9.2.

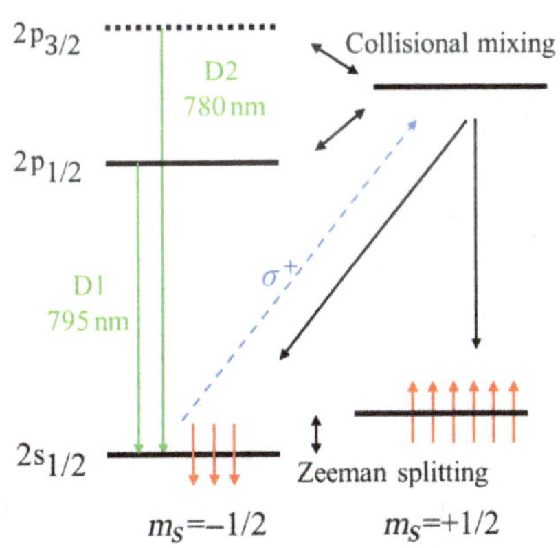

Figure 9.2 Electron levels in 85Rb atom, assuming I_{Rb}=0. The vertical axis is not drawn to scale

The optically pumped transport rate γ_{OPT} of alkali metal atom is defined as

$$\gamma_{opt} = \int \frac{I(v)}{hv} \sigma(v) dv \tag{9.5}$$

where $I(v)$ is the incident optical power density, the unit is W cm^{-2} Hz^{-1}; $\sigma(v)$ is photon absorption cross-section.

In a pure Rb-polarized cavity, the electron spin polarization relaxation (depolarization) of Rb atom mainly comes from absorption of unpolarized light; collision with impurity embedded in the inner wall of the polarization cavity; collisions with 3He, N_2, and other unpolarized Rb atoms. Ignoring the first two interactions (because the cross section is very small), the electron spin relaxation ratio of Rb atom Γ_{SD} is [51]

$$\Gamma_{SD} = \Gamma_{Rb-3He} + \Gamma_{Rb-Rb} + \Gamma_{Rb-N_2} \tag{9.6}$$

where $\Gamma_{Rb\text{-}3He}$, $\Gamma_{Rb\text{-}Rb}$, and $\Gamma_{Rb-N_2}\Gamma$ are the relaxation rate of Γ_{Rb-N_2} Rb atom with 3He, Rb, and N_2 respectively, and the unit is s^{-1}.

When the number density of each gas filled in the polarized cavity is [3He]=1 amg, [N_2]=0.1 amg (1 amg=2.6874×1 019 cm^{-3}, which represents the number density of gas at a standard atmospheric pressure and temperature T=273.5 K), then Γ_{SD}~488 s^{-1}.

For a spin-1/2 particle, which has two spin states (N_+ and N_-), the spin hyperpolarization is defined as the fractional difference between those two states:

$$P = \frac{N_+ - N_-}{N_+ + N_-} \tag{9.7}$$

So the spin hyperpolarization of Rb atom is

$$P(t) = \frac{\gamma_{opt}}{\gamma_{opt} + \Gamma_{SD}} \left(1 - e^{-(\gamma_{opt} + \Gamma_{SD})t}\right) \tag{9.8}$$

And

$$P(\infty) = \frac{\gamma_{opt}}{\gamma_{opt} + \Gamma_{SD}} \sim 99.9\% \tag{9.9}$$

Rb atoms can reach its maximum hyperpolarization within millisecond; therefore, when polarizing 3He, it can be considered that Rb atoms are fully polarized in the cavity.

9.2.2.3 Spin exchange

There are two ways to transfer spin-polarized state: (1) binary collision, as shown in Figure 9.3, particle A transfers its spin polarization state to particle B through collision with particle B; (2) van der Waals molecules are formed between the alkali metal atoms and the inert gas atoms in a short time, then the spin-polarized state would be transferred. In the polarizing of 3He by SEOP method, the spin

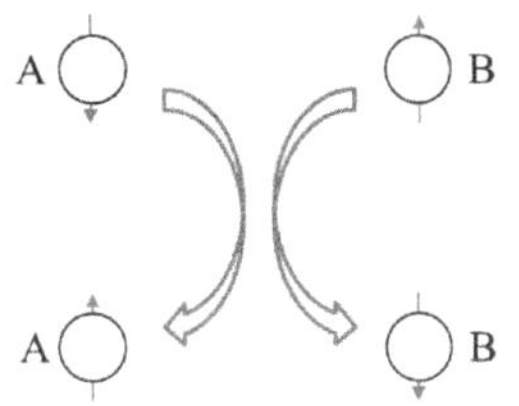

Figure 9.3 A atom and B atom exchange spins through a binary collision

exchange is mainly achieved through binary collisions, and the van der Waals molecular interaction could be ignored [52].

The spin-exchange efficiency between Rb and 3He (the ratio of the spin-exchange rate to the spin relaxation rate) is

$$\eta_{SE} = \frac{\gamma_{\mathrm{SE}}[\mathrm{3He}]}{[\mathrm{Rb}]\Gamma_{Rb}} \tag{9.10}$$

where γ_{SE} is spin-exchange rate, Γ_{Rb} is spin relaxation rate of Rb atom. The spin-exchange efficiency of Rb depends on the Rb number density and the spin-exchange rate coefficient. For Rb atom, the spin-exchange efficiency is only $\eta_{\mathrm{SE}}^{\mathrm{Rb-He}} = 0.02$ at T=453 K, which implies that 50 polarized Rb atoms are required to produce one polarized 3He nuclear.

9.2.2.4 Hybrid spin exchange

Traditionally, SEOP cells contained only Rb, which resulted in maximum 3He polarizations around 40%. However, it has been noted that other alkali metals might be more efficient spin-exchange partners and lead to a higher 3He polarization. In addition to the spin-exchange efficiency, the photon efficiency is useful for evaluating the efficiency of SEOP for polarizing a 3He nuclear. Despite having comparable spin-exchange rate coefficients, the spin-destruction rate of K is smaller than Rb. In general, the heavier alkali metals have higher spin-exchange and spin-destruction rates, but the spin-destruction rates increase more significantly. The spin-exchange efficiency $\eta_{\mathrm{se}}^{\mathrm{K-He}} = 0.1$ at T=508 K, which implies that just ten polarized K atoms are required to produce one polarized 3He nuclear.

The slower spin-relaxation rate and higher efficiency suggest that K would be a better spin-exchange partner for 3He than Rb; however, the close spacing of the D1 and D2 lines in the K spectrum prevent direct optical pumping of K given current diode laser technology. An alternative is to implement a hybrid spin-exchange method, where both Rb and K are present in the cell and Rb is optically pumped as described in the previous section. The Rb atoms will then exchange spins with K with very high efficiency (~99.8%) while both Rb and K will spin exchange with 3He. As the alkali density ratio increases, the efficiency approaches that of a K-only cell.

9.2.2.5 Hyperpolarization of 3He

The 3He polarization depends on the average alkali hyperpolarization, the spin-exchange rate between the 3He atom and the alkali, and the relaxation rate of 3He depolarized. Then, 3He hyperpolarization is

$$P(t) = P_A \frac{\gamma_{SE}}{\gamma_{SE} + \Gamma_{He}} \left(1 - e^{-(\gamma_{SE} + \Gamma_{He})t}\right) \tag{9.11}$$

where γ_{SE} is the total spin-exchange rate between 3He and the alkali, Γ_{He} is the 3He relaxation rate. The maximum 3He hyperpolarization is

$$P(\infty) = P_A \frac{\gamma_{SE}}{\gamma_{SE} + \Gamma_{He}} \tag{9.12}$$

which will approach the average alkali polarization if Γ_{He} is minimized.

The relaxation rate, Γ_{He}, includes all sources of relaxation not related to spin exchange. It can be measured by monitoring the polarization decay in the absence of optical pumping and spin exchange with the lasers off and the alkali at room temperature. The generally acknowledged sources of this relaxation in 3He target cells are the 3He–3He magnetic dipole–dipole interaction, inhomogeneities in the magnetic field, and collisions with the walls of the cell. Consequently, the relaxation rate can be written as

$$\Gamma_{He} = \Gamma_{dip} + \Gamma_B + \Gamma_{wall} \tag{9.13}$$

9.2.3 SEOP instrumentation

The polarized process consists of two main steps. First, the cells will be filled with a noble gas, nitrogen, and an alkali–metal, then the cells are polarized in the optical pumping system.

9.2.3.1 Pumping system

For different applications, the polarized cavity has different structural designs. In the electron depth non-scattering experiment, the polarization cavity is mostly designed as a double-cavity structure. In medical imaging applications, the polarization chamber is usually designed as a single chamber and connected with a valve to remove the polarized 3He gas.

The setup for polarizing 3He in our lab is schematically presented in Figure 9.4. The process requires heating the alkali so that the desired vapor number density and number density ratios are reached. The cell is oriented in a forced-air oven so that the pumping chamber could be heated. The alkali atoms are continual optical pumping while the 3He atoms in the pumping chamber become polarized through spin exchange with the polarized alkali.

A window in the front of the oven allows laser light to enter, while a window in the back allows the laser spectrum to be monitored by a fiber-coupled high-resolution spectrometer. The oven is between one set of Helmholtz coils. The coils provide a uniform holding field along the direction of laser propagation direction.

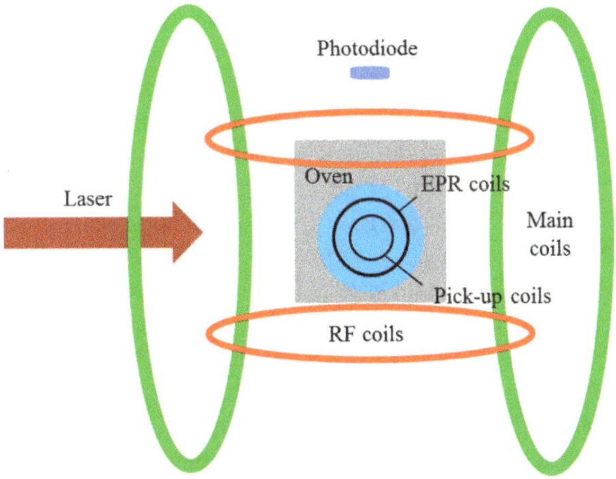

Figure 9.4 The cell, shown in blue, is centered between the Helmholtz coils while the pumping chamber is heated inside the oven. The main coils provide a uniform holding field, the RF coils create an oscillating field for NMR measurements, the pickup coils on the side of the oven and along the target chamber are used for detection during NMR and the EPR coil provides the RF excitation

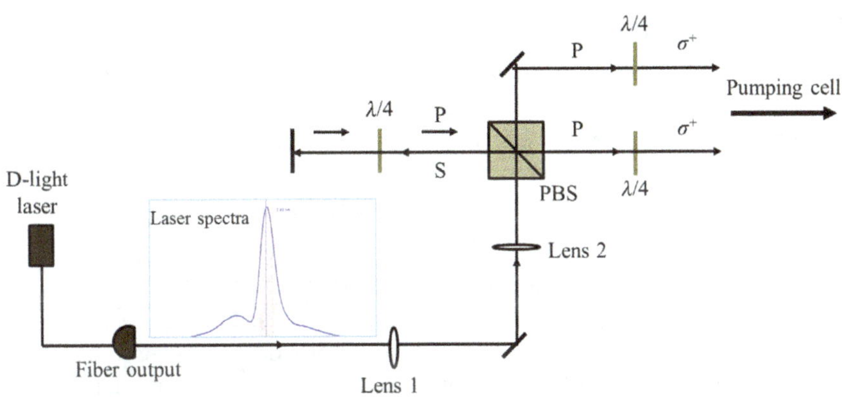

Figure 9.5 Schematic of the optics which is used to produce circularly polarized σ^+ light

The voltage supplied to the coils is controlled by a function generator connected to the main power supply and the current in the coils is monitored by an ammeter. The field is maintained at approximately 28 G during optical pumping in our lab.

9.2.3.2 The polarization optics

Figure 9.5 shows the optics used to produce circularly polarized laser light for optical pumping of Rb. The laser system consists of one diode lasers with a wavelength of approximately 795 nm corresponding to the Rb D1 transition. The maximum output power of laser is approximately 30 W and can be adjusted by changing the diode current. The width of the narrowed laser is a closer match to the absorption cross-section of the Rb D1 transition under typical conditions, which increases the pumping rate and results in higher polarization.

In the optical path, the linearly polarized light from the laser will be converted into a uniform circularly polarized laser (right-handed circularly polarized light or left-handed circularly polarized light), then pumping the polarization cavity. Changing the distance between the pair of lenses allows the diameter of the beam to be adjusted to match the diameter of the pumping chamber for optimal optical pumping. The beam splitter resolves the laser light into horizontal (P) and vertical (S) polarizations. The portion of the beam reflected by the beam splitter is S-polarized. It passes through a $\lambda/4$ plate then retro-reflects through the wave-plate again so that the S-polarization is converted to P-polarization. Then this beam now passes through the beam splitter cube, and along with the portion of the beam that originally passed through the cube, is directed through another $\lambda/4$ plate so that both beams are right-circularly polarized. The two beams are approximately parallel to each other and to the holding field.

9.2.3.3 Polarimetry system

There are two independent methods to measure the polarization of the 3He gas: the nuclear magnetic resonance (NMR) method and electron paramagnetic resonance (EPR) method. The NMR method is based on the inductive voltage generated in the surrounding coils of the 3He nucleus during the spin-flip process, and the signal amplitude proportional to the polarization of 3He gas. EPR is based on the Zeeman splitting of alkali metal by the effect of a weak magnetic field, which comes from polarized 3He gas. Both measurement processes are based on the adiabatic fastness process (AFP) [53].

NMR polarimetry

The main function of the AFP method is to adjust the spin direction of 3He nucleus to make it parallel or antiparallel to the direction of the holding magnetic field. In the magnetic field, the spin direction of 3He nuclear does not keep exactly consistent with the direction of holding magnetic field, instead, occurs Larmor precession around the main magnetic field at a certain deflection angle in the laboratory system (x, y, z), selecting the direction of the holding magnetic field as the z-axis direction. When RF field perpendicular to the z-axis is applied along the y-axis direction, the spin-flip of the 3He nucleus will occur in the *yoz* plane. At this point, an induced voltage proportional to the hyperpolarization of 3He will be generated in the picking coil whose surface is perpendicular to the x-axis, and the spin-flip of 3He atoms will change the magnetic flux in the pickup coil. Then a phase-locked amplifier is used to read the voltage signal in the coil to obtain the 3He hyperpolarization and is

$$S_x = \mu\rho PAf \tag{9.14}$$

where ρ is 3He gas density, μ is nuclear magnetic moment, P is the hyperpolarization of 3He, A is a constant (depends on the coil geometry) and f is the frequency of RF field.

In the process of AFP, the change rate of the effective magnetic field (generated by the RF field coupling with the holding magnetic field) should be as low as possible to ensure the spin following of 3He and needs to be much faster than the depolarization rate of 3He.

In addition to the precession around the effective magnetic field, the magnetization is subjected to the relaxation processes. There are two main types of relaxation: the T_1 relaxation is the relaxation of the longitudinal magnetization component back to thermal equilibrium levels, along the z-axis; the T_2 relaxation describes the decay of the transverse magnetization component to zero.

Figure 9.6 shows the schematics of the NMR electronics. A static magnetic field that is produced by a set of Helmholtz coils defines the z-axis. The other two sets of axes are defined by the RF coils and the NMR receiver coils.

The AFP signal from both receiver coils was added up and amplified in a preamplifier. As the receiver coils were not perfectly perpendicular to the RF coils, they picked up not only the AFP signal but also some residual driving RF field, which was produced by amplifying the output of a function generator. However, the RF pickup signal was nearly 180° phase-shifted in the two NMR coils. By adding the signals from the two coils, the RF pickup should have been canceled completely. In reality, the cancelation was not perfect, and there was still a small residual RF signal in the output of the preamplifier. A lock-in amplifier, an

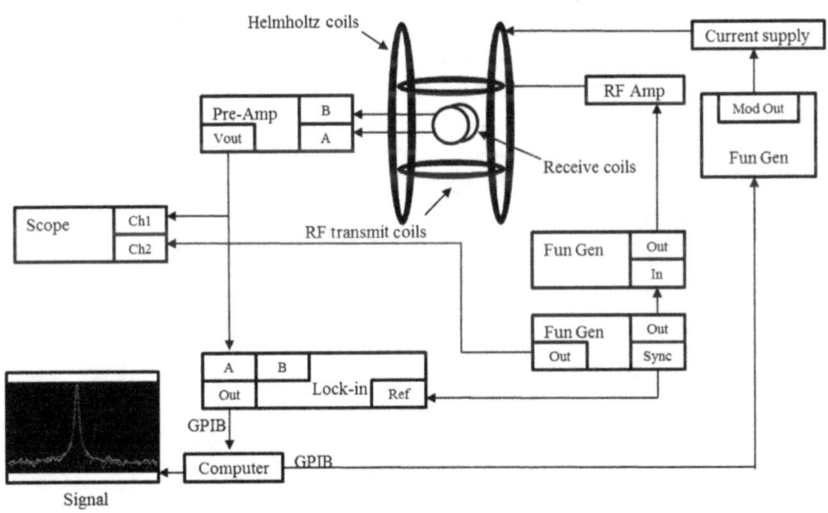

Figure 9.6 Electronic circuitry for NMR detection. The voltages induced in the pickup coils and read by the lock-in amplifier as the 3He spins are flipped

oscilloscope and a function generator with an adjustable amplitude and phase and with frequency locked to the RF were used to cancel the residual RF pickup field.

A LabView program and a function generator controlled the field sweep, which resulted in two spin flips and, therefore, two AFP signals. The resulting signal, Lorentz peak–shaped signal spectrum, was recorded by the computer and displayed in LabView.

Hyperpolarized gas EPR polarimetry

Polarized 3He atoms have a spin magnetic moment, so a weak magnetic field is generated around them. The magnetic field causes the Zeeman level splitting of the alkali metal, resulting in a shift in EPR frequency. The frequency shift of EPR is proportional to the polarization of 3He.

Due to the effect of hyperfine structure in ^{85}Rb atom, the ground state S is divided into two energy levels: **F**=3 and **F**=2. Under the action of a weak magnetic field generated by polarized 3He, energy level **F**=3 is divided into seven sub-energy levels, which are m_F=−3,...,3; and **F**=2 is divided into five sub-energy levels, which are m_F=−2,... and 2. The resonance frequency of EPR is the resonance frequency between m_F=3↔2 or m_F=−3↔−2 on the level **F**=3. The frequency is mainly determined by the main magnetic field and the 3He polarized magnetic field. In order to extract the effect of the polarization field of 3He, the effect of the main magnetic field was eliminated by the spin-flip of 3He. The 85Rb is eventually transported to m_F=−3 or m_F=3 on the ground state **F**=3 by the laser pumping. Using the EPR coil to induce a resonance transition between m_F=−3↔ −2 or m_F=3↔2 state, the electron is excited to the state m_F=−2 or m_F=2. The electrons on the ground state **F**=3 with m_F=−2 or m_F=2 will be polarized to the P state by absorbing laser, and about 3%–5% of the electrons in the P state will be de-excited to the m_F=−3 or m_F=3 in the ground state **F**=3 by emitting D1 and D2 light, the rest of the electrons will be de-excited to the ground state through the quenching process with N_2. The photodiode is used to detect the light intensity of D2, and when the light intensity reaches the peak, it indicates that the EPR process has occurred. The frequency of D1 light is the same as pumping laser, so a D1 filter should be added at the front of the photodiode used for filtering D1 light. By monitoring the intensity of D2 transitions as a function of RF, it would be able to detect the EPR.

The relationship between EPR frequency shift and hyperpolarization of 3He [55] is

$$\Delta v = v_1 - v_2 = \frac{d_v(F, m_F)}{d_B}\frac{8\pi}{3}\kappa_0[3\mathrm{He}]P_{\mathrm{He}} \tag{9.15}$$

where κ_0 is a frequency shift enhancement factor, which is related to temperature, [3He] is 3He gas number density, P_{He} is a polarization of 3He and $d_v(F,m_F)/d_B$ is the differential of EPR frequency shift to a magnetic field, please refer to the literature [54,56].

However, instead of monitoring the intensity of D2 fluorescence, we monitored the *changes* in the D2 fluorescence while frequency modulating the EPR excitation signal. The EPR electronics setup is schematically presented in Figure 9.7. The frequency-modulated D2 signal was detected by a lock-in amplifier

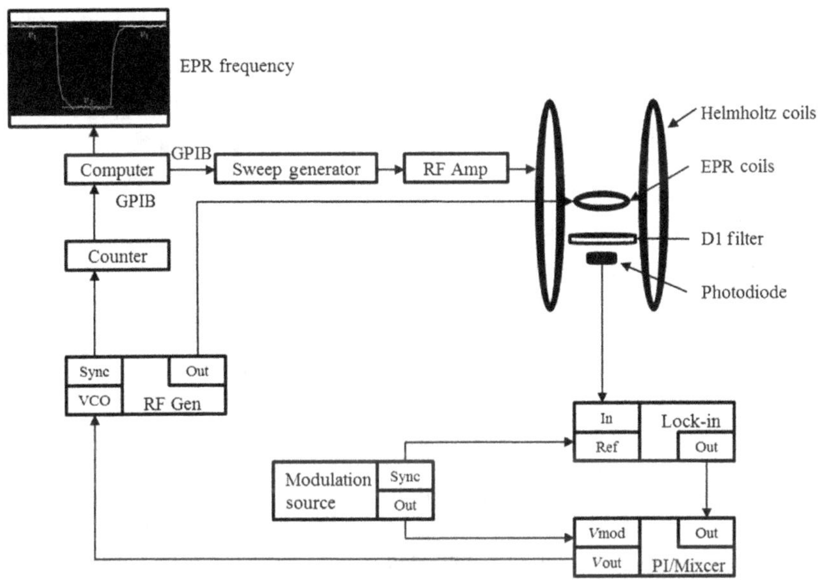

Figure 9.7 Electronic circuitry for EPR detection and the lock-in signal of resonance frequencies (v_1 and v_2)

that was referenced to the modulation source. The lock-in amplifier's output was a DC signal that was proportional to the RMS (root-mean square) voltage of the modulated D2 fluorescence.

The derivative of the D2 resonance served as a feedback signal to trace shifts in the central frequency of the EPR curve. When the frequency of excitation matches the EPR resonance, the derivative and thus the feedback signal are zero. When the frequency is less than the resonant frequency, the derivative is a positive signal. If this positive signal is converted into a positive frequency shift, the RF could be shifted back to the resonance. The output of the mixer that adds the modulation signal, and the feedback was sent to a voltage-controlled oscillator (VCO) input of an RF function generator. The VCO converted the amplitude of the input signal into a frequency offset. A counter was used to read off the frequency from the RF function generator, while the value would be recorded by a LabView program.

9.2.4 Storage, transfer of hyperpolarized gas

Besides ensuring its biological compatibility and safe administration, the most important considerations for using HP gas involve experimental design to maximize nuclear spin polarization and agent throughput, achieve efficient HP agent delivery, and maintain polarization levels as much as possible throughout the study.

First, any contributors to hyperpolarization destruction need to be addressed within and "downstream" of the polarization chamber. Although the lifetime of a given gas's polarization is physically capped by its intrinsic T_1 relaxation rate, this source of spin destruction is often small compared to extrinsic sources of polarization loss while transporting and delivering HP gas for imaging. Indeed, gas polarizations can be unintentionally destroyed via a number of ways in an experimental setup, including paramagnetic relaxation, diffusion through magnetic field gradients, and movement of the gas through magnetic "zero-field" crossings. Paramagnetic relaxation can be mitigated first by ensuring that all polarizer materials that can come in contact with the HP gas have minimal magnetic impurities, and that gas lines are well evacuated and/or purged with ultrapure gases to minimize O_2 exposure. When it comes to HP gas MRI on aerobic organisms, oxygen exposure will be unavoidable, but the addition of O_2 to create breathable admixtures with HP gas should be performed only at the last possible step prior to agent administration. For the 3He atoms, it is important to choose glass with minimal paramagnetic impurities (e.g., GE180) [57].

Permanent magnets or smaller auxiliary fields are sometimes used to accumulate or transport gases to avoid field relaxation. Particularly for 3He, minimizing field gradients using homogeneous fields [58] can be important for minimizing polarization losses. During the transfer of a prepared HP gas sample to a subject, special attention needs to be placed toward keeping the applied magnetic field as uniform as possible and avoiding areas of zero-field crossings. For 3He cells, degaussing may need to be performed [59] on occasion to remove weak permanent fields that have developed owing to impurities embedded in the glass. Automation of gas hyperpolarizers is highly desirable for maximizing throughput, maintaining reproducibility, and minimizing errors during HP gas preparation and delivery, but fields produced by some solenoid valve designs can be problematic [60]. Transit through a given gas's phase diagram can also be a source of relaxation. For example, the T_1 of solid 129Xe at liquid-N_2 temperature (77 K) can be several hours [61,62], but only if is kept from warming too close to the Xe melting point (where the T_1 can drop to seconds). Polarized solid xenon needs to be maintained in a strong field (0.500 Gs) in order to suppress (1) dipolar relaxation from lattice vacancy hopping [63] and (2) thermal mixing with fast relaxing 131Xe present in the lattice. Freezing or dissolving quadrupolar gases result in immediate loss of hyperpolarization because of subsecond T_1s in condensed phases unless at cryogenic temperatures. Thus, in addition to the fact that hyperpolarization processes themselves need to be monitored for a consistent production of HP substances, the seemingly endless ways to destroy hard-won polarization necessitates that polarizers are designed to include in situ polarimetry for quality assurance of the HP agent.

Importantly, HP gases are relatively easy to physically separate from auxiliary substances found in polarizers that may be toxic or otherwise undesirable if administered in a significant dosage to a patient. Additionally, HP gases are relatively easy to administer to a living subject via inhalation.

9.2.5 T_1 *Decay*

Having polarized a sample, the next challenge is storing it and delivering it to the NMR system. The T_1 of the sample depends strongly upon the physical environment. For example, pure 3He gas has minimal spin–lattice interactions and in the limit has T_1 that represents the dipole–dipole interaction and is extremely long (>700 h at 1-atm pressure). This opens up the possibility of transporting the polarized gas large distances from polarization source to NMR site. Brownian diffusion of HP gases in the presence of macroscopic B_0 field gradients will reduce the T_1 [64], as will microscopic field perturbations experience during collisional contact of the gas with magnetic impurities in the walls of the storage cells. Furthermore, mixing with a paramagnetic gas such as oxygen will radically reduce the T_1 (T_1 of 3He in air ~20 s) [65].

9.2.6 *In vivo administration of 3He*

Having polarized the 3He, it is typically mixed with a larger volume of nitrogen and delivered to the subject for inhalation either by manual means from a sealed plastic bag or by an automated respirator device. The volume of 3He used directly affects the signal-to-noise ratio (SNR) of the acquired images, with gas polarized to 30%, 300 mL of 3He typically provides sufficient SNR for a complete imaging sequence at 1.5 T.

Another very important factor that should be considered is patient safety during breath-hold imaging exams. All subjects have been imaged with full vital signs monitoring. The blood oxygen saturation levels tend to take a dip toward the end of a long breath-hold (20 s) whilst this can be preempted by prewashing the lungs with a high concentration of oxygen in patients without signs of emphysema. This measure can however degrade the SNR in the images by virtue of the T_1 shortening effect of oxygen [66]. In studies that compared the patient's vital signs when gas was delivered as an anoxic 1-L dose from a bag or as a bolus via the respirator device chased with room air, it was observed that the latter mode of delivery prevented the blood O_2 saturation from falling [67].

9.2.7 *MRI hardware considerations for HP 3He*

9.2.7.1 B_0 field strength

The common commercial MRI is based on hydrogen proton (1H) imaging in the organism, so soft tissue has good image resolution. When the organism is exposed in a uniform magnetic field, the hydrogen proton in the organism will split into two sub-energy levels due to the Zeeman effect, and the energy level difference between them is

$$\Delta E = E_{\downarrow} - E_{\uparrow} = |\gamma|\hbar B \tag{9.16}$$

The hyperpolarization is used to denote the difference in the number of particles between two sublevels, which is defined as

$$P = \frac{n_{\uparrow} - n_{\downarrow}}{n_{\uparrow} + n_{\downarrow}} = \tanh\frac{|\gamma|\hbar B}{2k_B T} \approx \frac{|\gamma|\hbar B}{2k_B T} \tag{9.17}$$

According to (9.17), increasing the magnetic field intensity or decreasing the temperature will polarize the particles, which is called thermal polarization. γ is the rotational magnetic ratio, for 1H, γ=2.67×108 rad s^{-1} T^{-1}; ħ is the reduced Planck constant, which is 1.05457266×10^{-34} J s; k_B is the Boltzmann constant, and k_B=1.3806488×10^{-23} J K^{-1}; B is the magnetic field strength with unit tesla (T); T is the temperature in Kelvin. If B=3 T and T=298.15 K, then the hyperpolarization of 1H is about 0.001% with thermal polarization. Fortunately, the human body is a water-rich structure, so it can provide a strong enough magnetic resonance signal. 3He is gaseous, if thermal polarization is also chosen, a strong enough signal cannot be provided for MRI.

The magnetic field of clinical MRI equipment has reached 3.0 T, and some research institutions have started to use 7.0-T MRI equipment. In order to improve image resolution in MRI, the methods commonly used are (1) to improve the sensitivity of the receiving coil; (2) magnetic shielding is used to further reduce noise and improve SNR; (3) introducing contrast agent containing gadolinium; (4) improve the magnetic field strength of MRI equipment, because the polarization of 1H is proportional to the magnetic field strength, the stronger the magnetic field strength, the higher the polarization of 1H, then the stronger the magnetic resonance signal. Therefore, MR images in high magnetic fields have higher spatial resolution than those in low magnetic fields. It is undoubtedly the most direct way to improve the image spatial resolution by enhancing the magnetic field intensity. However, due to the limitations of technology and physiological safety, the magnetic field intensity should not be enhanced blindly.

At present, when using commercial MRI equipment to carry out pulmonary MRI of polarized gas, there is an error in the correspondence between disease and image. As the permeability of the lung is very uneven, when the external magnetic field is strengthened, the local induced gradient field will be generated, and the intensity of the gradient field is directly proportional to the intensity of the external magnetic field. The inductive gradient field will destroy the imaging information of the lung and form image artifacts. In traditional MRI, the polarization of 1H is enhanced by a strength magnetic field, then the NMR signal that can be used for imaging is obtained. The strength of the signal is proportional to the strength of the magnetic field. However, for 3He gas, it is polarized by the SEOP method, and the polarization of 3He is independent of the magnetic field. When MRI is performed with 3He-polarized gas, as long as the polarized gas is introduced into the examined site, there is no need for thermal polarization as in 1H. Therefore, an MRI of polarized gas can be performed at a low magnetic field.

9.2.7.2 Radio-frequency hardware

Although non-proton imaging is possible on commercial MRI spectrometers, at the time of writing none of the major vendors offer an integrated complete hardware solution for 3He MRI. Thus, the interested party will either have to build their own transmit–receive switches and transmit–receive coils or purchase from a third party vendor. The resonant frequencies of 1H and 3He are different. Under the 1.5-T magnetic field, the resonant frequencies of 1H, 3He, and 129Xe are

$$f_{1H} = 63.87 \text{ MHz} \tag{9.18}$$

$$f_{3He} = 48.65\,\text{MHz} \tag{9.19}$$

$$f_{129Xe} = 17.67\,\text{MHz} \tag{9.20}$$

Transceiver coils for HP gas MRI need to be large enough to cover the field of view (FOV) of the adult lungs and airways (approximately 30×30×18 cm^3) without subject discomfort. Furthermore, the coils must be able to function safely and efficiently. Transceiver coils can be designed as birdcage coils with a uniform internal magnetic field, or phased array coils used for parallel imaging with a high imaging rate. When transmitting RF pulse signal, its power must be controlled. The energy generated by RF pulse in the RF coil is composed of two kinds of energy: coil stored and consumed. The consumed energy will be radiated in the space around the coil in the form of heat energy, and this part of the energy will act on the human body to raise the temperature and generate RF power precipitation (SAR). Most whole-body systems are fitted with integrated proton body transmitting coils and therefore resonant coupling between this volume resonator and the HP volume coil needs to be considered in the design process. Other design constraints include portability and minimization of scanner downtime due to hardware changes between 1H and HP nuclear imaging exams. From an application perspective, HP gas MRI is very sensitive to flip angle by virtue of the nonrenewable polarization; thus, the transmit coil must provide a uniform excitation angle across the whole of the lungs for a range of flip angles. A large volume resonator such as an insert birdcage provides a solution to many of these requirements [68].

A close-fitting transmit coil will invariably have a poorer B1 spatial homogeneity and may also pose problems with SAR and burning at the skin. A solution may be to use a volume coil with a dedicated 3He receiver array for increased sensitivity and also opens up the opportunity for parallel receiver imaging with 3He [69].

9.2.7.3 3He imaging pulse sequence considerations

The main problem of using polarized 3He to carry out lung imaging is how to obtain the high SNR MR images in a short time with limited hyperpolarization. During imaging, if the inhaled 3He gas is mixed with O_2, the longitudinal relaxation time T_1 of 3He will decrease rapidly [70], and the breath-holding time of the patient should be considered, which is generally 15 s [71]. Therefore, the pulse sequence used for polarized gas imaging must be designed to be short enough in time. In pulse designing, it should be taken into account the fact that the lung is a magnetic heterogeneous medium. There is about a 9-ppm magnetic coefficient difference between the solid tissue and the air in lung. During MRI, the magnetic coefficient difference will generate image artifacts and then lead to misjudgment [72].

Performing lung MRI with polarized 3He, the NMR signal is derived from the transverse relaxation of polarized 3He. Turning off the RF pulse, the transverse magnetization of polarized 3He decreases, and T_2 is the main parameter to evaluate the transverse relaxation. The transverse relaxation is caused by the uncorrelation of spin at different Larmor frequencies, while the inconsistency of Larmor frequencies is caused by local magnetic field differences. The causes of local magnetic field changes are as follows: (1) nonuniform external magnetic field; (2) in a magnetic field, the spin of a particle produces a magnetic moment, which affects the spin of its neighbors, known as spin–spin interaction. According to the distribution of particle spin density, the local magnetic field induced by particle spin is different at different locations; (3) spin particles will diffuse under the action of gradient field, and the local magnetic field generated by spin is a variable with time.

During lung MRI, the gas diffusion also makes inert gas imaging more difficult. The diffusion motion caused by the gradient field will destroy the MR signal and limit the highest resolution of the MR image.

9.2.7.4 Polarization usage

For a spoiled gradient echo (SPGR) sequence built up with a series of $n=1$ to N, RF views of constant flip angle α, the transverse magnetization during a breath-hold HP gas acquisition decays as

$$M_{xy}(n) = M_0 \sin\alpha(\cos\alpha)^{n-1}\exp\left[\frac{-t}{T1(\mathrm{pO_2})}\right] \tag{9.21}$$

where T_1 depends on the regional oxygen partial pressure, pO_2, which itself changes during the breath-hold [73]. This polarization depletion from view to view using a spoiled gradient echo (SPGR) sequence imposes a k-space filter on the data in the RF-encoding dimension [74] that can cause blurring or signal attenuation. As such the choice of RF-encoding trajectory is closely related to the flip angle used. For a Cartesian (spin-warp) SPGR sequence with a fixed flip angle, acentric encoding order will provide a higher SNR at the expense of blurring in the image, while as sequential ordering will result in a lower SNR in the images whilst preserving the fine structure. A partial Fourier acquisition that exploits the phase conjugate symmetry in the higher spatial frequencies represents a compromise that relies on less RF pulses. As the number of RF views is reduced either by partial Fourier methods [75], parallel imaging with receive coil arrays [76], or radial under-sampling [77], the flip angle can be increased in order to use up the polarization with less pulses. This provides the interesting possibility with HP gas MRI of SNR that is independent of the number of RF-encoding steps (N), a paradox with the familiar SNR∞N relation that holds for conventional thermally polarized MRIA variable flip angle (VFA) approach can also be used in SPGR imaging with HP gases [78]; here the flip angle is increased from view to view to maintain a constant transverse magnetization thus minimizing the k-space filtering effect. The flip angle for the nth RF view is given by

$$a(n) = \tan^{-1}\left[\frac{1}{\sqrt{(N-n)}}\right] \tag{9.22}$$

The VFA approach is potentially the optimum strategy for SPGR imaging of 3He; however, the idealized constant magnetization profile can diverge if there is slight miscalibration in the RF transmit amplitude. Similarly, in 2D SPGR imaging the distribution of flip angles across the 2D slice profile [79] can cause similar problems of divergence [80]. An alternative to spoiling the precious transverse magnetization from view to view is to recycle it using steady-state [81], EPI [82], or CPMG [83] based refocusing strategies. All these approaches allow a potentially increased SNR by using a higher excitation flip angle and subsequently refocusing residual transverse magnetization with the finite longitudinal magnetization. However, any sequence that employs refocusing is constrained by the effect of diffusion attenuation of the transverse magnetization that is considerable for 3He in the lungs. The diffusion-related signal loss is quantified by the signal attenuation at the center of the readout echo by the expression $\exp(-b(t)D)$, where

$$b(\tau) = \int_0^\tau |k(t)|^2 dt \tag{9.23}$$

b being the time-dependent b-value derived from the gradient integral with time, where

$$k(t) = \gamma \int_0^t G\left(t'\right) dt' \tag{9.24}$$

and G is the time-varying imaging gradient waveform.

This is most beneficial when imaging with small FOVs [84] or where diffusion is considerable such as in the upper airways [85]. The same constraint of diffusion dephasing imposed by the imaging gradients applies to EPI sequences where the echo train length and spatial resolution are limited. Nevertheless, single-shot EPI provides an attractive means of rapidly tracking gas flow dynamics and has been used to estimate global lung ventilation volume with time during exhalation. Diffusion dephasing also limits the minimum slice thickness in 2D imaging; when striving for a high resolution images, a 3D sequence is less prone to this source of attenuation in the slice direction and gives a higher SNR for a given spatial resolution. A secondary effect in 2D imaging is the mixing of gas polarization by diffusion between the slice being excited and the adjacent volume of gas; this is mitigated by keeping the sequence repetition time (TR) to a minimum and imaging slices in an interleaved fashion. This slice mixing effect is quantified by the following expression that describes the dissipation of the slice profile $f(z)$ with time due to diffusion with a Gaussian distribution:

$$f(z,t) = \frac{1}{2\sqrt{\pi D t}} \int_{-\infty}^{+\infty} f_0\left(z'\right) \exp - \frac{\left(z - z'\right)^2}{4\pi D t} dz' \tag{9.25}$$

As well as mitigating the effect of diffusion dephasing, non-Cartesian sequences such as spiral and radial offer the use of less RF pulses to sample k-space by angular under-sampling in either 2D or 3D.

9.3 Hyperpolarized 3He gas MR imaging

The following section will focus on how 3He images can be used to probe lung function, including how to sensitize the MR pulse sequences to different aspects of lung physiology and microstructure, and how to quantify the results with image processing.

9.3.1 Ventilation imaging

The obvious use for HP 3He imaging is to visualize ventilation distribution and homogeneity. For this purpose high-resolution images at breath-hold are needed and most groups still favor the robust 2D multi-slice SPGR sequence with Cartesian encoding [86]. Ventilation homogeneity can be expressed qualitatively with radiological scoring procedures. The degree of ventilation heterogeneity can potentially be further quantified by texture analysis [87] and lacunarity scoring that have been used in HRCT. A more quantitative approach is the evaluation of regional ventilation volumes [88]. For the latter approach the dark space from 1H lung MRI adds additional information on the potentially viable ventilated volume and can be used in tandem with the 3He MRI ventilation images to calculate an index of percentage-ventilated volume.

One aspect worth considering, especially in studies designed to assess the effects of respiratory medication, is the baseline repeatability of the ventilation imaging that depends on the respiratory maneuverer and redistribution of ventilation defects that have been shown to change with time and posture in healthy normal people [89].

Lung ventilation volume from 3He MRI has been shown to correlate both with spirometry in normal and in patients with the disease and with lung volumes from plethysmography in people. Since the images supply spatially resolved data, it is a shame to sacrifice the regional ventilation sensitivity by summing up all ventilated pixels into a global index of lung-ventilated volume.

9.3.2 Dynamic imaging

HP gas MRI is not constrained by the saturation recovery of the signal, so we can image with very short TR at a high SNR. This opens up the possibility of imaging gas flow dynamics, wash in and washout, and time-resolved processes such as air trapping. To date, humans work has largely focused on using very rapid time-resolved 2D sequences such as partial Fourier Cartesian SPGR [90], spiral [91], and radial sequences. The non-Cartesian methods oversample the center of *k*-space and can be readily adapted to sliding window reconstruction; thus, it seems to be particularly effective for 2D dynamic imaging. These sequences provide a 2D planar view of the lungs with very fast temporal resolution and have been used to elucidate rates of gas flow in the major airways and periphery. The time series of images obtained can be used to fit parametric maps of the signal kinetics such as the rise time, integrated total signal, and gas flow rate on a pixel-by-pixel basis. By modulating the flip angle used with respect to the rate of inhalation, the images can be weighted according to a gas flow rate in order to delineate the major airways where the gas flux is highest.

Dynamic imaging sequences can potentially be run directly after a volumetric breath-hold exam in order to investigate the gas clearance rate [92]. With the advent of faster volumetric imaging sequences that use state-of-the-art under-sampling and parallel imaging techniques, the possibility also exists for high temporal resolution 3D imaging of ventilation [93].

An alternative approach to image the rapid influx of signal is to monitor the slower wash-in of signal in a fashion, which is similar to that used in nuclear medicine ventilation studies. In this approach, the regional fractional ventilation of gas exchanged per breath is derived as an index of regional gas ventilation. A final dynamic imaging approach is to exploit the phase-contrast sensitivity to steady flow provided by MRI. Work in this field has used the methodology developed for phase contrast MR angiography, the preliminary results look useful for the mapping of flow profiles and turbulence in the upper airways [94].

9.3.3 Measurement of regional oxygen uptake with T_1

The T_1 decay of HP 3He is strongly affected by the effect of mixing with oxygen in the air. When paramagnetic oxygen mixes with polarized 3He in the lungs, a marked reduction in the 3He T_1 arises through the electron-nuclear spin dipolar coupling. Saam *et al.* quantified the dependence of the 3He T_1 on oxygen concentration [65]; the longitudinal relaxation rate ($1/T_1$) is given by $\Gamma O_2(t)=pO_2(t)/\xi$, where the coefficient ξ was determined empirically as 2.61 bar $\times$ s at 310 K temperature. This pO_2 dependence of the 3He T_1 was subsequently used for in vivo quantification of pO_2 in a series of breath-hold experiments on pigs and humans [66]. In breath-hold studies of HP 3He, the image signal intensity, A_n, in a time series of n images acquired with N RF views per image, can be derived as

$$A_n = A_0(\cos\alpha)^{nN}\exp\left\{-\frac{1}{\xi}\int_0^{t_n} pO_2(t)dt\right\} \tag{9.26}$$

Thus, by acquiring time series of images with different inter-image delay times, the RF depletion and T_1 (pO_2) effects can be separated to give an estimate of the regional $pO_2(t)$. The method relies on the assumption that oxygen uptake in the human lung can be approximated by a linear rate constant, $pO_2(t)=p_0-Rt$, which could represent a short timescale approximation to the exponential behavior recently reported in rat lungs with 3He T_1 measurements [95]. Practically, these in vivo experiments used images that can be acquired from whole lung projections (very thick 2D slices) with two sets of weightings—either different flip angles or different inter-image delays. The dual-scan approach is 3He intensive and prone to registration and breath-hold irreproducibility, as such single breath-hold versions of the method have recently been proposed. For accurate fitting of the decay curve, an SNR needs to be high so spatial resolution in the images is less paramount. Furthermore, the effect of inter-slice diffusion of gas during the significant inter-image delay time (typically up to 7 s) can introduce erroneous decay rates that can be circumvented by using a 3D-imaging sequence.

Whilst perhaps the most powerful tool with which to measure regional lung function, the pO_2 method still remains the least evaluated in a clinical setting and a robust solution that gives accurate data in a reasonable breath-hold duration remains to be fully evaluated.

9.3.4 Diffusion measurement

One of the most powerful and proven aspects of HP 3He MRI is its sensitivity to gas diffusion (random Brownian motion of the atoms). In air at STP, the diffusion coefficient (D) for helium-3 is on the order 0.88 $cm^2\ s^{-1}$ [96], and it can travel RMS distances of millimeters within times of milliseconds as calculated from the solution to the 1D diffusion equation $\bar{x} = \sqrt{2Dt}$. For example, in an experimental time-frame of 5 ms, the gas atoms can travel an RMS distance of $\approx$1 mm. Considering the smallest confining structure in the lungs to be an alveolus, which is approximately 0.3 mm in diameter, the gas atoms can encounter the tissue walls multiple times during a typical MR sequence TR, which is typically 5 ms. The confinement by the walls leads to a "restriction" in gas diffusion and hence the measured ADC is much smaller in healthy lungs than for diffusion in free space. Typical MRI measurements reveal that the helium-3 ADC is between 0.1 and 0.2 $cm^2\ s^{-1}$ in healthy lungs [97], whereas in free space it is 0.88 $cm^2\ s^{-1}$ when mixed with room air (see Figure 9.8).

9.3.5 Measuring diffusion: time-length scale dependence

Diffusion acts to attenuate irreversibly the MR signal whenever a magnetic field gradient is present as discussed earlier. Hence, MRI sequences can be used to measure diffusion by using pulsed or static gradients after the application of the excitation RF pulse. The most commonly employed method is the pulsed-gradient-spin-echo

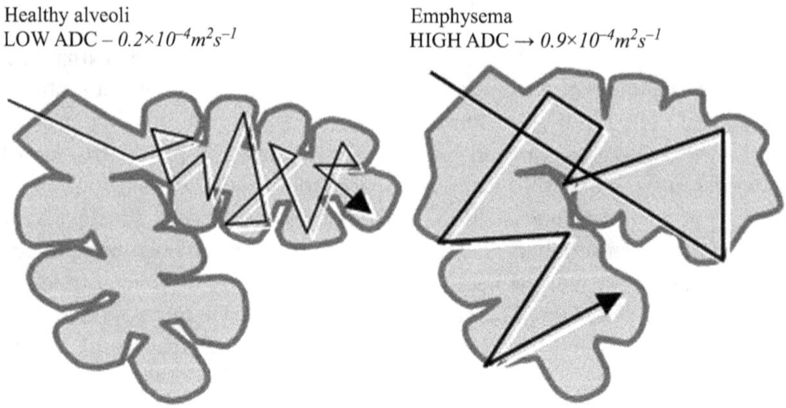

Figure 9.8 Schematic of a healthy alveolar and emphysematous alveolus

(PGSE) technique. It is easily implemented, robust, and, most importantly, it can be incorporated into fast sequences that can be encompassed within a breath-hold. The standard PGSE method utilizes two pulsed gradients separated by a timeΔ, and a 180° refocusing pulse, all situated after the slice-selection gradient and (usually) before the phase encode step of the sequence. The same diffusion measurement can also be undertaken without the 180° refocusing. However, this essentially limits experimentation to shorter durations of Δ, since T_2* causes signal attenuation. Furthermore, the refocusing pulse can mitigate some of the measurement errors due to the superposition of background gradients. The simplified PSGE method is incorporated within a standard gradient echo (SPGR) sequence block. This sequence is best run in an interleaved mode where the acquisition of each line of *k*-space is repeated: the first interleave has no diffusion weighting (reference scan at matched time-to-echo (TE)), while the subsequent interleaves incorporate bipolar gradient waveform of different *b*. Interleaving in this fashion ensures a reduced sensitivity to motion artifacts and greatly reduces any flip angle, and T_1 relaxation bias in the measured ADC. However, it is crucial that each interleave has the same TE and TR.

The first reported measurements of 3He diffusion were by Mugler [98] at a field strength of 1.5 T. Measurements were made using a bipolar gradient waveform (PGSE), with four *b*-values of 0.4, 0.8, 1.2, and 1.6 cm s^{-1}. The ADC values were calculated on a pixel-by-pixel basis using a linear, least-squares fit to yield a single average ADC value for all four *b*-values. The overall mean ADC value over all healthy volunteers was found to 0.25 cm s^{-1}, almost a factor of four times smaller than unrestricted diffusion in free space.

Here, diffusion was encoded using only two *b*-values: for the healthy volunteers the values were b=0 cm s^{-1}, and b=2.75 cm s^{-1}; for the emphysema patients a lower *b*-value of 1.375 cm s^{-1} was selected. Diffusions in both experiments were encoded with a relatively long diffusion time of 7.5 ms. The results from the healthy volunteers yielded an average ADC value of 0.20 cm s^{-1}, whereas the ADC values from the emphysema patients were greatly elevated, yielding an average of 0.50 cm s^{-1}. The results clearly demonstrated that a destruction of the lung tissue leads to the higher ADC values, closer to the unrestricted diffusion coefficient. Salerno *et al.* conducted a study in 16 healthy volunteers, and 11 patients suffering from emphysema. The encoding methods were identical to those of Mugler *et al.* Here, the ADC was on average 0.23 cm s^{-1} for healthy volunteers, and 0.45 cm s^{-1} for the patients with emphysema. In addition, the ADC values were compared to spirometry measurements taken before each scan. The ADC values were found to correlate strongly with the forced-expiratory-volume within 1 s (FEV1). This was an important finding since spirometry is routinely used to assess disease severity. Various groups have since used PGSE sequences such as these to elucidate early emphysematous changes in smokers (see Figure 9.9), growth of alveoli with age, postural and anatomical gradients within the lung, and subtle changes in asthma. PGSE 3He ADC results have been shown to match well with the alveolar dimensions measured results from histological sections in experiments made in animal lungs and more recently in human lungs [99].

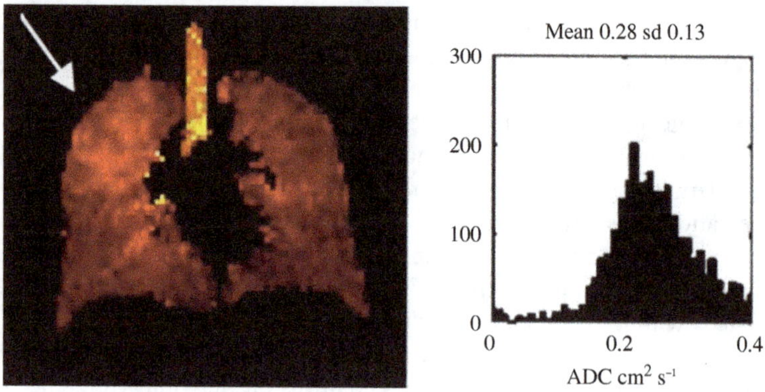

Figure 9.9 ADC map and histogram from a patient with emphysema; a hot spot of elevated ADC is clearly seen in the upper right lobe. Images acquired with a PGSE SPGR sequence

The mean ADC value is clearly an indicator of the alveolar size and hence disease severity in the case of emphysema; however, the interconnected nature of the alveolar microstructure imposes a time-length scale dependence on the ADC that depends upon the diffusion weighting gradient strengths and timings. In simple terms, if we give the gas a longer time to diffuse, there is more chance of it hitting a wall and encountering a restriction thus giving a lower ADC.

This sequence timing dependence of the ADC means that care should be taken when making a direct comparison of ADC results measured at different sites with sequences with different diffusion weightings and international consensus on standardization of *b*-value for 3He ADC measurement would be worthwhile.

The time dependence of the PGSE sequence also indicates that with longer diffusion times, we can potentially probe longer-range diffusion in the lungs that represents interacinar connectivity and disease processes that lead to different gas mixing washout times. The problem with extending the diffusion time Δ to the tens of milliseconds needed to probe longer length scales is that T_2* decay (approximately 25 ms for 3He in the lungs at 1.5 T) can attenuate the signal before application of the second gradient pulse. To address this, the diffusion-encoded magnetization can be stored in the longitudinal direction (with a flip back RF pulse of the opposite phase, i.e., a stimulated echo sequence) where the longer T_1s (~20 s) allow longer diffusion times, the magnetization being read-out with a third pulse with the same phase as the original excitation pulse.

Various manifestations of sequence for measurement of long-timescale diffusion have been proposed; all give ADC values approximately an order of magnitude less than those measured with PGSE, which indicates that we are measuring gas mixing by convection/diffusion through collateral connectivity over a longer length scale. Whether this is more or less sensitive than the shorter timescale measurements to different aspects of lung microstructure in healthy and diseased lungs remains to be fully investigated but preliminary comparison shows differences in sensitivity.

Much work has been performed in modeling the effect of diffusion inside geometrical models that mimic the lung microstructure; this is an area of theoretical study in its own right and the reader is referred to the papers from the various groups active in this field who have proposed analytical and numerical models of restricted diffusion.

9.3.6 Transverse relaxation time T_2*

As mentioned earlier, the lungs are a magnetically inhomogeneous medium due to the magnetic susceptibility difference between air and parenchyma (9-ppm volume susceptibility difference) creating microscopic field gradients. The diffusion of 3He in these gradients gives rise to a microscopic (sub-pixel) T_2*, which can be measured at breath-hold with interleaved SPGR sequence blocks of different TE. The T_2* could thus provide an additional means of exploring the lung physiology with sensitization to both the susceptibility differences in the perfused micro-vasculature and anatomical gradients in the T_2* within the lung having been reported [100].

9.4 Examples of current and future applications of HP gas MRI

9.4.1 Hyperpolarized 3He gas MRI studies of pulmonary disease

9.4.1.1 Introduction

Although pathological descriptions of COPD date back to the seventeenth century, we still do not know the entirety of disease origins or pathogenesis, nor do we have any treatments or therapies that can reduce mortality rates in individuals with COPD. What is well understood, however, is the significant burden of the disease on those individuals affected. According to estimates from the World Health Organization, over 60 million people are affected with COPD [101]. Recent estimates also report that COPD is responsible for approximately 3.0 million deaths globally and is the fourth leading cause of death worldwide [102].

A number of methods have been introduced for COPD assessment over recent years, including plethysmography for measuring lung volumes, the forced oscillation technique, the multiple breath washout technique [103], and markers of airway inflammation are also used, but, again, these tests provide only global assessments of pulmonary function. Therefore, other measurement tools that can identify and quantify these underlying mechanisms or phenotypes of the disease are required. Due to the lack of direct, noninvasive, and regional methods capable of assessing disease phenotypes, the development, and application of medical imaging technologies for the assessment of COPD has gained a great deal of attention in the COPD research community.

CT of the lung has undoubtedly provided investigators and clinicians with valuable structural information since its introduction in the early 1970s [104–106].

While CT typically does not provide functional information, structural information related to both the airways and lung parenchyma [107] can be obtained that are highly correlated with pathology and other physiological parameters [108,109]. Importantly, CT also provides important information on patient-centered outcomes in COPD, including mortality, disease progression, exacerbations, and treatment response. CT measurements have been shown to be independent predictors of all-cause mortality in patients with COPD [110] and to be associated with decline in pulmonary function [111,112] and exacerbations [113]. CT emphysema measurements have been shown to identify a subgroup of patients with better responses following lung-volume-reduction surgery [114] and endobronchial-valve implantation [115,116]. However, many studies investigating responses to interventions in COPD patients require serial investigations, and although low-dose protocols are utilized by many multicenter cohort studies of COPD, the ionizing radiation dose to research participants remains an understandably significant concern. Furthermore, questions remain regarding the utility of CT for assessing early or mild emphysema [117], and CT has obvious limitations for assessing the morphology of the small airways due to resolution limits. Therefore, interest in other nonradiation-based imaging modalities that can provide information related to emphysema and airway disease has been an active area of research over recent years.

MRI does not use ionizing radiation and therefore, in contrast to X-ray based imaging modalities, allows for more intensive serial investigations and longitudinal studies. However, it is important to note that although MRI is the imaging modality of choice and the clinical standard for many organ systems, MRI is not used in the clinical assessment of respiratory disease. MRI of the lung is challenged by a number of factors, including low 1H density, differences in magnetic susceptibilities at the alveolar–air interfaces, and respiratory and cardiac motion. Despite these limitations, a number of novel approaches have been introduced and are still under development, with potential for COPD evaluation, such as ultrashort echo time MRI measurements, Fourier Decomposition MRI, and oxygen-enhanced MRI.

However, among these MRI pulmonary imaging approaches that have emerged, the introduction of HP noble gas MRI has made the greatest impact to date on the respiratory imaging field. Albert *et al.* were the first to recognize the potential to use HP noble gases for MRI lung imaging in 1994. Using a polarization process called SEOP, the MRI SNR is increased approximately 10^5 times above the thermal equilibrium value and therefore when the subject inhales the HP gas, the distribution of the gas within the lung can be visualized. Since its inception, HP noble gas MRI has proven to be a powerful technique for assessing a number of respiratory diseases, including COPD.

The following will provide a background on the underlying COPD disease phenotypes, an introduction to the HP 3He MRI approaches and measurements developed to investigate these disease phenotypes, and an overview of some of the early HP noble gas MRI work performed for investigating COPD. Finally, there will be a discussion of the most recent HP 3He MRI studies and the impact of the application of this technique on the COPD patient.

9.4.1.2 Emphysema

Emphysema is "a condition of the lung characterized by abnormal, permanent enlargement of airspaces distal to the terminal bronchiole, accompanied by the destruction of their walls, and without obvious fibrosis" [118].

Although pathological studies of emphysema are important for investigating disease pathogenesis, these studies involve lung tissue that has been obtained ex vivo, either postmortem or following surgical intervention, and are therefore limited for improving our understanding of COPD pathogenesis and response to treatment. The following sections will introduce the HP 3He MRI ADC measurement and discuss the application of this measurement for assessing emphysema.

Hyperpolarized noble gas diffusion-weighted MRI

During the inhalation of 3He gas, the gas passes through the mouth, pharynx, larynx, trachea, and follows more than 20 generations of airway branching before it enters into the alveolar ducts and sacs. Once the 3He gas atoms are within the lung microstructure, the displacement of the atoms over time is determined by the atom's diffusion coefficient; the diffusion coefficient of helium in the air is 0.88 $cm^2\ s^{-1}$. By allowing the gas atom to diffuse for very short diffusion times, on the order of milliseconds, the lung microstructure can be probed. For example, if an individual gas atom is permitted to diffuse for 2 ms, it will travel approximately 590 μm. It has been estimated that the mean diameter of an alveolus is roughly 200 μm [119], and therefore the walls of the alveolar structures will act as barriers by restricting the gas atoms' motion or displacement. For the 2-ms time interval, an ADC can be derived that will be proportional to the RMS displacement in one direction of the atom diffused and thus indicates the level of restriction to diffusion present within the alveolar ducts and sacs. The ADC therefore reflects the restricted space within which the gas atoms may travel. Accordingly, in the airspaces of healthy volunteers, the HP 3He gas atoms travel shorter distances, and therefore low ADC values are measured. In emphysema, which is characterized by enlarged airspaces, the HP 3He gas atoms travel further distances and this is reflected by the greater ADC values measured. Furthermore, slightly elevated 3He ADC values can be observed in smokers with normal lung function, suggesting early evidence of lung structural abnormalities.

An advantage of HP 3He diffusion-weighted MRI is that it is not limited to a certain set of image acquisition parameters, and by adjusting these parameters we can probe different features of the lung microstructure. As described before, for the 3He gas atom to probe the alveolar microstructure where it resides during the breath-hold, short diffusion times are used such that the 3He gas remains restricted within a single acinus. However, if the diffusion time is increased, the 3He gas atoms are permitted to diffuse farther distances, and, in subjects with more severe disease, the 3He gas atoms may make use of the collateral channels that are known to be enlarged and more numerous in regions of the lung with severe emphysematous tissue destruction [120–122]. Furthermore, more detailed information regarding the geometrical parameters at the alveolar level can be obtained by changing different imaging parameters and obtaining HP 3He diffusion-weighted MR images at multiple different *b*-values [123–125].

9.4.1.3 Airway disease

Hogg *et al.* [126] found that small airways disease, the resultant ventilation and gas exchange abnormalities, could be present and progress might be undetected by direct measurements of airway resistance, or indirectly using spirometry, and, most recently, Hogg provided evidence that the narrowing and loss of the small airways may precede the development of emphysema [127]. Therefore, there is great interest in evaluating small airway disease in the very early disease stages—before disease changes are detected by spirometry—and using this information to phenotype patients and stratify them for preventative treatment. The following sections will introduce HP 3He MRI static ventilation imaging and discuss the applications of 3He MRI for evaluating gas distribution abnormalities in COPD.

Hyperpolarized 3He MRI static ventilation imaging

In subjects with COPD, airflow limitation due to both emphysematous tissue destruction and narrowing and obstruction of the small airways leads to differences in regional time constants for lung filling and emptying, and, consequently, regional and heterogeneous abnormalities in ventilation. When a subject inhales the HP 3He gas and holds their breath during MRI, the regional distribution of the gas within the lung can be directly visualized.

In addition to directly visualizing the regions of the lung that receive the HP 3He gas, in patients with COPD we can also directly visualize the regions of the lung where the flow of the 3He gas has been obstructed. Identifying the lung regions where airflow is obstructed has clear advantages as it provides an opportunity to better understand which parts of the lung may or may not be functional, which may be useful for guiding COPD treatment.

Before using HP 3He static ventilation MRI to evaluate the treatment and other patient-centered outcomes, we need to develop methods to quantify regional gas distribution abnormalities visualized using HP 3He MRI. Early investigations to quantify HP 3He MRI gas distribution used ventilation defect counting or scoring. Woodhouse *et al.* use the ratio of 3He MRI ventilation volume and the 1H MRI thoracic cavity volume to calculate the "percentage-ventilated lung volume."

Tustison *et al.* [128] used a seeded region-growing algorithm to quantify the regions of poor ventilation. The lung shape can be quantified indirectly by using a principle component analysis as described by Tustison *et al.* [129]. Alternatively, the thoracic cavity can be quantified directly by acquiring conventional 1He MRI in addition to 3He MRI and performing 1H–3He coregistration and segmentation [130].

There are other technologies used for HP 3He MRI segmentation. Approaches that can correct for the magnetic RF field inhomogeneity and intensity similarity between the vasculature and the 3He MRI ventilation defects signal have been described. When performing 1H–3He image registration and segmentation, an approach that simultaneously segments the 1H–3He MR images has also been introduced. Finally, the development of hybrid MRI allows for a simultaneous acquisition of 1H and 3He MRI in the same breath-hold. However, there is currently no standard approach for HP 3He MRI gas distribution analysis.

9.4.1.4 Discussion and future

HP 3He MRI has shown great promise for evaluating COPD over the last two decades. Measurements derived from HP 3He diffusion-weighted and static ventilation MRI have been clinically validated, are reproducible, associated with exacerbations, symptoms, and exercise limitation, and have demonstrated utility in evaluating the effects of various COPD treatments. However, it must be acknowledged that there are several barriers to the wider adoption and clinical translation of this technology.

One of the most important setbacks to the translation of HP 3He MRI is the fact that it requires 3He gas, which is very expensive and in limited supply globally, and the fact that specialized coils and polarization equipment are required in order to obtain 3He MR images. While this means that the technique is not currently widely available, polarizer systems can be purchased commercially, and other noble gases, such as HP 129Xe, can be utilized. While the image quality was not as high with HP 129Xe MRI as 3He MRI during initial investigations in the 1990s, improvements in xenon polarizers and imaging techniques now allow for comparable image quality. Similar to 3He MRI, 129Xe MRI can provide images of the 129Xe gas distribution in the lung using static ventilation MRI with quantitative approaches already being introduced, as well as the lung microstructure using diffusion-weighted MRI. In contrast to 3He gas that is inert, 129Xe gas is tissue soluble and therefore 129Xe MRI can also provide information on gas exchange in the lung. Therefore, transitioning to 129Xe gas will aid in the broader clinical translation and adoption of HP noble gas MRI.

Another important drawback that should be mentioned is the lack of studies comparing 3He MRI between sites. Large-scale, multicenter studies, which could be possible with 129Xe MRI, are important for clinical translation because they allow for external validity. Furthermore, because patients from different geographical areas can be evaluated, the findings from multicenter studies are more generalizable to the broader population. Additionally, the standardization of imaging protocols as well as the standardization of measurements and analysis tools is required in order for wider adoption and translation of this technology.

HP noble gas MRI has great potential to be used clinically to guide treatment decisions, which makes a difference in the lives of patients with COPD.

9.4.2 Hyperpolarized gas MRI of radiation-induced lung injury

9.4.2.1 Introduction

Lung cancer is the leading cause of cancer death in the world. Approximately 80% of all lung cancers are non-small cell lung carcinoma (NSCLC) and are often treated with thoracic radiotherapy (RT). Unfortunately, the lung is a very radiosensitive organ and RILI is a frequent consequence limiting the effectiveness of thoracic RT. The severity of RILI is closely related to the lung volume that exceeds the lung radiation tolerance. Radiation pneumonia is a kind of acute RILI, which has two manifestations: early acute radiation and late radiation. Acute radiation pneumonia is the earliest complication of RILI. It usually appears within 4–12 weeks after radiation therapy and is accompanied by symptoms such as inflammation, cough, fever, shortness of breath, and redness of the skin at the radiation site. Pulmonary fibrosis is a second-stage complication of RILI that usually occurs within 6–24 months of radiotherapy and results in reduced lung compliance and volume. The incidence of RILI is reported to be 37% and of this population, 20% are diagnosed with moderate-to-severe RILI [131]. Coughing, fever, and dyspnea have also been reported in 5%–50% of the RILI population [132]. RILI can lead to temporary or permanent loss of lung function and, in extreme cases, death [133].

Clinical assessment and management of RILI utilize both pulmonary function tests (PFTs) and imaging techniques. Persistence of hypoxia as measured by the partial pressure of oxygen in arterial blood (paO_2) has been reported post-radiation therapy [134,135] and recent studies suggest that it may further exacerbate lung injury. However, PFTs are whole-lung measurements and cannot identify regional deficiencies in lung function, which presumably reduces the sensitivity of PFTs to an early injury. Imaging of RILI is typically performed using planar X-ray and CT. Although CT changes have been observed before the onset of clinical RILI [136], these anatomical changes (e.g., lung density) often do not occur before clinical symptoms manifest [137,138]. CT imaging of late-stage RILI is currently the gold standard for discerning fibrosis from lung tumor recurrence but is often too late (months) to effect any change in therapy to mitigate RILI. In a previous study, RILI was detected using CT in roughly 75% of patients undergoing RT but was not detected earlier than 4 weeks post-RT [139]. An imaging method sensitive to early (weeks) changes associated with RILI would be valuable to identify radiosensitive individuals and adjust therapy accordingly.

Nuclear medicine imaging techniques such as single-photon emission computed tomography (SPECT) and PET can be used when functional lung information such as perfusion is required. Functional imaging with SPECT can provide ventilation and perfusion maps of the lung postinjection of Technetium-99m. Studies have demonstrated a dose-dependent reduction in perfusion and ventilation at 3–4 months post radiation therapy [140,141]. However, correlations between these metrics and whole-lung function assessed by pulmonary function testing (i.e., FEV1 and diffusing capacity for carbon monoxide) are weak and additional work is required to assess regional injury [142]. Additionally, SPECT imaging is limited in spatial resolution, lacks specificity, and provides ~3 mSv of extra whole-body radiation dose to the patient [143], which is approximately three times the annual background dose (~1 mSv) and 60% of the annual radiation worker limit (~5 mSv). PET imaging with fluorodeoxyglucose (18F-FDG) has shown an increased uptake of 18F-FDG associated with RILI in lung cancer patients [144]; however, the technique is heavily dependent on a tissue uptake of 18F-FDG and is susceptible to a high false positive rate [145]. In particular, a high uptake of 18F-FDG is associated with both inflammation and tumor growth and no clear separation of RILI and cancer has been demonstrated [146,147]. As with SPECT, PET requires an acquisition time of approximately an hour and also incurs additional radiation dose to the patient (~15% of the annual radiation worker limit).

In contrast to X-ray and nuclear medicine imaging methods, MRI provides an approach for probing lung anatomy and function without the use of ionizing radiation, which may be particularly well suited for tracking the progression and regression of the early stage of RILI. Conventional MRI approaches aimed at the detection of RILI have been performed previously through the measurement of regional perfusion and the T_2 relaxation times of lung tissues. However, proton MRI is challenging in the lung due to low proton signal as it contains only approximately 20% soft tissue. This low signal is further diminished by the presence of microscopic magnetic field nonuniformities arising from susceptibility differences at the gas/tissue interface. Furthermore, respiratory motion can be problematic, leading to image blurring and other artifacts.

The issue of low MRI signal in the lung has recently been addressed by the advent of SEOP techniques, which can boost the signal of certain inhaled noble gases (3He and 129Xe) by up to five orders of magnitude. High spatial resolution imaging of the airways and alveoli can be achieved from the gas phase of either 3He or 129Xe, within a single breath-hold. Lung dysfunction from obstructive pulmonary disease can be inferred by regions of signal dropout (or defect). This form of imaging can also be applied to animals, including mice and rats. A unique morphological lung measurement is possible using HP gas MRI, namely, the ADC, a surrogate for alveolar size. Additionally, 129Xe dissolves in both the parenchymal tissue and red blood cell compartments of the lung and reflects changes in sizes and gas exchange associated with these compartments. Several of these measures have been investigated in patients with COPD, asthma [148], and cystic fibrosis, as well as in animal models of lung disease.

The following reviews the current state of HP gas MRI in the context of a mechanistic picture of RILI pathogenesis. And applications of HP 3He to models of RILI are summarized. Finally, limitations and future directions of HP gas MRI for detection of RILI are presented.

9.4.2.2 Pathogenesis of RILI

Following acute radiation damage, the inflammatory cascade associated with RILI consists of two main phases: (1) an early phase characterized by RP and (2) a later phase characterized by tissue remodeling and fibrosis [149,150], though one can occur without the other. The RP stage, typically lasting days to several weeks, is initiated by an overwhelming inflammatory response believed to be triggered by cytokines released by activated resident leukocytes (i.e., macrophages), signaling migrating leukocytes (e.g., macrophages and neutrophils) to adhere to, and penetrate the injured epithelial and endothelial layers [151]. Immunohistochemical analysis of RP in animal models reveals underlying cellular changes, including increases in alveolar macrophages, inflammatory cytokines, and type II pneumocytes [152,153]. These changes are observed both within and outside the region of conformal RT [154,155] and persist up to 4-week postirradiation in rats [156]. If injury to the alveolar epithelium is significant and/or unrepaired, chronic fibrosis will result (months). This can lead to progressive lung function loss and ultimate organ failure, affecting about 50% of individuals with severe lung injury.

Detection of RILI and its severity in the RP stage, before irreversible fibrosis, could potentially alter the course of RT fractionation and/or initiate adjuvant therapy earlier to mitigate RILI and improve patient outcomes. A number of microanatomical and functional changes accompanying RP may be useful targets for HP gas MRI methods. The RP phase is marked by a loss of alveolar function due to flooding (i.e., edema) from epithelial damage, thickening of alveolar and capillary walls, and inactivation of surfactant leading to reductions in ventilation and perfusion, ultimately leading to hypoxia/ischemia, compromised gas exchange, and reduced lung compliance [157]. ADC of HP 3He and 129Xe MRI may be employed to detect the reduction of alveolar air space associated with RP and fibrosis while measurement of the time for 129Xe to diffuse through the alveolar wall can enable the detection of the thickening of alveolar walls due to RP and fibrosis.

9.4.2.3 Application of hyperpolarized 3He MRI in RILI

The strong signal and insolubility of 3He in tissues provides a powerful approach for the assessment of the lung airspace to probe both functional and micro-anatomical changes associated with RILI, using ventilation defects and ADC, respectively. HP 3He gas ventilation defects have been used for studies of later stage RILI, both in clinical subjects and animal models. These studies include the identification of ventilation defect progression, stasis, and decline correlated with the presence of RILI measured longitudinally [158,159], as well as approaches to register 3He images with CT images to enable computation of RT plans for the avoidance of functional lung deficits [160,161]. However, the presumption that ventilation defects reflect functional deficits solely due to RILI is likely not strictly true due to gross obstruction of gas by scarring and/or tumor recurrence in lung cancer patients. Furthermore, lung cancer patients often have other lung comorbidities, including COPD, which further confound ventilation defect patterns. Perhaps most importantly, early RILI may not result in changes in ventilation, thereby requiring a more sensitive measure of microstructural changes due to RP and fibrosis.

Mapping of ADC may be particularly useful for identifying microstructural changes associated with RP in the ventilated lung, as alveolar gas space decreases due to RP and fibrosis are opposite to the alveolar enlargement expected in emphysema, a common component of COPD. Decreases in 3He ADC corresponding to regions of fibrosis-related to radiation exposure have been reported in a rat model of RILI consisting of fractionated delivery of 40 Gy to the right lung. Increases in 3He ADC have also been reported in the contralateral lung of subjects undergoing unilateral RT of the lung suggesting that a compensatory effect may be occurring between the functional lung and an injured lung.

9.4.2.4 Discussion and future

RILI is an important limiting factor in the RT treatment of thoracic cancers, most notably NSCLC, responsible for 80% of lung cancers. Strategies to mitigate RILI, and especially subsequent and irreversible fibrosis, benefit from early detection of

RP, where the effects are most readily treated. MRI following inhalation of HP gases, specifically 3He and 129Xe, may offer a useful approach for the detection of RP. To the extent that these HP nuclei can be delivered to the injured portions of the lung, these approaches can offer valuable insight into the microanatomical and functional changes accompanying RILI. Irradiation of animal lungs, both whole-thorax and conformal delivery, can be useful for imaging RILI in a controlled fashion, particularly to study longitudinal effects and correlate with histological changes.

MRI of the apparent diffusion of HP gases is a powerful tool for quantifying regional microanatomical changes associated with RP as the diffusion lengths of these gases are sensitive to the morphometry of the terminal airways and alveoli. The use of both 3He and 129Xe ADC to investigate regional longitudinal changes, especially from conformal irradiation and fractionated delivery similar to that used clinically, will likely be fruitful areas of future research as each gas is sensitive to different diffusion length scales and can thus probe different microanatomical changes. MRI morphometry is also expected to benefit from emerging 3D histology approaches in order to validate microanatomical changes, which are inherently three-dimensional in nature.

Detection of early RP using HP gas MRI could allow monitoring of ongoing radiation therapy of breast cancer, esophageal cancer, and other thoracic cancers that may be susceptible to RILI. The information could be used as feedback for modification of the radiation therapy (or chemotherapy) plan or to determine whether anti-inflammatory drugs would help. Since every patient may have a slightly different physiological makeup, HP gas MRI could assist with personalized treatment where the pulmonary function of each patient could be mapped and used in the ongoing therapeutic intervention. The nonionizing nature of MRI also permits repeated scans for continuous monitoring of a patient, which may not be possible with PET and CT. Continuous monitoring may be important to track the evolution of both the tumor response and RP in cancer patients.

Early and regional detection of RP associated with RILI using these emerging imaging methods may play a significant role in the personalization of ongoing RT and adjuvant therapy, thereby improving outcomes.

9.4.3 Radiomics

9.4.3.1 Introduction

The prognosis of patients with lung cancer after radiotherapy is mainly based on the assessment of lung function and lung structure by imaging methods. However, at present, there is no practical method to identify the characteristics of lung tissue quantitatively and effectively in clinical practice. In terms of practicality, no matter CT, PET, or MRI, especially the latter two, a single examination is expensive; if used for a routine examination, it will cost a lot of money for patients. Especially for tumor patients, both energy and material resources will be under great pressure. Therefore, if an effective, accurate, and inexpensive evaluation method is found, its clinical value and social significance are self-evident.

With the development of imaging technology, CT, PET/CT, MRI, and other detection methods are playing an increasingly important role in the diagnosis, treatment, and efficacy evaluation of tumors. The present imaging examination can not only obtain the morphological characteristics of the tumor but also provide some biological characteristics of the tumor by means of functional imaging and hypoxia imaging. The application of digital image-processing technology and machine learning methods to the analysis of medical images has given rise to the emergence of radiomics. Radiomics is a high-throughput quantitative analysis method that extracts quantitative image features from areas of interest in medical imaging such as CT, PET/CT, and MRI. After screening and analysis, these characteristics will be used to describe the biological characteristics and heterogeneity of tumors.

In 2012, Lambin [162] proposed the concept of radiomics for the first time, which originated from the heterogeneity of tumors. The spatial and temporal heterogeneity of solid tumors at the levels of genes, proteins, cells, microenvironments, tissues, and organs limit the accuracy and representativeness of the results of invasive detection methods such as pathology and molecular techniques. Medical imaging can comprehensively, noninvasively, and quantitatively observe the overall morphology of tumors and monitor the development process and treatment response of tumors at any time, thus providing a reliable solution to the tumor heterogeneity. Radiomics hypothesized that microscopic changes in gene or protein patterns could be expressed on macroscopic imaging features. Therefore, Lambin [163] believes that radiomics is “the extraction of a large number of features from radiological images with high throughput and the conversion of imaging data into a minable data space with high resolution by automatic or semi-automatic analysis methods.” Kumar *et al.* [164] further extended the definition of radiomics as “the high-throughput extraction and analysis of a large number of advanced quantitative imaging features from CT, MRI, and PET.” Gillies [165] mentioned in the keynote report of the Radiological Society of North America Summit in 2014 that the microenvironment can be quantified and the degree of genetic heterogeneity of tumors can be predicted through in-depth analysis of images. He believes that compared with the traditional clinical medicine that only interprets medical images from the visual level, radiomics can dig into the biological nature of images and provide clinical decision support. In recent years, more and more scholars pay attention to radiomics and have made a lot of achievements in the diagnosis, treatment, and prognosis of tumors. Radiomics high-throughput features, extracted from different modal images and using data mining, can be used for tumor molecular typing, differential diagnosis, treatment plan selection, efficacy detection, and prognosis evaluation.

The radiomics process can be divided into distinct steps with definable inputs and outputs, such as image acquisition and reconstruction, segmentation, feature extraction and qualification, and analysis and model building [166]. The first step is to obtain high-quality and standardized images (CT, PET/CT, or MRI, etc.) for diagnosis and evaluation. Excessive heterogeneity should be avoided in the selection of cases in order to obtain desirable analytical results. At the same time, the same type of scanning machine should be selected as far as possible when collecting images, and reasonable parameters such as layer thickness, pixel size, and tube voltage should be selected. The second step is to delineate the tumor parenchyma (segmentation of the region of interest, ROI), from the acquired images, either by automatic, semiautomatic segmentation methods or by experienced radiation oncologists. At present, the commonly used segmentation algorithms include a graphic cutting method, active contour method, region growing method, and level set method. When drawing ROI, consider whether the image needs to be registered, and the ROI should not be too small. The third step is to extract radiomics features from ROI, including the description of intensity distribution, the spatial relationship between different intensity levels, the shape and heterogeneity of texture patterns, and the description of the relationship between tumor and surrounding tissues. The fourth step is to screen the image features according to the repeatability of the data and the correlation of other features, etc. and analyze the relationship between the selected features and treatment results or gene expression. Finally, accurate risk prediction was provided by including the radiomics features in the predictive model of treatment outcome and using additional information provided by common predictors to evaluate the radiomics features. Radiomics is derived from conventional imaging diagnosis, but it is different in that it can perform quantitative analysis of tissue characteristics that conventional imaging cannot. For each of the abovementioned steps, there are still unresolved issues, such as to what extent acquisition and reconstruction parameters may have an impact on the features [167,168]; what kind of segmentation is more precise among manual, semiautomatic, and automatic; what features are really stable and reproducible; how overfitting can be avoided; and what type of statistical analysis is more appropriate for model building [169].

Since pulmonary nodules are usually detected and followed up by CT, problems related to the variability in acquisition and reconstruction do exist but are limited to a small number of variables.

The high contrast resolution between pulmonary nodules and lung parenchyma makes them ideal candidates for volumetric segmentation. Radiomics features may include semantic qualitative features, such as shape, margins, density, and agnostic quantitative features mathematically extracted by different software [170]. The quantitative features may have different levels of complexity, such as describing lesion shape, intensity, texture, and wavelet. More specifically, first-order statistics features describe the distribution of individual voxel values without concern for spatial relationships. These are generally histogram-based methods and reduce an ROI to single values for mean, median, maximum, minimum, and uniformity or randomness (entropy) of the intensities on the image, as well as the skewness (asymmetry) and kurtosis (flatness) of the histogram of values. Shape features describe the shape and geometric properties of the analyzed volume, such as maximum diameter or the diameters along the three orthogonal directions, maximum surface, tumor compactness, and sphericity.

Second-order statistics features generally describe the so-called textural features, indicating the statistical relationships between voxels with similar (or dissimilar) values and take into account the spatial arrangement of the values [171]. Examples of these features belong to the category of the gray level co-occurrence matrix and gray level run length matrix. Higher-order statistics features are generated by statistical methods after imposing filter grids on the image to extract repetitive or non-repetitive patterns, such as fractal analyses, Minkowski functionals, wavelets, and Laplace transforms of Gaussian bandpass filters. As a result, the extraction of textural features may generate hundreds of variables, some of which may be redundant and require covariance evaluation [172,173].

Once features have been extracted, the next process in radiomics is establishing relationships between patterns of features and clinical variables, also known as data mining. This can vary from straightforward statistical analyses based on a priori hypotheses- to machine learning methods. Machine learning is a field of computer science that combines the study of pattern recognition and computational learning theory to construct algorithms that can learn from data and make predictions on outcomes as well as uncover hidden insights. Random forests are an example of a machine learning algorithm that works by constructing a collection of decision trees [174].

9.4.3.2 Radiomics and lung cancer

At present, it has carried out preliminary exploration in lung cancer, head and neck cancer, breast cancer, brain tumor, rectal cancer, esophageal cancer, prostate cancer, liver cancer, and other tumor diseases. Different from traditional medical image-assisted diagnosis, radiomics excavates image features from a large number of medical images as new biomarkers based on data analysis, which is helpful for the clinical selection of appropriate treatment regimens and monitoring of treatment effects.

Cunliffe *et al.* [175] studied the CT data of patients with esophageal cancer treated with radiotherapy and found that the texture characteristic values extracted by radiomics were closely related to the occurrence of radiation pneumonia. Huynh *et al.* [176], Hunter [177], and Mattonen *et al.* [178] all used radiomics to quantitatively evaluate the efficacy of radiotherapy for lung cancer. Huynh *et al.* found that the wavelet decomposition features were significantly correlated with the prognosis of distant metastases, and the overall survival was related to both conventional imaging features and radiomics features. Hunter *et al.* analyzed CT image data of NSCLC patients before radiotherapy by using quantitative image feature model and successfully predicted tumor regression after radiotherapy, which proposed a new index for tumor treatment evaluation and survival prediction. Mattonen conducted qualitative diagnosis and radiation oncology experts such as radiomics quantitative traits in lung cancer radiotherapy effect and recurrence prediction in comparison, and the results prove that radiomics prediction during the follow-up period and coincided basically with the clinical evaluation, but radiomics can detect early postoperative atypical recurrent lesions that are difficult for clinicians to detect. Vallières *et al.* [179] used fluorodeoxyglucose FDG-PET and MRI texture features to predict lung metastasis of soft tissue tumors, and the four texture features of FDG-PET/MRI fusion images obtained through logistic regression multivariate analysis had the best prediction effect. Coroller *et al.* [180] also used the radiomics method to evaluate the possibility of distant metastasis of lung adenocarcinoma. These studies suggest that radiomics can be used for the selection of treatment methods and monitoring of clinical efficacy, and it has guiding significance for the formulation of individualized treatment plans for lung cancer. Parmar *et al.* [181] believe that the phenotypic characteristics of quantitative CT can detect the metastatic or invasive ability of NSCLC, which is of great value in predicting tumor outcome and guiding clinical individualized treatment. Coroller *et al.* [182] extracted 635 features from CT images of lung adenocarcinoma patients using the radiomics method to predict distant metastasis and survival, of which 35 features were related to distant metastasis and 12 features were related to survival, among which the LoG feature could significantly improve the accuracy of prediction. Paul *et al.* [183] further extracted CT image features through the convolutional neural network, and the highest prediction accuracy of lung cancer prognosis reached 82.5% [184] by Hosny *et al.* during the prognosis of lung cancer through deep learning. Prognostic analysis of non-small cell lung cancer based on radiology was also carried out successively [185]. van Timmeren *et al.* [186] used FDG-PET/CT radiomics to evaluate early response to treatment in patients with NSCLC. Unfortunately, the radiomics model based on FDG-PET or CT did not produce a clinically relevant prognostic model.

Asai *et al.* [187] used 18F-FDGPET/CT radiomics to predict the local recurrence of patients with early non-small cell lung cancer after stereotactic body radiotherapy (SBRT). In NSCLC patients receiving SBRT, two radiomics features from 18F-FDGPET were independently associated with local control, and the established predictive model provided information related to local recurrence and could be used for clinical decision-making. Starkov *et al.* [188] used texture-based CT radiomics to predict the efficacy of SBRT in early non-small cell lung cancer. In this study, a survival prediction model for NSCLC patients was established based on the radiomics characteristics of CT images. van Timmeren *et al.* [189] conducted a longitudinal radiomics study on cone-beam CT (CBCT) images in patients with non-small cell lung cancer and assessed the prognostic overall survival rate and local recurrence. However, the final conclusion could not prove that the radiomics features extracted from longitudinal CBCT helped improve the prognostic information. Avanzo *et al.* [190] summarized the application of radiomics and deep learning in lung cancer and the latest progress of radiomics in lung cancer. Pulmonary malignancies have been extensively characterized by radiomics and deep learning. Through the three-dimensional characteristics of the lesions, CT- and PET-based radiomics feature models have been used to detect nodules, distinguish between malignant and benign lesions, and characterize their histology, staging, and genotype. Deep learning models have been used to automate the segmentation of organs at risk from lung cancer radiotherapy, to stratify patients according to the risk of local and distant recurrence, and to identify patients suitable for molecular targeted therapy and immunotherapy. In addition, radiomics has been successfully used to predict side effects, such as radiation and immunotreatment-induced pneumonia, and to distinguish between lung injury and recurrence. Radiomics can be further developed to optimize dose-volume data for radiotherapy planning. Chetan *et al.* [191] summarized the application of radiomics in the prediction of non-small cell lung cancer treatment response.

At present, there are only some sporadic lung MRI radiomics analyses, such as preoperative prediction of histological subtypes of patients with non-small cell lung cancer by using the radiomics characteristics of MRI [192]; lung diseases were classified by multiparameter MRI [193]; the prognosis of non-small cell lung cancer was predicted by the texture features of MRI and CT images [194]; clinical routine MRI and tumor heterogeneity index were used to evaluate the heterogeneity of primary lung tumors [195]. So far, although polarized inert gas has great potential in pulmonary MRI, radiomics analysis based on polarized inert gas has not been reported.

9.5 Conclusion

A number of HP gases are available for lung imaging and other in vivo imaging applications, including 3He, 129Xe, and 83Kr. A number of factors determine its in vivo availability and clinical effectiveness as a contrast agent for HP: (1) the availability and cost of the substances involved; (2) the cost and throughput of the HP equipment; (3) life of high-pressure gas state; (4) availability of appropriate MRI hardware. Historically, human lung MRI using 3He was first demonstrated, followed relatively quickly by lung MRI using 129Xe. While 3He has driven the initial feasibility of ventilation and diffusion imaging, the emergence of clinical scale production of HP 129Xe has led to the expansion of biomedical HP gas applications, including gas perfusion imaging, brown fat imaging, and brain imaging.

Despite scientific and technological breakthroughs, many clinical trials using HP 129Xe and 3HE have been successfully completed in human, and HP gas has not yet been used for clinical diagnostics. Therefore, the widespread clinical use of HP gas depends on addressing these transformation challenges. Although it is not yet clear which HP gas and type of hyperpolarization technology will be suitable for clinical use, it may require fundamental changes to the MR hardware to achieve clinical application. For example, for HP 129Xe or 3He, the upgrades of 1.5 or 3-T clinical scanners are expensive. As an alternative approach, dedicated low-field MRI scanners may have unique advantages as a platform for clinical adaptation of HP gas. Low-field MRI scanners are essentially cheaper than high-field superconducting MRI scanners; and low-field MRI can produce a higher SNR in HP applications; in addition, due to significantly lower specific absorption rates at lower RF frequencies and significantly higher patient throughput, low-field MRI provides greater patient safety.

In conclusion, the preparation and imaging techniques of HP gas are mature and have significant and positive effects on lung diagnosis. However, significant translational challenges remain to be addressed before this promising treatment can become a routine clinical practice.

References

[1] Ferlay J, Colombet M, Soerjomataram I, Parkin DM and Bray F. Cancer statistics for the year 2020: an overview. *Int J Cancer* 2021.

[2] American Cancer Society 2018 *Global Cancer Facts and Figures* 4th edn (Atlanta, GA: American Cancer Society).

[3] Jemal A, Miller KD, Ma J, Siegel RL and Thun MJ. Higher lung cancer incidence in young women than young men in the United States. *N Engl J Med* 2018;378(21):1999–2009.

[4] Jemal A, Center MM, DeSantis C and Ward EM. Global patterns of cancer incidence and mortality rates and trends. *Cancer Epidemiol Biomarker Prev* 2010;19:1893–907.

[5] Ferlay J, Colombet M, Soerjomataram I, *et al.* Cancer incidence and mortality patterns in Europe: estimates for 40 countries and 25 major cancers in 2018. *Eur J Cancer* 2018;103:356–87.

[6] Chen WQ, Zhang SW, Zou XN and Ping Z. Cancer incidence and mortality in china, 2013. *Chin J Cancer Res* 2011;23(001):3–9.

[7] Chen W, Zheng R, Baade PD, *et al.* Cancer statistics in China, 2015. *CA Cancer J Clin* 2016;66(2).

[8] Parkin DM. International variation. *Oncogene* 2004;23:6329–40.

[9] Yang L, Parkin DM, Ferlay J, Li L and Chen Y. Estimates of cancer incidence in China for 2000 and projections for 2005. *Cancer Epidemiol Biomarker Prev* 2005;14:243–50.

[10] Ferlay J, Ervik M, Lam F, *et al.* Global cancer observatory: Cancer tomorrow [Internet], 2018. (Lyon, France: International Agency for Research on Cancer). Available from: https://gco.iarc.fr/tomorrow.

[11] GBD Tobacco Collaborators 2017 Smoking prevalence and attributable disease burden in 195 countries and territories, 1990–2015: a systematic analysis from the Global Burden of Disease Study 2015. *Lancet* 2015;389:1885–906.

[12] Peto R, Lopez A D, Boreham J, Thun M and Heath Jr.C. 1994 *Mortality From Smoking in Developed Countries 1950–2000* (Oxford: Oxford University Press).

[13] Lewis DR, Check DP, Caporaso NE, Travis WD and Devesa SS. Us lung cancer trends by histologic type. *Cancer* 2015;120(18):2883–92.

[14] Lortet-Tieulent J, Soerjomataram I, Ferlay J, Rutherford M, Weiderpass E and Bray F. International trends in lung cancer incidence by histological subtype: adenocarcinoma stabilizing in men but still increasing in women. *Lung Cancer* 2014;84(1):13–22.

[15] Kinoshita FL, Ito Y and Nakayama T. Trends in lung cancer incidence rates by histological type in 1975–2008: a population-based study in Osaka, Japan. *J Epidemiol* 2016;26:579–86.

[16] CDC 2004 *Surgeon General's 2004 Report: The Health Consequences of Smoking* (Rockville, MD: US Department of Health and Human Services).

[17] Miller KD, Nogueira L, Mariotto AB, Rowland JH and Siegel RL. Cancer treatment and survivorship statistics, 2019. *CA Cancer J Clin* 2019;69(5).

[18] American Cancer Society 2019 *Cancer Facts and Figures* (Atlanta, GA: American Cancer Society).
[19] Oken MM, Hocking WG, Kvale PA, Andriole GL and Berg CD. Screening by chest radiograph and lung cancer mortality: the Prostate, Lung, Colorectal, and Ovarian (PLCO) randomized trial. *JAMA* 2011;306(17):1865–73.
[20] Kim SK, Allen-Auerbach M, Goldin J, Fueger BJ and Schiepers C. Accuracy of PET/CT in characterization of solitary pulmonary lesions. *J Nucl Med* 2007;48(2):214–20.
[21] Bauman G, Luetzen U, Ullrich M, *et al.* Pulmonary functional imaging: qualitative comparison of Fourier decomposition MR imaging with SPECT/CT in porcine lung. *Radiology* 2011;260:551–9.
[22] Baert AL, Knauth M and Sartor K. 2009 *MRI of the Lung* (Germany: Springer);3–4:179.
[23] Donnelly LF, MacFall JR, McAdams HP, *et al.* Cystic fibrosis: combined hyperpolarized 3He-enhanced and conventional proton MR imaging in the lung-preliminary observation. *Radiology* 1999;212:885–9.
[24] Muller HE, Chen XJ, Saam B, *et al.* MRI of the lungs using hyperpolarized noble gases. *Magn Reson Med* 2002;47(6):1029–51.
[25] Larson PEZ, Bok R, Kerr AB, *et al.* Investigation of tumor hyperpolarized [1-13C]-pyruvate dynamics using time-resolved multiband RF excitation echo-planar MRSI. *Magn Reson Med* 2010;63(3):582–91.
[26] Couch MJ, Ball IK, Fox MS, *et al.* Pulmonary ultrashort echo time 19F MR imaging with inhaled fluorinated gas mixtures in healthy volunteers: feasibility. *Radiology* 2013:904–8.
[27] Kastler A. Some suggestions concerning the production and detection by optical means of inequalities in the populations of levels of spatial quantization in atoms. Application to the Stern and Gerlach and magnetic resonance experiments. *J Phys Radium* 1950;11(11).
[28] Walker TG and Happer W. Spin-exchange optical pumping of noble-gas nuclei. *Rev Mod Phys* 1997;69(2):629.
[29] Colegrove FD, Schearer LD and Walters GK. Polarization of He 3 gas by optical pumping. *Phys Rev* 1963;132(6):2561.
[30] Albert MS, Cater GD, Driehuys B, *et al.* Biological magnetic resonance imaging using laser-polarized 129Xe. *Nature* 1994;370:199–201.
[31] MacFall JR, Charles HC, Black RD, *et al.* Human lung air spaces: potential for MR imaging with hyperpolarized He-3. *Radiology* 1996;200:553–8.
[32] Kauczor HU, Hofmann D, Kreitner KF, Nilgens H and Thelen M. Normal and abnormal pulmonary ventilation: visualization at hyperpolarized He-3 MR imaging. *Radiology* 1996;201:564–8.
[33] Mugler JP 3rd, Driehuys B, Brookeman JR, *et al.* MR imaging and spectroscopy using hyperpolarized 129Xe gas: preliminary human results. *Magn Reson Med* 1997;37:809–15.
[34] Tastevin G and Nacher P. NMR measurements of hyperpolarized 3He gas diffusion in high porosity silica aerogels. *J Chem Phys* 2005;123(6):064506:1–12.

[35] Donnelly LF, MacFall JR, McAdams HP, *et al.* Cystic fibrosis: combined hyperpolarized 3He-enhanced and conventional proton MR imaging in the lung-preliminary observation. *Radiology* 1999;212:885–9.
[36] Mayo JR and Hayden ME. Hyperpolarized helium 3 diffusion imaging of the lung. *Radiology* 2002;222:8–11.
[37] Jing C, Mclawhorn R, Altes TA, Lange ED and Ke S. Helical tomotherapy planning for lung cancer based on ventilation magnetic resonance imaging. *Med Dosim* 2011;36:389–96.
[38] Lutey BA, Lefrak SS, Woods JC, *et al.* Hyperpolarized 3He MR imaging: physiologic monitoring observations and safety considerations in 100 consecutive subjects. *Radiology* 2008;248:655–61.
[39] Miranda K, Mohammadreza H, Andrew W, *et al.* Evaluating bronchodilator effects in chronic obstructive pulmonary disease using diffusion-weighted hyperpolarized helium-3 magnetic resonance imaging. *J Appl Physiol* 2012;112:651–7.
[40] Ireland RH, Bragg CM, McJury M, *et al.* Feasibility of image registration and intensity-modulated radiotherapy planning with hyperpolarized helium-3 magnetic resonance imaging for non–small-cell lung cancer. *Int J Radiat Oncol Biol Phys* 2007;68(1):273–81.
[41] Tseng CH, Wong GP, Pomeroy VR, *et al.* Low-field MRI of laser polarized noble gas. *Phys Rev Lett* 1998;81(17):3785–8.
[42] Bermuth J, Merle P, Carasco C, *et al.* The neutron charge form factor and target analyzing powers from 3He (e→, e′n) scattering. *Phys Lett B* 2003;564(3):199–204.
[43] Gast KK, Eberle B, Schmiedeskamp J and Kauczor HU. Magnetic resonance imaging using hyperpolarized 3 He-gas 1. *Acad Radiol* 2003;10(10):1119–31.
[44] Ebert M, Grossmann T, Heil W, *et al.* Nuclear magnetic resonance imaging with hyperpolarised helium-3. *Lancet* 1996;347(9011):1297–9.
[45] Walker TG. Fundamentals of spin-exchange optical pumping. *J Phys* 2011;294(1):012001.
[46] Larson B, Häusser O, Delheij PPJ, Whittal DM and Thiessen D. Optical pumping of Rb in the presence of high-pressure He 3 buffer gas. *Phys Rev A* 1991;44(5):3108.
[47] Kastler A. Optical methods of atomic orientation and of magnetic resonance. *JOSA* 1957;47(6):460–5.
[48] Babcock E, Nelson I, Kadlecek S, *et al.* Hybrid spin-exchange optical pumping of He 3. *Phys Rev Lett* 2003;91(12):123003.
[49] Romalis MV. Laser-polarized (3) He target used for a precision measurement of the neutron spin structure. 1997.
[50] Baranga ABA, Appelt S, Romalis MV, Erickson CJ and Happer W. Polarization of 3 He by spin exchange with optically pumped Rb and K vapors. *Phys Rev Lett* 1998;80(13):2801.
[51] Chen WC, Gentile TR, Walker TG and Babcock E. Spin-exchange optical pumping of He 3 with Rb–K mixtures and pure K. *Phys Rev A* 2007;75 (1):013416.

[52] Tsai LL, Mair RW, Rosen MS, Patz S and Walsworth RL. An open-access, very-low-field MRI system for posture-dependent 3 He human lung imaging. *J Magn Reson* 2008;193:274–85.

[53] Abragam A. *The principles of nuclear magnetism*, 1961. (London: Oxford University Press).

[54] Schaefer SR, Cates GD, Chien TR, *et al.* Frequency shifts of the magnetic-resonance spectrum of mixtures of nuclear spin-polarized noble gases and vapors of spin-polarized alkali-metal atoms. *J Phys Rev A* 1989; 39(11): 5613–23.

[55] Romalis MV and Cates GD. Accurate 3He polarimetry using the Rb Zeeman frequency shift due to the Rb-3He spin-exchange collisions. *Phys Rev A* 1998;58:3004–11.

[56] Barton AS, Newbury NR, Cates GD, *et al.* Self-calibrating measurement of polarization-dependent frequency shifts from Rb-3 He collisions. *J Phys Rev A* 1994; 49(4): 2766–70.

[57] Chen WC, Gentile TR, Ye Q, Walker TG and Babcock E. On the limits of spin-exchange optical pumping of 3He. *J Appl Phys* 2014;116:014903.

[58] Barker JR. New coil systems for the production of uniform magnetic fields. *J Sci Instrum* 1949;26:273–5.

[59] Jacob RE, Morgan SW, Saam B and Leawoods JC. Wall relaxation of He3 in spin-exchange cells. *Phys Rev Lett* 2001;87:143004.

[60] Nikolaou P, Coffey AM, Walkup LL, *et al.* XeNA: an automated 'open-source' 129Xe hyperpolarizer for clinical use. *Magn Reson Imaging* 2014;32:541–50.

[61] Cates GD, Benton DR, Gatzke M, Happer W, Hasson KC and Newbury NR. Laser production of large nuclear-spin polarization in frozen xenon. *Phys Rev Lett* 1990;65:2591–4.

[62] Gatzke M, Cates GD, Driehuys B, Fox D, Happer W and Saam B. Extraordinarily slow nuclear spin relaxation in frozen laser-polarized 129Xe. *Phys Rev Lett* 1993;70:690–3.

[63] Driehuys B, Cates G, Miron E, Sauer K, Walter D and Happer W. High-volume production of laser-polarized 129Xe. *Appl Phys Lett* 1996;69:1668–70.

[64] Schearer LD and Walters GK. Nuclear spin-lattice relaxation in the presence of magnetic-field gradients. *Phys Rev A* 1965;139:1398–402.

[65] Saam B, Happer W and Middleton H. Nuclear relaxation of 3He in the presence of O_2. *Phys Rev A* 1995;52(1):862–5.

[66] Deninger AJ, Eberle B, Bermuth J, *et al.* Quantification of regional intra-pulmonary oxygen partial pressure evolution during apnea by (3)He MRI. *J Magn Reson* 1999;141(2):207–16.

[67] Woodhouse N, Mills GH, Flemming S, Fichele S and van Beek EJ. Comparison of hyperpolarized 3-He administration methods in healthy as diseased subjects. *Proc ISMRM* 2006;2006:1288.

[68] Zanche ND, Chhina N, Teh K, *et al.* Asymmetric quadrature split birdcage coil for hyperpolarized 3He lung MRI at 1.5 T. *Magn Reson Med* 2008; 60(2):431–8.

[69] Lee RF, Johnson G, Grossman RI, *et al.* Advantages of parallel imaging in conjunction with hyperpolarized helium – a new approach to MRI of the lung. *Magn Reson Med* 2006;55(5):1132–41.

[70] Saam B, Happer W and Middleton H. Nuclear relaxation of He 3 in the presence of O 2. *Phys Rev A* 1995;52(1):862.

[71] Mata JF, Altes TA, Cai J, *et al.* Evaluation of emphysema severity and progression in a rabbit model: comparison of hyperpolarized 3He and 129Xe diffusion MRI with lung morphometry. *J Appl Physiol* 2007; 102(3):1273–80.

[72] Wild JM, Fichele S, Woodhouse N, *et al.* Assessment and compensation of susceptibility artifacts in gradient echo MRI of hyperpolarized 3He gas. *Magn Reson Med* 2003;50(2):417–22.

[73] Deninger AJ, Eberle B, Bermuth J, *et al.* Quantification of regional intra-pulmonary oxygen partial pressure evolution during apnea by (3)He MRI. *J Magn Reson* 1999;141(2):207–16.

[74] Wild JM, Schmiedeskamp J, Paley MNJ, *et al.* MR imaging of the lungs with hyperpolarized helium-3 gas transported by air. *Phys Med Biol* 2002;47(13): N185–90.

[75] Wild JM, Fichele S, Woodhouse N, *et al.* Assessment and compensation of susceptibility artifacts in gradient echo MRI of hyperpolarized 3He gas. *Magn Reson Med* 2003;50(2):417–22.

[76] Lee RF, Johnson G, Grossman RI, *et al.* Advantages of parallel imaging in conjunction with hyperpolarized helium – a new approach to MRI of the lung. *Magn Reson Med* 2006;55(5):1132–41.

[77] Wild JM, Paley MN, Kasuboski L, Swift A and Beek EJRV. Dynamic radial projection MRI of inhaled hyperpolarized 3He gas. *Magn Reson Med* 2003;49(6):991–7.

[78] Zhao L, Mulkern R, Tseng CH, *et al.* Gradient-echo imaging considerations for hyperpolarized 129Xe MR. *J Magn Reson B* 1996;113:179–83.

[79] Wild JM, Paley MNJ, Viallon M, Schreiber W, Beek EJRV and Griffiths P. k-space filtering in 2D gradient-echo breath-hold hyperpolarized He-3 MRI: spatial resolution and signal-to-noise ratio considerations. *Magn Reson Med* 2002;47(4):687–95.

[80] Teh K, Lee KJ and Wild JM. Slice profile effects in variable flip angle hyperpolarized 3He MRI. *Proc Int Soc Magn Reson Med* 2007;15:1297.

[81] Wild JM, Teh K, Woodhouse N, *et al.* Steady-state free precession with hyperpolarized 3He: experiments and theory. *J Magn Reson* 2006; 183(1):13–24.

[82] Saam B, Yablonskiy DA, Gierada DS and Conradi MS. Rapid imaging of hyperpolarized gas using EPI. *Magn Reson Med* 1999;42(3):507–14.

[83] Durand E, Guillot G, Darrasse L, *et al.* CPMG measurements and ultrafast imaging in human lungs with hyperpolarized helium-3 at low field (0.1 T). *Magn Reson Med* 2002;47(1):75–81.

[84] Driehuys B, Walker J, Pollaro J, Cofer GP and Johnson GA. 3He MRI in mouse models of asthma. *Magn Reson Med* 2007;58(5):893–900.

[85] Wild JM, Woodhouse N, Paley MN, *et al.* Comparison between 2D and 3D gradient-echo sequences for MRI of human lung ventilation with hyperpolarized 3He. *Magn Reson Med* 2004;52(3):673–8.

[86] Van Beek EJ, Hill C, Woodhouse N, *et al.* Assessment of lung disease in children with cystic fibrosis using hyperpolarized 3-helium MRI: comparison with Shwachman score, Chrispin-Norman score and spirometry. *Eur Radiol* 2007;17(4):1018–24.

[87] Al-Kadi OS and Watson D. Texture analysis of aggressive and non-aggressive lung tumor CE CT images. *IEEE Trans Biomed Eng* 2008; 55(7):1822–30.

[88] Woodhouse N, Wild JM, Paley MN, *et al.* Combined helium-3/proton magnetic resonance imaging measurement of ventilated lung volumes in smokers compared to never-smokers. *J Magn Reson Imaging* 2005;21(4):365–9.

[89] Mata J, Altes T, Knake J, Mugler J, Brookeman J and de Lange E. Hyperpolarized 3He MR imaging of the lung: effect of subject immobilization on the occurrence of ventilation defects. *Acad Radiol* 2008;15(2):260–4.

[90] Schreiber WG, Weiler N, Kauczor HU, Markstaller K and Thelen JM. Ultrafast MRI of lung ventilation using hyperpolarized helium-3. *Rofo* 2000;172(2):129–33.

[91] Salerno M, Altes TA, Brookeman JR, Lange EED and Iii JPM. Dynamic spiral MRI of pulmonary gas flow using hyperpolarized (3)He: preliminary studies in healthy and diseased lungs. *Magn Reson Med* 2001;46(4):667–77.

[92] Holmes JH, Korosec FR, Du J, *et al.* Imaging of lung ventilation and respiratory dynamics in a single ventilation cycle using hyperpolarized He-3 MRI. *J Magn Reson Imaging* 2007;26(3):630–6.

[93] Holmes JH, O'Halloran RL, Brodsky EK, Jung Y, Block WF and Fain SB. 3D hyperpolarized He-3 MRI of ventilation using a multi-echo projection acquisition. *Magn Reson Med* 2008;59(5):1062–71.

[94] De Rochefort L, Maitre X, Fodil R, *et al.* Phase-contrast velocimetry with hyperpolarized 3He for in vitro and in vivo characterization of airflow. *Magn Reson Med* 2006;55(6):1318–25.

[95] Cieslar K, Alsaid H, Stupar V, *et al.* Measurement of nonlinear pO_2 decay in mouse lungs using 3He-MRI. *NMR Biomed* 2007;20(3):383–91.

[96] Liner J and Weissman S. Determination of the temperature dependence of gaseous diffusion coefficients using gas chromatographic apparatus. *J Chem Phys* 1972;56:2288–90.

[97] Fain SB, Panth SR, Evans MD, *et al.* Early emphysematous changes in asymptomatic smokers: detection with 3He MR imaging. *Radiology* 2006;239(3):875–83.

[98] Mugler JP, Brookemann JR, Knight-Scott J, Maier T, De Lange EE and Bogorad PL. Regional measurement of the 3He diffusion coefficient in the human lung. *Proc Int Soc Magn Reson Med* 1998;(6).

[99] Woodhouse N, Mills GH, Flemming S, Fichele S and van Beek EJ. Comparison of hyperpolarized 3-He administration methods in healthy as diseased subjects. *Proc ISMRM* 2006;2006:1288.

[100] Ajraoui S, Ireland R, Lee KJ, Woodhouse N and Wild JM. Anatomical trends in coregistered ADC and T2* maps of 3He gas in the lungs of healthy normals. *Proc Int Soc Magn Reson Med* 2008;1.

[101] World Health Organization 2008 *The Global Burden of Disease: 2004 Update* (Geneva: WHO).

[102] Oostveen E, MacLeod D, Lorino H, *et al.* The forced oscillation technique in clinical practice: methodology, recommendations and future developments. *Eur Respir J* 2003;22:1026–41.

[103] Downie SR, Salome CM, Verbanck S, Thompson B, Berend N and King GG. Ventilation heterogeneity is a major determinant of airway hyperresponsiveness in asthma, independent of airway inflammation. *Thorax* 2007;62:684–9.

[104] Gevenois PA, De Vuyst P, de Maertelaer V, *et al.* Comparison of computed density and microscopic morphometry in pulmonary emphysema. *Am J Respir Crit Care Med* 1996;154:187–92.

[105] Gevenois PA, de Maertelaer V, De Vuyst P, Zanen J and Yernault JC. Comparison of computed density and macroscopic morphometry in pulmonary emphysema. *Am J Respir Crit Care Med* 1995;152:653–7.

[106] Turner MO, Mayo JR, Muller NL, Schulzer M and FitzGerald JM. The value of thoracic computed tomography scans in clinical diagnosis: a prospective study. *Can Respir J* 2006;13:311–16.

[107] Nakano Y, Muro S, Sakai H, *et al.* Computed tomographic measurements of airway dimensions and emphysema in smokers. Correlation with lung function. *Am J Respir Crit Care Med* 2000;162:1102–8.

[108] Hruban RH, Meziane MA, Zerhouni EA, *et al.* High resolution computed tomography of inflation-fixed lungs. Pathologic-radiologic correlation of centrilobular emphysema. *Am Rev Respir Dis* 1987;136:935–40.

[109] Kuwano K, Matsuba K, Ikeda T, *et al.* The diagnosis of mild emphysema. Correlation of computed tomography and pathology scores. *Am Rev Respir Dis* 1990;141:169–78.

[110] Johannessen A, Skorge TD, Bottai M, *et al.* Mortality by level of emphysema and airway wall thickness. *Am J Respir Crit Care Med* 2013;187: 602–8.

[111] Vestbo J, Edwards LD, Scanlon PD, *et al.* Changes in forced expiratory volume in 1 second over time in COPD. *N Engl J Med* 2011;365:1184–92.

[112] Nishimura M, Makita H, Nagai K, *et al.* Annual change in pulmonary function and clinical phenotype in chronic obstructive pulmonary disease. *Am J Respir Crit Care Med* 2012;185:44–52.

[113] Coxson HO, Dirksen A, Edwards LD, *et al.* The presence and progression of emphysema in COPD as determined by CT scanning and biomarker expression: a prospective analysis from the ECLIPSE study. *Lancet Respir Med* 2013;1:129–36.

[114] Han MK, Kazerooni EA, Lynch DA, *et al.* Chronic obstructive pulmonary disease exacerbations in the COPDGene study: associated radiologic phenotypes. *Radiology* 2011;261:274–82.

[115] Fishman A, Martinez F, Naunheim K, *et al.* A randomized trial comparing lung-volume-reduction surgery with medical therapy for severe emphysema. *N Engl J Med* 2003;348:2059–73.

[116] Sciurba FC, Ernst A, Herth FJ, *et al.* A randomized study of endobronchial valves for advanced emphysema. *N Engl J Med* 2010;363:1233–44.

[117] Gompelmann D, Eberhardt R, Michaud G, Ernst A and Herth FJ. Predicting atelectasis by assessment of collateral ventilation prior to endobronchial lung volume reduction: a feasibility study. *Respiration* 2010;80:419–25.

[118] Snider GL, Kleinerman JL, Thurlbeck WM and Bengali ZH. The definition of emphysema-report of a national-heart-lung-and-blood-institute, division of lung-diseases workshop. *Am Rev Respir Dis* 1985;132:182–5.

[119] Ochs M, Nyengaard JR, Jung A, *et al.* The number of alveoli in the human lung. *Am J Respir Crit Care Med* 2004;169:120–4.

[120] Woods JC, Yablonskiy DA, Choong CK, *et al.* Long-range diffusion of hyperpolarized 3He in explanted normal and emphysematous human lungs via magnetization tagging. *J Appl Physiol* 2005;99:1992–7.

[121] Conradi MS, Yablonskiy DA, Woods JC, *et al.* The role of collateral paths in long-range diffusion of 3He in lungs. *Acad Radiol* 2008;15:675–82.

[122] Bartel SE, Haywood SE, Woods JC, *et al.* Role of collateral paths in long-range diffusion in lungs. *J Appl Physiol* 2008;104:1495–503.

[123] Yablonskiy DA, Sukstanskii AL, Leawoods JC, *et al.* Quantitative in vivo assessment of lung microstructure at the alveolar level with hyperpolarized 3He diffusion MRI. *Proc Natl Acad Sci USA* 2002;99:3111–16.

[124] Yablonskiy DA, Sukstanskii AL, Woods JC, *et al.* Quantification of lung microstructure with hyperpolarized 3He diffusion MRI. *J Appl Physiol* 2009;107:1258–65.

[125] Quirk JD, Lutey BA, Gierada DS, *et al.* In vivo detection of acinar microstructural changes in early emphysema with (3)He lung morphometry. *Radiology* 2011;260:866–74.

[126] Hogg JC, Macklem PT and Thurlbeck WM. Site and nature of airway obstruction in chronic obstructive lung disease. *N Engl J Med* 1968;278:1355–60.

[127] McDonough JE, Yuan R, Suzuki M, *et al.* Small-airway obstruction and emphysema in chronic obstructive pulmonary disease. *N Engl J Med* 2011;365:1567–75.

[128] Tustison NJ, Altes TA, Song G, de Lange EE, Mugler III JP and Gee JC. Feature analysis of hyperpolarized helium-3 pulmonary MRI: a study of asthmatics versus nonasthmatics. *Magn Reson Med* 2010;63:1448–55.

[129] Tustison NJ, Avants BB, Flors L, *et al.* Ventilation-based segmentation of the lungs using hyperpolarized (3)He MRI. *J Magn Reson Imaging* 2011;34:831–41.

[130] Kirby M, Heydarian M, Svenningsen S, *et al.* Hyperpolarized He-3 magnetic resonance functional imaging semiautomated segmentation. *Acad Radiol* 2012;19:141–52.

[131] Mathew L, Vandyk J, Etemad-Rezai R, Rodrigues G and Parraga G. Hyperpolarized (3)He pulmonary functional magnetic resonance imaging prior to radiation therapy. *Med Phys* 2012;39(7):4284–90.

[132] Marks LB, Yu X, Vujaskovic Z, Small Jr. W, Folz R and Anscher MS. Radiation-induced lung injury. *Semin Radiat Oncol* 2003;13(3):333–45.
[133] Gross NJ. The pathogenesis of radiation-induced lung damage. *Lung* 1981;159(3):115–25.
[134] Emirgil C and Heinemann H. Effects of irradiation of chest on pulmonary function in man. *J Appl Physiol* 1961;16(2):331–8.
[135] Siemann DW and Hill RP. Quantitative changes in the arterial blood gases of mice following localized irradiation of the lungs. *Radiat Res* 1983; 93(3):560–6.
[136] Robbins ME, Brunso-Bechtold JK, Peiffer AM, Tsien CI, Bailey JE and Marks LB. Imaging radiation-induced normal tissue injury. *Radiat Res* 2012;177(4):449–66.
[137] Movsas B, Raffin TA, Epstein AH and Link Jr. CJ. Pulmonary radiation injury. *Chest* 1997;111(4):1061–76.
[138] Ghafoori P, Marks LB, Vujaskovic Z and Kelsey CR. Radiation-induced lung injury. Assessment, management, and prevention. *Oncology (Williston Park)* 2008;22(1):37–47 discussion 52–3.
[139] Ikezoe J, Takashima S, Morimoto S, *et al.* CT appearance of acute radiation-induced injury in the lung. *AJR Am J Roentgenol* 1988;150(4):765–70.
[140] Boersma LJ, Damen E, de Boer RW, *et al.* Recovery of overall and local lung function loss 18 months after irradiation for malignant lymphoma. *J Clin Oncol* 1996;14(5):1431–41.
[141] Theuws J, Seppenwoolde Y, Kwa SL, *et al.* Changes in local pulmonary injury up to 48 months after irradiation for lymphoma and breast cancer. *Int J Radiat Oncol Biol Phys* 2000;47(5):1201–8.
[142] Petersson J, Sanchez-Crespo A, Larsson SA and Mure M. Physiological imaging of the lung: single-photon-emission computed tomography (SPECT). *J Appl Physiol* 2007;102(1):468–76.
[143] McCurdy MR, Castillo R, Martinez J, *et al.* 18F-FDG uptake dose-response correlates with radiation pneumonitis in lung cancer patients. *Radiothe Oncol* 2012;104(1):52–7.
[144] Moon DH, Maddahi J, Silverman D, Glaspy JA, Phelps ME and Hoh CK. Accuracy of whole-body fluorine-18-FDG PET for the detection of recurrent or metastatic breast carcinoma. *J Nucl Med* 1998;39(3):431–5.
[145] Ishimori T, Saga T, Nagata Y, *et al.* 18F-FDG and 11C-methionine PET for evaluation of treatment response of lung cancer after stereotactic radiotherapy. *Annal Nucl Med* 2004;18(8):669–74.
[146] Hicks RJ, Mac Manus MP, Matthews JP, *et al.* Early FDG-PET imaging after radical radiotherapy for non small-cell lung cancer: inflammatory changes in normal tissues correlate with tumor response and do not confound therapeutic response evaluation. *Int J Radiat Oncol Biol Phys* 2004;60(2):412–18.
[147] Ogasawara N, Suga K, Karino Y and Matsunaga N. Perfusion characteristics of radiation-injured lung on Gd-DTPA-enhanced dynamic magnetic resonance imaging. *Invest Radiol* 2002;37(8):448–57.

[148] Tsoutsou PG and Koukourakis MI. Radiation pneumonitis and fibrosis: mechanisms underlying its pathogenesis and implications for future research. *Int J Radiat Oncol Biol Phys* 2006;66(5):1281–93.

[149] Hill RP, Zaidi A, Mahmood J and Jelveh S. Investigations into the role of inflammation in normal tissue response to irradiation. *Radiothe Oncol* 2011;101(1):73–9.

[150] Johnston CJ, Piedboeuf B, Baggs R, Rubin P and Finkelstein JN. Differences in correlation of mRNA gene expression in mice sensitive and resistant to radiation-induced pulmonary fibrosis. *Radiat Res* 1995;142(2):197–203.

[151] Rodemann HP and Bamberg M. Cellular basis of radiation-induced fibrosis. *Radiothe Oncol* 1995;35(2):83–90.

[152] Khan MA, Hill RP and Van Dyk J. Partial volume rat lung irradiation: an evaluation of early DNA damage. *Int J Radiat Oncol Biol Phys* 1998; 40(2):467.

[153] Khan MA, Van Dyk J, Yeung IW and Hill RP. Partial volume rat lung irradiation; assessment of early DNA damage in different lung regions and effect of radical scavengers. *Radiothe Oncol* 2003;66(1):95–102.

[154] Calveley VL, Khan MA, Yeung IW, Vandyk J and Hill RP. Partial volume rat lung irradiation: temporal fluctuations of in-field and out-of-field DNA damage and inflammatory cytokines following irradiation. *Int J Radiat Biol* 2005;81(12):887–99.

[155] Ding K, Bayouth JE, Buatti JM, Christensen GE and Reinhardt JM. 4D CT-based measurement of changes in pulmonary function following a course of radiation therapy. *Med Phys* 2010;37(3):1261–72.

[156] Ghobadi G, Bartelds B, van der Veen SJ, *et al.* Lung irradiation induces pulmonary vascular remodelling resembling pulmonary arterial hypertension. *Thorax* 2012;67(4):334–41.

[157] Allen AM, Albert M, Caglar HB, *et al.* Can Hyperpolarized Helium MRI add to radiation planning and follow-up in lung cancer? *J Appl Clin Med Phys* 2011;12(2):3357.

[158] Ireland RH, Din OS, Swinscoe JA, *et al.* Detection of radiation-induced lung injury in non-small cell lung cancer patients using hyperpolarized helium-3 magnetic resonance imaging. *Radiother Oncol* 2010;97(2): 244–8.

[159] Mathew L, Gaede S, Wheatley A, Etemad-Rezai R, Rodrigues GB and Parraga G. Detection of longitudinal lung structural and functional changes after diagnosis of radiation-induced lung injury using hyperpolarized 3He magnetic resonance imaging. *Med Phys* 2010;37(1):22–31.

[160] Ireland RH, Bragg CM, McJury M, *et al.* Feasibility of image registration and intensity-modulated radiotherapy planning with hyperpolarized helium-3 magnetic resonance imaging for non-small-cell lung cancer. *Int J Radiat Oncol Biol Phys* 2007;68(1):273–81.

[161] Mathew L, Wheatley A, Castillo R, *et al.* Hyperpolarized (3)He magnetic resonance imaging: comparison with four-dimensional X-ray computed tomography imaging in lung cancer. *Acad Radiol* 2012;19(12):1546–53.

[162] Lambin P, Rios-Velazquez E, Leijenaar R, *et al.* Radiomics: extracting more information from medical images using advanced feature analysis. *Eur J Cancer* 2012; 48(4): 441–6.

[163] Aerts HJWL, Velazquez ER, Leijenaar RTH, Parmar C and Lambin P. Decoding tumour phenotype by noninvasive imaging using a quantitative radiomics approach. *Nat Commun* 2014;5:4006.

[164] Kumar V, Gu Y, Basu S, Erglund A, Eschrich S. Radiomics: the process and the challenges. *Mag Reson Imaging* 2012; 30(9): 1234–48.

[165] Gillies R J, Kinahan P E and Hricak H. Radiomics: images are more than pictures, they are data. *Radiology* 2015;278(2):563–77.

[166] Rizzo S, Botta F, Raimondi S, *et al.* Radiomics: the facts and the challenges of image analysis. *Eur Radiol Exp* 2018;2:36.

[167] Rizzo S, Kalra MK, Schmidt B, *et al.* CT images of abdomen and pelvis: effect of nonlinear three-dimensional optimized reconstruction algorithm on image quality and lesion characteristics. *Radiology* 2005;237:309–15.

[168] Dalal T, Kalra MK, Rizzo S, *et al.* Metallic prosthesis: technique to avoid increase in CT radiation dose with automatic tube current modulation in a phantom and patients. *Radiology* 2005;236:671–5.

[169] Aerts H, Velazquez ER, Leijenaar R, Parmar C and Lambin P. Decoding tumour phenotype by noninvasive imaging using a quantitative radiomics approach. *Nat Commun* 2014;5(1):4006.

[170] Larue R, Timmeren JV, Jong ED, *et al.* Influence of gray level discretization on radiomic feature stability for different CT scanners, tube currents and slice thicknesses: a comprehensive phantom study. *Acta Oncol* 2017;56:1544–53.

[171] Balagurunathan Y, Kumar V, Gu Y, Kim J and Gillies RJ. Test-retest reproducibility analysis of lung CT image features. *J Digit Imaging* 2014;27(6).

[172] de Jong EEC, van Elmpt W, Rizzo S, *et al.* Applicability of a prognostic CT-based radiomic signature model trained on stage I-III non-small cell lung cancer in stage IV non-small cell lung cancer. *Lung Cancer* 2018;124:6–11.

[173] Rizzo S, Raimondi S, de Jong EEC, *et al.* Genomics of non-small cell lung cancer (NSCLC): association between CT-based imaging features and EGFR and K-RAS mutations in 122 patients-An external validation. *Eur J Radiol* 2019;110:148–55.

[174] Wilson R and Devaraj A. Radiomics of pulmonary nodules and lung cancer. *Transl Lung Cancer Res* 2017;6:86–91.

[175] Cunliffe A, Armato SG, Castillo R, Pham N, Guerrero T and Al-Hallaq HA. Lung texture in serial thoracic computed tomography scans: correlation of radiomics-based features with radiation therapy dose and radiation pneumonitis development. *Int J Radiat Oncol Biol Phys* 2015;91(5):1048–56.

[176] Huynh E, Coroller TP, Narayan V, *et al.* CT-based radiomic analysis of stereotactic body radiation therapy patients with lung cancer. *Radiother Oncol* 2016;120(2):258–66.

[177] Hunter LA, Chen YP, Zhang L, *et al.* NSCLC tumor shrinkage prediction using quantitative image features. *Comput Med Imaging & Graphics*, 2016;49:29–36.

[178] Mattonen SA, Palma DA, Johnson C, *et al.* Detection of local cancer recurrence after stereotactic ablative radiation therapy for lung cancer: physician performance versus radiomic assessment. *Int J Radiat Oncol Biol Phys* 2016;94(5):1121–8.

[179] Vallières M, Freeman CR, Skamene SR and El Naqa I. A radiomics model from joint FDG-PET and MRI texture features for the prediction of lung metastases in soft-tissue sarcomas of the extremities. *Phys Med Biol* 2015;60(14):5471–96.

[180] Coroller TP, Grossmann P, Hou Y, *et al.* CT-based radiomic signature predicts distant metastasis in lung adenocarcinoma. *Radiother Oncol* 2015;114(3):345–50.

[181] Parmar C, Grossmann P, Bussink J, Lambin P and Aerts HJWL. Machine learning methods for quantitative radiomic biomarkers. *Sci Rep* 2015;5:13087.

[182] Coroller TP, Grossmann P, Hou Y, *et al.* CT-based radiomic signature predicts distant metastasis in lung adenocarcinoma. *Radiother Oncol* 2015;114(3):345–50.

[183] Paul R, Hawkins SH, Schabath MB, Gillies RJ, Hall LO and Goldgof DB. Predicting malignant nodules by fusing deep features with classical radiomics features. *J Med Imaging (Bellingham)* 2018;5(1):011021.

[184] Hosny A, Parmar C, Coroller TP, *et al.* Deep learning for lung cancer prognostication: a retrospective multi-cohort radiomics study. *PLoS Med* 2018;15(11):e1002711.

[185] Zhang Y, Oikonomou A, Wong A, Haider MA and Khalvati F. Radiomics-based prognosis analysis for non-small cell lung cancer. *Sci Rep* 2017;7:46349.

[186] van Timmeren JE, Carvalho S, Leijenaar RTH, *et al.* Challenges and caveats of a multi-center retrospective radiomics study: an example of early treatment response assessment for NSCLC patients using FDG-PET/CT radiomics. *PLoS One* 2019;14(6):e0217536.

[187] Asai B, Baba O, Maruoka K, Rieken Y and Honda D. Pre-treatment 18F-FDG PET/CT parameters in non-small-cell lung cancer patients treated with stereotactic radiotherapy. *J Nucl Med* 2020;61(6).

[188] Starkov P, Aguilera TA, Golden DI, *et al.* The use of texture-based radiomics CT analysis to predict outcomes in early-stage non-small cell lung cancer treated with stereotactic ablative radiotherapy. *Br J Radiol* 2019;92 (1094):20180228.

[189] van Timmeren JE, van Elmpt W, Leijenaar RTH, *et al.* Longitudinal radiomics of cone-beam CT images from non-small cell lung cancer patients: evaluation of the added prognostic value for overall survival and locoregional recurrence. *Radiother Oncol* 2019;136:78–85.

[190] Avanzo M, Stancanello J, Pirrone G and Sartor G. Radiomics and deep learning in lung cancer. *Strahlenther Onkol* 2020;196(10):879–87.

[191] Chetan MR and Gleeson FV. Radiomics in predicting treatment response in non-small-cell lung cancer: current status, challenges and future perspectives. *Eur Radiol* 2020.

[192] Tang X, Xu X, Han Z, *et al.* Elaboration of a multimodal MRI-based radiomics signature for the preoperative prediction of the histological subtype in patients with non-small-cell lung cancer. *Biomed Eng Online* 2020;19(1):5.

[193] Wang X, Wan Q, Chen H, Li Y and Li X. Classification of pulmonary lesion based on multiparametric MRI: utility of radiomics and comparison of machine learning methods. *Eur Radiol* 2020;30(8):4595–605.

[194] Mahon RN, Hugo GD and Weiss E. Repeatability of texture features derived from magnetic resonance and computed tomography imaging and use in predictive models for non-small cell lung cancer outcome. *Phys Med Biol* 2019.

[195] Hu N, Yin S, Li Q, *et al.* Evaluating heterogeneity of primary lung tumor using clinical routine magnetic resonance imaging and a tumor heterogeneity index. *Front Oncol* 2021;10:591485.

Chapter 10

Acoustic imaging and treatments methods in biomedical

Fadıma Gülsever Aksoy[1], *Volkan Akdoğan*[2] *and Muharrem Karaaslan*[2]

Imaging has an important place in the diagnosis and treatment of diseases. Biomedical imaging technologies have been developed to scan inside the body with noninvasive methods. Within the scope of this chapter, currently used advanced biomedical imaging technologies; magnetic resonance imaging (MRI), ultrasound (US) imaging, and US treatment methods have been studied. The advantages, disadvantages, and application areas of these techniques are presented in detail in this chapter.

Medical science is being developed to understand and interpret the structure and function of the human body in all health, disease, and injury situations. Utilizing the images of the human body to generate information about biological and medical processes is also used in clinical medicine and in biomedical research areas that support medicine. For this reason, developments in biomedical imaging have accelerated with the advances in current electronics and computer technology. Medical images are produced by the penetration of various sources such as X-ray, gamma-ray, ultraviolet, optical, radio frequency, magnetic field and US into the human body, and their interaction with tissues. As technology develops, biological processes have been visualized in detail, so imaging has become an important element in the detection, diagnosis, treatment planning, and monitoring of treatment response.

10.1 Magnetic resonance imaging

MRI is a method that does not involve ionizing radiation. With this method, cross-sectional imaging is provided by using magnets and radio waves. When the patient is placed in a fixed magnetic field, the protons in the body rotate in parallel and antiparallel alignment in the direction of the vector of the magnet. Then, radio

[1]Audiology Department, Cappadocia University, Nevşehir, Turkey
[2]Electrical-Electronics Engineering, Iskenderun Technical University, İskenderun, Turkey

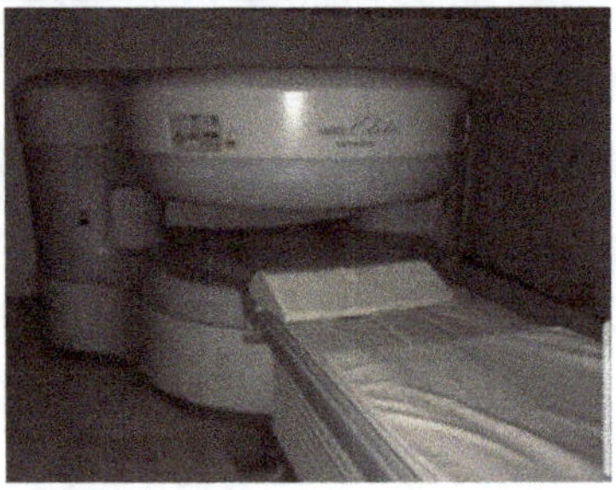

Figure 10.1 Open magnetic imaging

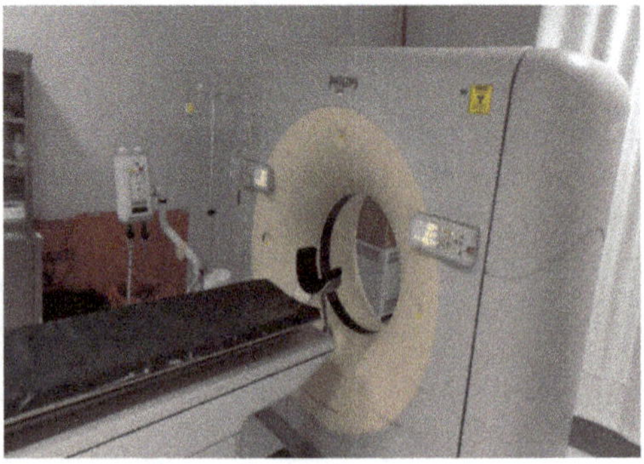

Figure 10.2 Closed magnetic imaging

waves are sent to provide deviations in the hydrogen atoms in the tissues. When the radio waves are interrupted, the protons return to their former positions in the direction of the magnet and return the energy they receive while returning. This energy is converted into a signal through a receiver [1] (Figures 10.1 and 10.2).

As seen in Figures 10.1 and 10.2, there are two types of MRI. Open MRI and closed MRI. Since the deviation that occurs for each texture is different, the time to return to their previous positions will be different. Images are created with these signal differences. MRI creates images by measuring the signal originating mainly from 1H protons in water and oil molecules. Hydrogen atoms are abundant in tissues containing water and the human body contains high amounts of water and fat. The signal level is strong in MRI because water is present in high amounts (in the molar range) in the body. Since the hydrogen atom is the most abundant atom in water and fat, MRI is used effectively in the evaluation of solid organs such as the brain, musculoskeletal system, and abdominal organs [2].

MRI is preferred over others due to having the highest soft tissue contrast resolution power. Separating the soft tissues that make up the majority of the body under high contrast resolution makes it easier to reveal their internal structures better. Multiplane images can be obtained with MRI without changing the patient position. Since there is no risk of ionizing radiation, it can be used in childhood and pregnant women, which can be repeated over and over in the same patient. Nevertheless, MRI is contraindicated in patients with devices such as pacemakers, neurostimulators, and infusion pumps. These devices will become inoperable by being affected by the magnetic field and may endanger the patient life [3,4].

Since the signals in MRI mainly depend on the proton density, sufficient signals cannot be obtained from some tissues or formations and it becomes difficult to evaluate these tissues. Cortical bone, calcification, and lung tissues can be given as examples for insufficient signal receiving. The central nervous system constitutes the majority of the use of MRI in daily practice. The rest consists of the musculoskeletal system and the rest of the abdomen, pelvic, and thorax examinations [3–6].

As mentioned earlier, not only anatomical details can be illustrated with MRI, but also functional images can be obtained. Contrast materials can be applied in MRI, and gadolinium-containing chelates are used in routine applications for functional imaging. MR contrast substances are increasing in use in diagnosing patients as they contribute to better disease detection, characterization, and monitoring. Therefore, they become an important part of disease management and they also play an important role in the evaluation of tumor angiogenesis. Within the advances in functional MRI (fMRI), organ-specific contrast substances developed after conventional extracellular gadolinium chelates [7].

In cases where the diagnosis is uncertain, MR-spectroscopy (MRS) technique that shows the biochemical structure and character of the tissues spectrally can be used. MRS data is obtained based on the principle that protons have different oscillation frequencies in different environments such as water, lactate, and oil. The obtained each spectral peak is proportional to the amount of chemical metabolite and represents how much of each chemical metabolite is present. The change in these peaks is used to clarify the etiology of the lesion, usually whether or not it is a tumor. *N*-Acetyl aspartate (NAA), choline (Co), creatinine (Cr), lactate (Lac), and glutamine (Glu) can be given as examples to evaluation parameters in MRS [8].

Aneurysms and vascular malformations can be detected by MRI. Especially in the detection of aneurysms, besides classical imaging sequences, MRI technique is also used. Two- or three-dimensional MR applications called time of flight and phase contrast (PC) can illustrate intracerebral main arteries and veins without intervention [9,10] (Figures 10.3 and 10.4).

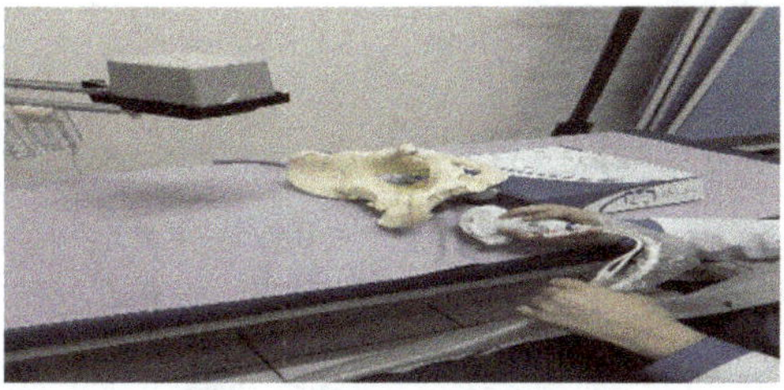

Figure 10.3 Fusion imaging technique

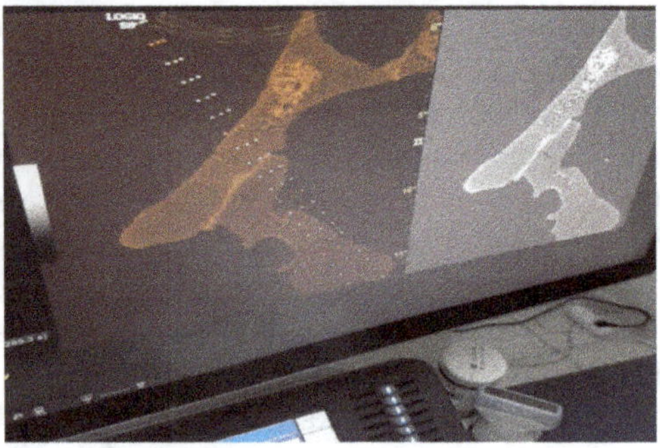

Figure 10.4 2D Demonstration of Fusion imaging technique

10.1.1 MRI spectroscopy

MRS (MRI spectroscopy) provides information on various tissue metabolites and is a complement to diagnostic MRI examinations. Protons (hydrogen nuclei) have magnetic properties in a strong magnetic field and are the source of signals in both MRI and MRI spectroscopy methods. All protons in a water molecule will have equal magnetic properties and will be the most important signal source in MRI.

Protons in different molecules have slightly different magnetic properties, and this difference means that small molecules in the body can be detected by MRI spectroscopy. Therefore, an MRI spectrum will show molecules in tissues, provided the molecules are mobile and are present in a measurable amount (>1 mmol/l). In addition to this, some diseases can be characterized by MRI spectroscopy. Therefore, diseases have been detected by identifying molecules that are not normally seen in healthy tissues or by the concentration of metabolites different from that seen in similar healthy tissues [11,12].

Some diseases can also be diagnosed by detecting the concentration of metabolites different from those seen in healthy tissues. MRI spectroscopy can be used to detect metabolites such as creatinine and choline. With this method, the diagnosis of brain tumors without the use of interventional methods can be detected, and then tumor treatment can be started [11,13].

Protons of water and oil generate signals in MR and other metabolites do not contribute to the image in MRI as their proportions are very low. MRS is a method of measuring the ratio of these metabolites in small amounts [13].

10.1.2 Functional MRI

fMRI can be described as a noninvasive brain function imaging method. Increase in regional blood flow and oxygenation are observed in neuronal activity. fMRI detects these changes in oxygenation and shows neural activation. It measures specific brain function, and neurological function assessment and it is a method that can be used in pre-neurosurgery risk assessment [14–16].

fMRI is an imaging method that allows the display of changes in cerebral blood supply dependent on blood oxygen level at rest or during function. These changes are called BOLD (blood oxygen level dependent). Perfusion of neural tissues with activation and temporal changes of these processes can be visualized with this method [17].

This technique can be used for various purposes such as planning before a brain surgery or a radiation therapy, mapping brain to identify regions associated with critical functions, detecting diseases such as Alzheimer and autism, and measuring drug effects [18].

The fMRI method is based on the changes of the MR signals depending on the oxygen level of the blood in the brain. Instead of directly measuring neural activity, it measures perfusion signals; therefore it is mostly used in researches rather than clinical settings [19].

10.1.3 4D flow MRI

Traditional flow PC methods show the 2D unidirectional flow of a single slice, while 4D flow MRI allows us to visualize complex flow patterns in a 3D volume and measure the temporal evolution of the model. The improvement of the methodologies provides the opportunity to view the vascular structures one by one and access the 4D MR flow data covering the vascular regions in a short time.

Various methodological improvements allow the acquisition of 4D flow MRI data within reasonable scan times, covering individual vascular structures and entire vascular regions such as the heart, adjacent aorta, carotid arteries, abdominal, or peripheral vessels [20].

Its importance has increased recently due to new developments in MR methodology and data analysis capabilities. It has the potential to provide a comprehensive vascular assessment and can be used for future cardiac and vascular diagnoses [21].

10.2 Ultrasound

US is an imaging method that has been used for more than half a century for diagnostic purposes, and it is one of the most widely used imaging methods among imaging technologies in medicine today. US is more cost-efficient and portable than other methods and provides a cross-sectional anatomical view simultaneously (Figure 10.5) [22].

US waves in the range of 1–20 MHz are used in medical applications and high-frequency US waves produce images with high axial resolution. Increasing the number of compression and dilution waves can more accurately distinguish between two separate structures along the axial plane [23].

High-frequency waves are more useful for imaging outer tissues because of their greater attenuation. Conversely, low-frequency waves (long wavelength) provide lower resolution images but can penetrate deeper structures due to the a

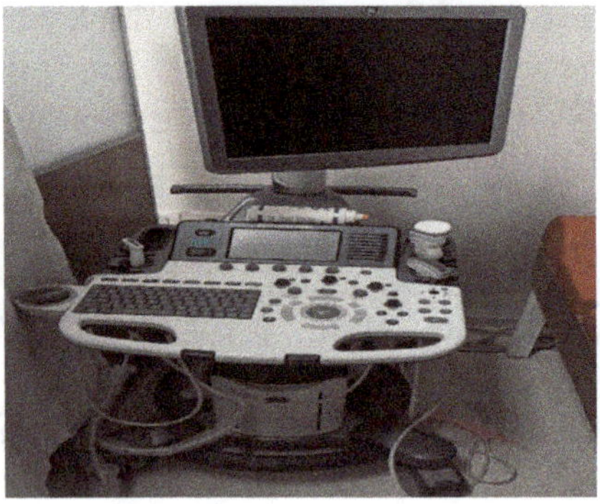

Figure 10.5 Ultrasound device

lower degree of attenuation. Therefore, it is best to use high-frequency converters in medical applications [24].

US waves are usually generated in pulses (intermittent pressure sequences) consisting of two or three sound loops of the same frequency. The pulse repetition frequency (PRF) indicates the number of pulses emitted per unit time produced by the transducer. In medical devices, PRF should be given between 1 and 10 kHz to allow the signal to reach the target and return as an echo before producing the next pulse.

While US waves are partially transmitted to deep tissues and reflected back to the transducer, they are partially converted to heat and some are scattered. In medical imaging, images are composed using echoes reflected in the transducer. The amount of echo returned after hitting a tissue interface is determined by a tissue property called acoustic impedance [24].

Acoustic impedance is a unique physical feature of an environment, and it is defined as the density of the environment times the velocity of propagation of the US wave in the environment. Organs containing air, such as lungs, have the lowest acoustic impedance, while dense organs have very a high acoustic impedance. The intensity of the reflected echo can be measured by the impedance difference between the two environments. If the impedance difference of the tissues is small, echo cannot be produced. Similar tissues have lower echo density differences. Contrary, a large impedance difference occurs between soft tissues and bones and strong echoes are produced. US is often used as an aid and guide for interventional applications. Its fields of usage are increasing in pain relief procedures [24,25].

10.2.1 Doppler ultrasonography

Doppler US is a medical imaging method used in many evaluations, from fetal and pregnancy evaluations and flow patterns in heart valves to blood flow in the brain. Doppler US provides simultaneous information and is portable, including high-performance models. It can be used to subjectively visualize anatomy or the presence of flow or to quantitatively evaluate physiological features. In clinical practice, Doppler US is a method based on frequency shift and frequency alteration due to the movement of the echo-forming object. For example, blood flow velocity is determined by frequency shift [26].

The waves are sent to the vein at a certain angle and the signal is formed by penetrating the vessel wall and directly hitting the blood cells. Then the waves are reflected by the blood cells and the intensity of the reflected sound decreases or increases according to the direction of movement [27].

The most important reflector in this method is erythrocyte, the velocity of which can be calculated using Doppler. Flow direction can be determined by color determination, current to the transducer direction is coded in red, and flow in the opposite direction is coded in blue [28,29].

Ultrasonography provides information about the size, location, and boundaries of a lesion, and whether it tends to spread to surrounding tissues [20]. Doppler ultrasonography is a method that provides analysis of total blood flow characteristics, including arterial and venous flow in the target organ [30,31].

10.2.2 Therapeutic ultrasound

It has been known for years that US waves cause changes on the tissue, and its usage for diagnosis, treatment, and surgical purposes has been still investigated. The US intensity to be applied for imaging is in the range of 0.005–0.5 W/cm^2 and the US intensity used for surgical purposes is in the range of 0.2–10,000 W/cm^2. Therapeutic US waves are used in the range of 0.5–3 W/cm^2 [32–36].

Therapeutic US has been in use for a long time, and its use in the clinic has changed significantly during this time. Although it was used primarily for its thermal effect in the past, it is now more widely used for its nonthermal effects such as tissue repair and wound healing. US is almost the most widely used therapy among electrophysical agents in the clinic today (Figure 10.6).

When US passes through the tissue, it is absorbed and causes heat generation in the treated tissue. The rate of absorption varies according to the nature of the tissue, the degree of vascularization, and the frequency of applied US. Tissues with high protein content are more absorbed than tissues with fat content. Biologically significant thermal effect can be achieved if the temperature of the tissue is raised

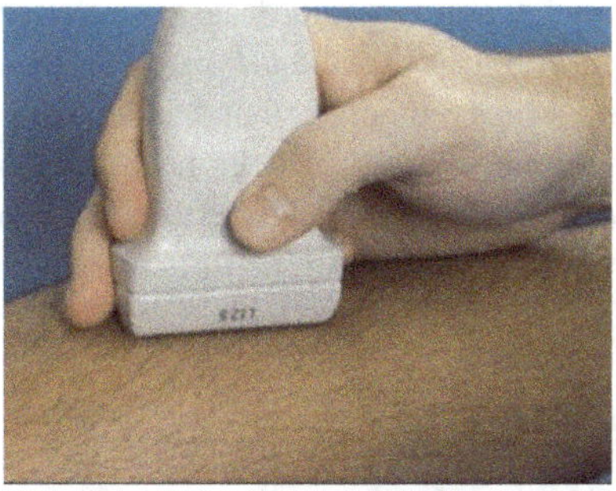

Figure 10.6 Application of ultrasound therapy to skin

to between 40°C and 45°C. A minimum of 5 min of controlled warming can provide positive effects such as reduced joint stiffness, relief of pain, and increased local blood flow [37–39].

The changes on tissues instigated by the therapeutic US by increasing the temperature are called thermal effects. The thermal effect is obtained by absorbing US energy by the tissues and converting it into heat energy [31,32]. This temperature increase in the tissues induces changes in collagen distribution, blood flow velocity, pain threshold, enzyme activity, inflammatory reactions, and nerve conduction velocity [40,41].

The thermal effect created on the tissues varies according to the US intensity, frequency, duration, size of the treatment area, and tissue type. The effect of US on tissues independent of temperature change is called a nonthermal effect. Although it is nonthermal, a minimum temperature increase may occur due to energy absorption during application, and this increase is known as microthermal effect. Since the therapeutic effect is not connected to this temperature increase, it is called nonthermal [42].

Physical mechanisms called cavitation and physical flow play an important role in the formation of the nonthermal effect. There are experimental studies showing that the acoustic flow effect is more effective in tissue regeneration. Cavitation is an application that has multiple effects on the skin; however, the most common area of its application is regional slimming. Gas particles in liquids form bubbles with the ambient pressure decrease during the relaxation of sound waves. During the compression phase of sound waves, the bubbles disperse in the liquid and then coalesce and grow. This behavior is called cavitation effect. These bubbles may combine and cause cell destruction, and cell destruction may cause necrosis, bleeding, and hemolysis. Therefore, attention should be paid to the US dose and probe should not be kept in the same place for a long time [43–45].

10.2.2.1 High-intensity focused ultrasound

High-intensity-focused US (HIFU) has the potential to be used as a treatment modality, as it can noninvasively ablate a targeted tumor beneath the skin surface and subsequently enhance host tumor immunity. In this way, it can provide micrometastatic control and long-term tumor resistance for cancer patients. HIFU therapy is an emerging therapeutic modality that uses US waves propagating through the tissue environment as energy carriers. HIFU technology has potential for use in tumor ablation, thrombolysis, and targeted drug/gene delivery [46].

US reaches the target point in the body through an environment of interfering tissues and noninvasively raises temperature and induces biological interactions. If US is properly positioned and focused, it does not create any negative biological effects. This therapy method has attracted the attention of clinicians because it is noninvasive and can provide almost complication-free treatment [46].

Catheter-based ultrasound

Intravascular catheters increase thrombus dissolution with the aid of an US transducer with mHz frequency placed near the tip. The catheter is placed in a deep vein thrombus and guided into the thrombus. US enhances the effect of thrombolytic drugs, so infusion doses and treatment times of drugs can be greatly reduced [47].

10.2.2.2 Low-intensity pulsed ultrasound

Low-intensity pulsed US (LIPUS) has attracted strong attention due to having potential on adjunctive therapy for fast fresh fracture healing. The LIPUS is utilized on cells and molecules in these healing operations. LIPUS has therapeutic applications to accelerate healing and union of bone fractures [45]. The process appears to be effective and safe but it is slow and limited to the treatment of nonhealing fractures. Therapeutic applications are noninvasive physical stimulus [46]. LIPUS protects the transmission of acoustic energy to the target tissue and has a little thermal effect due to its low density and pulsed output mode [48–50].

10.2.2.3 Sonophoresis

Sonophoresis is a procedure that increases the absorption of topical compounds (transdermal application) into the skin. In the sonophoresis method, US waves stimulate the vibrations in the skin epidermis and increase the kinetic energy of the molecules of the drug applied to the skin. It is widely used in hospitals when administering drugs through the skin [51].

When pharmacists apply medication, they mix it with a binding substance such as an ointment or gel, which transfers ultrasonic energy from the transducer to the skin. All these increase transdermal drug delivery by increasing skin permeability and allowing large molecules to pass through. A correct selection of parameters such as US frequency, energy dose, transducer distance from the skin is important for the sonophoresis process. Low-frequency sonophoresis increases skin permeability to a variety of low and high molecular weight drugs, including insulin and heparin [51].

10.2.2.4 Molecular ultrasound imaging (contrasted ultrasound)

Contrast-enhanced US is the application of the contrast mechanism in the US imaging system. The contrast material increases the intensity of the signal returning to the transducer, and it is small enough to pass through the gas-filled system and can be injected into the vein. Owing to the high difference in echogenicity of the contrast material with soft tissues, the intensity of the signal returning to the transducer boosts in this operation. Ultrasonographic contrast substance should be able to reveal normal, increased or decreased vascularity, vascular stenosis, and occlusion. In addition, ultrasonographic contrast materials should provide neoplasm segregation [52,53].

This substance should be able to intravenously injected, must be smaller than 7 μm in order to pass through the pulmonary, cardiac, and capillaries, and must not contain a toxic substance. It should be able to last for a period of time to allow the examination of the targeted environment without the need for a second injection [52].

10.2.2.5 Focused ultrasound

Using the thermal effect created by a focused US (FUS) transducer, deep soft tissue tumors can be treated with an incisionless surgical method. FUS is a procedure that can be applied when there is no air or bone in the lesion path. This method, when applied in combination with MRI, allows monitoring of localization and the temperature that US gives to the tissue. The advantage of this method is that it reduces the cost by shortening the recovery time compared to traditional surgery [54].

The FUS method does not damage the tissue or upper tissues surrounding the focal point, and its ability to induce cell death in tissue volume away from the US source makes it a noninvasive method for surgical use. While applying US, some of its energy is converted into heat and if the heating rate is higher than the cooling rate, it heats the area. Cellular growth stops if the temperature is kept above 43°C for 60 min or longer. Above the 56°C threshold, rapid thermal toxicity can occur and cause irreversible cell death through coagulation necrosis. If applied above the 56°C threshold for 1 s, rapid thermal toxicity can occur and cause irreversible cell death via coagulation necrosis [55].

10.3 Acoustic imaging methods

10.3.1 Vibroacoustography

The purpose of the vibroacoustography method is to separate healthy tissues from diseased tissues using tissue elasticity. Acoustic waves carry momentum, and radiation force is produced by varying their energy densities. Using US radiation, the soft tissue is deformed in a noninvasive way and the mechanical response of the tissue is obtained by applying US radiation [56].

Vibroacoustography is an imaging technique that measures the objects dynamic response to low-frequency vibrational force. The intensity of the FUS beam is changed, and the resulting radiation force is oscillated at the desired frequency [57,58].

The vibration of the tissue creates an acoustic field, the signal amplitude of this area is detected with the help of the hydrophone, and the brightness of each corresponding point on the image is determined by using this signal amplitude information. In this method, images are obtained by using low- and high-frequency records, and low frequency is applied by US using acoustic radiation force. The dynamic response of the treated areas to low frequencies is obtained with vibroacoustography, and this observation distinguishes vibroacoustic from US. Hard and soft tissues can also be distinguished by using vibroacoustography. Vibroacoustography can be used to detect microcalcifications, calcified arteries, and mass lesions in breast imaging [59,60].

If resources are limited, maternal perception of fetal movements in response to vibroacoustic stimulation can be a useful alternative to prescreening for high-risk pregnancies [61].

10.3.2 Ultrasound elastography

US elastography (USE) is an imaging technology that is sensitive to tissue stiffness. Elastography is a method used by measuring the elasticity of soft tissue resulting from changes in pathological or physiological processes. The elasticity of solid tumors and tissues around the tumor is substantially different from each other. Fibrosis in chronic liver diseases causes hardening of the liver compared to normal

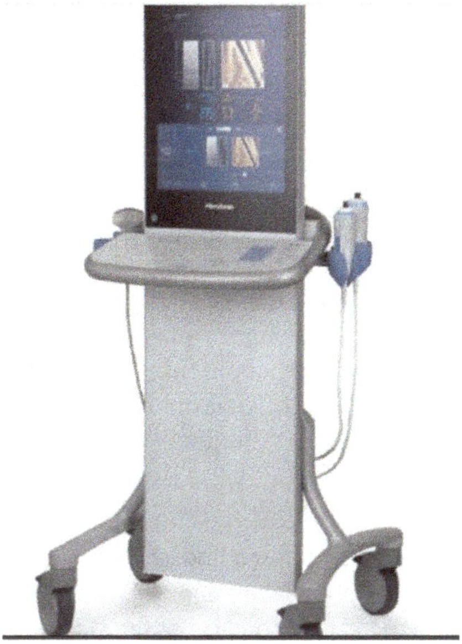

Figure 10.7 Ultrasound elastography device

tissues. In such cases, USE is used for diagnosis. USE can be used as a complement to US by providing measurable properties such as elasticity data to US data [62,63] (Figure 10.7).

10.3.2.1 Strain elastography

Strain elastography can be further subdivided by the method of excitation.

The US transducer can apply manual compression to the tissue, or internal physiological movements can be performed by holding the US transducer stationary. While manual application works in organs near skin, imaging can be performed in deeper organs when the transducer is kept in a fixed position [64].

In elastography, abdominal fluid accumulation or subcutaneous fat layer reduces the spread of external stimulus applied to the surface; in obesity, measurements may become invalid. While there are limits in manual palpation used by physicians, elastography can detect the presence of tumoral formation at deeper levels [65,66].

10.3.2.2 Shear-wave elastography

Shear-wave elastography (SWE), also called dynamic elastography, is used in the evaluation of musculoskeletal system. SWE is an imaging method that allows the user-independent and quantitative measurement of tissue elasticity. The acoustic propagation strength of conventional US waves propagates in the transverse plane perpendicular to the US waves during the interaction of the sound waves with the tissue. SWE generates waves that cause small displacements in tissues, and displacement maps of these tissues are obtained with the Speckle tracking algorithm. Shear waves travel faster in hard tissues and slower in soft tissues. Also, it is practical and repeatable and does not require manual compression [67–69].

10.3.2.3 Transient elastography

Shear-wave is a variant of elastography that measures the shear rate in tissue, and it is applied through the instrument that applies external vibration. In this method, vibration is given for a short time to distinguish the reflected waves formed in the tissue from the precursor waves, and it is generally used in liver examinations [70].

When comparing magnetic resonance elastography and USE, MRI elastography has many advantages. For example, it can stage hepatic fibrosis by measuring liver elasticity and stiffness. MR elastography can also be used in patients who are obese or with abdominal acid buildup [70,71].

10.3.3 Harmonic motion imaging

Harmonic motion imaging (HMI) is a method of estimating relative tissue stiffness by noncontact palpation using a pulsating acoustic radiation force generated by an US beam without the need for any contact or interference. HMI is a method of estimating relative tissue stiffness by contactless palpation using a pulsating acoustic radiation force generated by an US beam without the need for any contact or interference [72].

HMI is an elasticity imaging technique but differs from quasi-static elastography by not requiring direct contact. HMI stimulates the local vibration of tissues with US beam radiation force and reveals the mechanical properties of the tissue.

The mechanical properties of tissues alter in the event of pancreatic cancer, and tissues become stiff, and this situation causes the tissue to be displaced. The HMI system can determine the amplitude of stiffness-related displacement and the location of the tumor. It has an advantage over similar methods with its low cost, not having ionizing radiation effect, noninvasiveness, and estimation of tissue stiffness [72–76].

10.3.4 Acoustic radiation force imaging

Acoustic radiation force imaging (ARFI) is a diagnostic technique that is applied without any compression using US acoustic radiation, which allows the assessment of tissue hardness by evaluating the wave propagation rate. This technique performs staging of fibrosis noninvasively without the use of liver biopsy and can provide information about whether the liver is cirrhotic. ARFI assesses deep tissue stiffness using a conventional probe in the US scanner without the need for external compression. This practice and assessment reduces operator dependency and provides potentially useful supplementary information for diagnosis [77–79].

10.3.5 Acoustic emission

Acoustic emission frequencies are in the range of 150–300 kHz. Creep, fracture, and crack formation can be detected and localized by the acoustic emission method.

Preliminary information can be obtained before a bone fracture occurs with this technique. While the fracture healing process can be observed with this method, the healing decision in other methods is subjective and based on the experience of the physician. In this method, acoustic emission sensors are placed around the broken limb and the patient is asked to make movements such as walking, sitting, and standing. If the acoustic emission event cannot be detected, it can be decided that it has healed and it is objectively determined that the bone is mechanically healed [80,81].

10.3.6 Photoacoustic imaging

Photoacoustic imaging (PAI) is a mixed imaging method that combines optoacoustic imaging, illumination, and US. Optical imaging methods cause optical scattering and high resolution cannot be maintained, but the ability to obtain high-resolution images in deep tissues in biological tissues has made PAI more suitable for clinical imaging [82,83].

In PAI, a nanosecond-pulsed laser is often used to illuminate the biological sample. Molecules absorb optical energy and convert it into heat, creating a temperature increase, and with this increase, thermoelastic expansion occurs, which produces acoustic waves with ultrasonic transducers. Since sound scatters less than light, the acoustic signal propagates much longer without much attenuation in biological tissues [84,85].

PAI is a radiation-free technique and is very economical compared to other methods. It is also called optoacoustic or thermoacoustic imaging. It can display animal or human organs such as breast and brain with both high contrast and high spatial resolution.

PAI can be configured by using three methods according to optical signal applications methods and acoustic sensing methods. These are tomography, microscopy systems, and mesoscopy. Common photoacoustic tomography utilizes wide-field lightening and senses the acoustic signals with a single or an array of transducer. The utilization of single-element transducer is to provide time focusing and static imaging. This property makes it insufficient in vivo clinical imaging process.

In the case of multiple transducers for sensing, the provided acoustic signals can be collected at various angles and therefore it is better for real-time observation of the imaging area with higher obtainment velocity.

10.4 Conclusion

Biomedical imaging techniques introduce new and remarkable technologies for unraveling and understanding the complexity of biological systems, providing technological contributions to basic, surgical and clinical medical sciences, and the improvement of healthcare and disease diagnosis and treatment. Recent advances in biomedical imaging have focused not only on visualizing structure and morphology, but also on visualizing individual biological processes underlying disease.

This study presents a review about acoustic imaging and ultrasonic treatment techniques and provides information about the working principles, development processes, benefits, and applications of these techniques. Among the imaging techniques, MRI, fMRI, US imaging, Doppler US, and ultrasonic treatment methods have been investigated. These acoustic imaging and treatment techniques have become indispensable in the medical world in diagnosis and physical therapy by virtue of their performances.

References

[1] Herek, D and Karabulut N. Manyetik rezonans görüntüleme. *TTD Toraks Cerrahisi Bülteni* 2010; 1.3: 214–222.
[2] Kemik K and Ada E Data analysis and reliability in functional magnetic resonance imaging. *Turkish Journal of Radiology* 2018; 37(3): 39–46.
[3] Oyar O. *Fundamental Physical Concepts in Radiology*. [in Turkish] Nobel Tıp Kitapevleri, İstanbul, 1998: 151–210.
[4] Zhu M, Dai J and Li S. Cerebral angiography and MR perfusion images in patients with ischemic cerebral vascular disease. *Chinese Medical Journal (England)* 2002; 115(11): 1687–1691.
[5] Yeşildağ A and Oyar O. Magnetic resonance imaging physics. [in Turkish] Oyar O and Gülsoy UK ed. *Tıbbi Görüntüleme Fiziği*. Tisamat Basım, Ankara, 2003: 281–372.
[6] Edelman RR, Wielopolski PA and Fast MRI. In: Edelman RR and Hessellink JR eds. *Clinical Magnetic Resonance Imaging*. Second ed. W.B Saunders Company, Philadelphia, PA, 1996: 302.
[7] Bellin M-F. MR contrast agents, the old and the new. *European Journal of Radiology* 2006; 60(3): 314–323.
[8] Ulmer S and Ahlhelm FJ. MR spectroscopy in neuroradiology. *Applications of NMR Spectroscopy*. United Arab Emirates: Bentham Science Publishers, 2015; 2: 93–120.
[9] Wilms G, Bosmans H, Demaerel P and Marchal G. Magnetic resonance angiography of the intracranial vessels. *European Journal of Radiology* 2001; 38(1): 10–18.
[10] Oyar O, Öztürk M and Yünten N. Magnetic resonance angiography (MRA). [in Turkish] *Nörolojik Bilimler Dergisi* 1993; 10(3–4): 283–289.
[11] Ross B and Bluml S. Magnetic resonance spectroscopy of the human brain. *The Anatomical Record* 2001; 265: 54–84.
[12] Bloch R, Hansen WW and Packard M. Nuclear induction. *Physiological Reviews* 1946; 69: 127.
[13] Oz G, Alger JR, Barker PB *et al.* Clinical proton MR spectroscopy in central nervous system disorders. *Radiology* 2014; 270: 658–79.
[14] Turner R, Howseman A, Rees GE, *et al.* Functional magnetic resonance imaging of the human brain: data acquisition and analysis. *Experimental Brain Research* 1998; 123(1–2): 5–12.
[15] Sabbah P, Simond G, Levrier O, *et al.* Functional magnetic resonance imaging at 1,5 T during sensorimotor and cognitive task. *European Neurology* 1995; 35(3): 131–136.

[16] Holdsworth SJ and Bammer R. Magnetic resonance imaging techniques: fMRI, DWI, and PWI. *Seminars in Neurology* 2008; 28(4): 395–406.

[17] Buxton RB, Wong EC and Frank LR. Dynamics of blood flow and oxygenation changes during brain activation: the balloon model. *Magnetic Resonance in Medicine* 1998; 39: 855–864.

[18] Subbaraju V, Sundaram S and Narasimhan S. Identification of lateralized compensatory neural activities within the social brain due to autism spectrum disorder in adolescent male. *European Journal of Neuroscience* 2018.

[19] Faro SH and Mohamed FB. Functional MRI: basic principles and clinical applications. *American Journal of Neuroradiology* 2006; 28(9): 1831–1832.

[20] Markl M, Frydrychowicz A, Kozerke S, Hope M and Wieben O. 4D flow MRI. *Journal of Magnetic Resonance Imaging* 2012; 36: 1015–1036.

[21] Prince MR. Is there replacement for percentage stenosis in characterizing occlusive vascular disease. *Radiology* 2007; 245: 617–618.

[22] Edler I and Lindstrom K. The history of echocardiography. *Ultrasound in Medicine and Biology* 2004; 30: 1565–1644.

[23] Lawrence JP. Physics and instrumentation of ultrasound. *Critical Care Medicine* 2007; 35: S314–S322.

[24] Kossoff G. Basic physics and imaging characteristics of ultrasound. *World Journal of Surgery* 2000; 24(2): 134–142.

[25] Chan V and Perlas A. Basics of ultrasound imaging. *Atlas of Ultrasound-Guided Procedures in Interventional Pain Management*. New York: Springer-Verlag, 2010.

[26] Evans DH, McDicken WN, Skidmore R and Woodcock JP *Doppler Ultrasound: Physics, Instrumentation and Clinical Applications*. Wiley, Chichester, 1989.

[27] McDicken WN and Anderson T. The difference between color-Doppler velocity imaging and power Doppler imaging. *European Journal of Echocardiography* 2002; 3: 240–244.

[28] Sofferman RA and Ahuja AT. Physics and principles of ultrasound. *Ultrasound of the Thyroid and Parathyroid Glands*. First ed. Springer, New York, NY, 2012: 9–19.

[29] Gunderman R. *Essential radiology: clinical presentation, pathophysiology, imaging*, 2nd ed. New York, NY, USA: Thieme, 2006.

[30] Gianfranco G, Eloisa F, Vito C, Raffaele G, Gianluca T and Umberto T. Color Doppler ultrasound in the diagnosis of oral vascular anomalies. *North American Journal of Medical Sciences* 2014; 6: 1–5.

[31] Tucunduva MJ, Tucunduva-Neto R, Saieg M, Costa AL and de Freitas C. Vascular mapping of the face: B-mode and Doppler ultrasonography study. *Medicina Oral, Patologia Oral, Cirugia Bucal* 2016.

[32] Cameron MH. *Physical Agents in Rehabilitation: From Research to Practice*. Philadelphia: Elsevier Health Sciences, 2012: 173–198.

[33] Ter Haar G. Therapeutic ultrasound. *European Journal of Ultrasound* 1999; 9: 3–9.

[34] Fellinger K and Schmidt J. *Klinik and Therapies des Chromischen Gelenkreumatismus*. Maudrich, Vienna, Austria, 1954: 549–552.

[35] Lehmann JF and DeLateur BJ. Therapeutic heat. Lehmann JF ed. *Therapeutic Heat and Cold*. Williams and Wilkins, Baltimore, MD, 1982.

[36] Coodley EL Bursitis and post-traumatic lesions: management with combined use of ultrasound and intra-articular hydrocortisone. *American Practitioner and Digest of Treatment* 1960; 11: 181–188.

[37] Watson T. Ultrasound in contemporary physiotherapy practice. *Ultrasonics* 2008; 48(4): 321–329.

[38] Mason TJ. Therapeutic ultrasound an overview. *Ultrasonics Sonochemistry* 2011; 18: 847–852.

[39] Robinson SE and Buono MJ. Effect of continuous-wave ultrasound on blood flow in skeletal muscle. *Physical Therapy* 1995; 75: 145–149.

[40] Öncü J, İlişer R, Yılmaz F and Kuran B. Efficacy of kinesio taping on symptoms, hand functions, and hand grip strength in carpal tunnel syndrome: a single-blind and randomized controlled study. *Türkiye Fiziksel Tıp ve Rehabilitasyon Dergisi* 2014; 60: 43–51.

[41] Fabrizio PA, Schmidt JA, Clemente FR, Lankiewicz LA, and Levine ZA. Acute effects of therapeutic ultrasound delivered at varying parameters on the blood flow velocity in a muscular distribution artery. *Journal of Orthopaedic & Sports Physical Therapy* 1996; 24: 294–302.

[42] NyoRc WL. *Physical Mechanisms for Biological Effects of Ultrasound*. US Department of Health, Education, and Welfare, Publication, 1977: 78.

[43] Mortimer AJ and Dyson M. The effect of therapeutic ultrasound on calcium uptake in fibroblasts. *Ultrasound in Medicine; Biology* 1988; 14: 499–506.

[44] Draper DO, Schulthies S, Sorvisto P, and Hautala AM. Temperature changes in deep muscles of humans during ice and ultrasound therapies: an in vivo study. *Journal of Orthopaedic Sports Physical Therapy* 1995; 21: 153–157.

[45] Sağol A. *The effects of therapeutıc ultrasound ın cortıcosteroıd ınduced achılles' tendinosis in rats*. [in Turkish] Uzmanlık tezi, Dokuz Eylül Üniviersitesi Tıp Fakültesi, İzmir, 2006: 51–53.

[46] Wu F, Zhou L and Chen WR. Host antitumour immune responses to HIFU ablation. *International Journal of Hyperthermia* 2007; 23(2): 165–171.

[47] Costantino TG, Parikh AK, Satz WA and Fojtik JP. Ultrasonography-guided peripheral intravenous access versus traditional approaches in patients with difficult intravenous access. *Annals of Emergency Medicine* 2005; 46(5): 456–461.

[48] Wei F-Y, Leung K-S, Li G, *et al.* Low intensity pulsed ultrasound enhanced mesenchymal stem cell recruitment through stromal derived factor-1 signaling in fracture healing. *PLoS One* 2014; 9(9): e106722.

[49] Miller DL, Smith NB, Bailey MR, Czarnota GJ, Hynynen K, Makin IRS and Bioeffects Committee of the American Institute of Ultrasound in Medicine Overview of therapeutic ultrasound applications and safety considerations. *Journal of Ultrasound in Medicine* 2012; 31(4): 623–634.

[50] Xin Z, Lin G, Lei H, Lue TF and Guo Y. Clinical applications of low-intensity pulsed ultrasound and its potential role in urology. *Translational Andrology and Urology* 2016; 5(2): 255–266.

[51] Pahade A, Jadhav VM and Kadam VJ. Sonophoresis: an overview. *International Journal of Pharmaceutical Sciences Review and Research* 2010; 3: 24–32.

[52] Robbin ML. Ultrasound contrast agents: a promising future. *Radiologic Clinics of North America* 2001; 39: 399–414.

[53] Robbin ML and Weber TM. The potential role of ultrasound contrast agents in the liver. *Applied Radiology* 1997; 26: 13–19.

[54] Cline HE, Hynynen K, Hardy CJ, Watkins RD, Schenck JF and Jolesz FA. MR temperature mapping of focused ultrasound surgery. *Magnetic Resonance in Medicine* 1994; 31(6): 628–636.

[55] Kennedy JE, Ter Haar GR and Cranston D High intensity focused ultrasound: surgery of the future? *The British Journal of Radiology* 2003; 76 (909): 590–599.

[56] Urban MW, Alizad A, Aquino W, Greenleaf JF and Fatemi M. A review of vibroacoustography and its applications in medicine. *Current Medical Imaging Reviews* 2011; 7(4): 350–359.

[57] Fatemi M and Greenleaf JF. Ultrasound stimulated vibro-acoustic spectroscopy. *Science* 1998; 280: 82–85.

[58] Fatemi M and Greenleaf JF. Vibro-acoustography: an imaging modality based on ultrasound-stimulated acoustic emission. *Proceedings of the National Academy of Sciences of the United* 1999; 96: 6603–6608.

[59] Alizad A, Fatemi M, Whaley DH and Greenleaf JF. Application of vibro-acoustography for detection of calcified arteries in breast tissue. *Journal of Ultrasound in Medicine* 2004; 23(2): 267–273.

[60] Alizad A, Whaley DH, Greenleaf JF and Fatemi M. Critical issues in breast imaging by vibro-acoustography. *Ultrasonics* 2006; 44: e217–e220.

[61] Nyman M, Arulkumaran S, Jakobsson J and Westgren M. Vibro-acoustic stimulation in high-risk pregnancies; maternal perception of fetal movements, fetal heart rate and fetal outcome. *Journal of Perinatal Medicine* 1992: 267–274.

[62] Gennisson JL, Deffieux T, Fink M and Tanter M. Ultrasound elastography: principles and techniques. *Diagnostic and Interventional Imaging* 2013; 94: 487–495.

[63] Kamaya A, Machtaler S, Safari Sanjani S, *et al.* New technologies in clinical ultrasound. *Seminars in Roentgenology* 2013; 48: 214–223.

[64] Ophir J, Cespedes I, Ponnekanti H, Yazdi Y and Li X. Elastography: a quantitative method for imaging the elasticity of biological tissues. *Ultrasonic Imaging* 1991; 13: 111–134.

[65] Morikawa H, Fukuda K, Kobayashi S, *et al.* Real-time tissue elastography as a tool for the noninvasive assessment of liver stiffness in patients with chronic hepatitis C. *Journal of Gastroenterology* 2011; 46: 350–358.

[66] Palmeri ML and Nightingale KR. What challenges must be overcome before ultrasound elasticity imaging is ready for the clinic? *Imaging in Medicine* 2011; 3: 433–444.
[67] Taljanovic MS, Gimber LH, Becker GW, *et al.* Shear-wave elastography: basic physics and musculoskeletal applications. *Radiographics* 2017; 37: 855–870.
[68] Drakonaki EE, Allen GM and Wilson DJ. Ultrasound elastography for musculoskeletal applications. *The British Journal of Radiology* 2012; 85: 1435–1445.
[69] Creze M, Nordez A, Soubeyrand M, Rocher L, Maître X and Bellin MF. Shear wave sonoelastography of skeletal muscle: basic principles, biomechanical concepts, clinical applications, and future perspectives. *Skeletal Radiology* 2018; 47: 457–471.
[70] Li Y and Snedeker JG. Elastography: modality-specific approaches, clinical applications, and research horizons. *Skeletal Radiology* 2011; 40: 389–397.
[71] Sandrin L, Fourquet B, Hasquenoph JM, *et al.* Transient elastography: a new noninvasive method for assessment of hepatic fibrosis. *Ultrasound in Medicine and Biology* 2003; 29: 1705–1713.
[72] Konofagou E. Harmonic motion imaging. *Ultrasound Elastography for Biomedical Applications and Medicine*. New Jersey, USA: Wiley, 2018: 264–283.
[73] Maleke C and Konofagou EE. In vivo feasibility of real-time monitoring of focused ultrasound surgery (FUS) using harmonic motion imaging (HMI). *IEEE Transactions on Biomedical Engineering* 2010; 57(1): 7–11.
[74] Maleke C, Pernot M and Konofagou EE. Single-element focused transducer method for harmonic motion imaging. *IEEE Ultrasonics Symposium* 2005; 2005: 17–20.
[75] Han Y, Wang S and Konofagou EE. Harmonic motion imaging for detection and focused ultrasound ablation monitoring of ex vivo human breast tumors, In: 15th International Symposium on Therapeutic Ultrasound. Utrecht, Netherlands, 2015.
[76] Fahey BJ, Palmeri ML and Trahey GE. The impact of physiological motion on tissue tracking during radiation force imaging. *Ultrasound in Medicine and Biology* 2007; 33: 1149–1166.
[77] Nightingale KR, Palmeri ML, Nightingale RW and Trahey GE. Acoustic radiation force impulse imaging of vulnerable plaques: a finite element method parametric analysis. *Journal of the Acoustical Society of America* 2001; 110: 625–634.
[78] D'Onofrio M, Crosara S, De Robertis R, *et al.* Acoustic radiation force impulse of the liver. *World Journal of Gastroenterology* 2013; 19(30): 4841–4849.
[79] Franke RP, Dorner P, Schwlbe HJ and Ziegler B. Acoustic emission measurement system for the orthopedic diagnostics of the human femur and knee joint. *Journal of Acoustic Emission* 2004; 22: 92–99.

[80] Claes LE and Cunningham JL. Monitoring the mechanical properties of healing bone. *Clinical Orthopaedics and Related Research* 2009; 467: 1964–1971 Symposium: Biomechanics of Bone Healing.

[81] Ntziachristos V and Razansky D. Molecular imaging by means of multispectral optoacoustic tomography (MSOT). *Chemical Reviews* 2010; 110(5): 2783–2794.

[82] Xu M and Wang LV. Photoacoustic imaging in biomedicine. *Review of Scientific Instruments* 2006; 77(4): 041101.

[83] Lengenfelder B, Mehari F, Hohmann M, *et al.* Remote photoacoustic sensing using speckle-analysis. *Scientific Reports* 2019; 9(1): 1057.

[84] Wang LV and Hu S. Photoacoustic tomography: in vivo imaging from organelles to organs. *Science (New York, NY)* 2012; 335(6075): 1458–1462.

[85] Salibi N and Brown MA. *Clinical MR Spectroscopy First Principles.* Siemens Medical System, Inc., 1998; 6: 151–164.

[86] Paiva FF, *et al.* Comparison of human brain metabolite levels using 1H MRS at 1.5 T and 3.0 T. *Dementia & Neuropsychologia* 2013; 7: 216–220.

Index